INTERNAL MEDICINE
Mastering The Boards and Clinical Examinations

RHEUMATOLOGY

A.B.R. Thomson

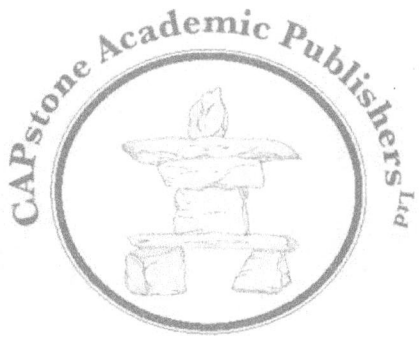

CAPstone (Canadian Academic Publishers Ltd) is a not-for-profit company dedicated to the use of the power of education for the betterment of all persons everywhere.

"The Democratization of Knowledge"

2016

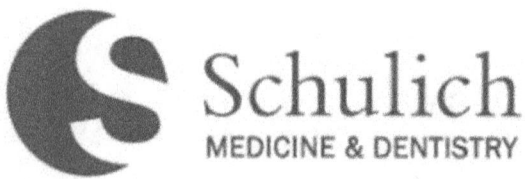 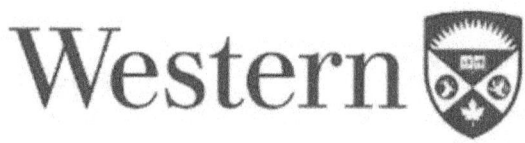

THE WESTERN WAY

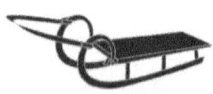

TABLE OF CONTENTS

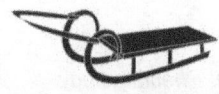

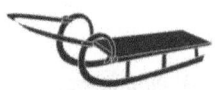

MASTERING THE BOARDS AND THE CANMED OBJECTIVES

Medical expert

The discussion of complex cases provides the participants with an opportunity to comment on additional focused history and physical examination. They would provide a complete and organized assessment. Participants are encouraged to identify key features, and they develop an approach to problem-solving.

The case discussions, as well as the discussion of cases around a diagnostic imaging, pathological or endoscopic base provides the means for the candidate to establish an appropriate management plan based on the best available evidence to clinical practice. Throughout, an attempt is made to develop strategies for diagnosis and development of clinical reasoning skills.

Communicator

The participants demonstrate their ability to communicate their knowledge, clinical findings, and management plan in a respectful, concise and interactive manner. When the participants play the role of examiners, they demonstrate their ability to listen actively and effectively, to ask questions in an open-ended manner, and to provide constructive, helpful feedback in a professional and non-intimidating manner.

Collaborator

The participants use the "you have a green consult card" technique of answering questions as fast as they are able, and then to interact with another health professional participant to move forward the discussion and problem solving. This helps the participants to build upon what they have already learned about the importance of collegial interaction.

Manager

The participants are provided with assignments in advance of the three day GI Practice Review. There is much work for them to complete before as well as afterwards, so they learn to manage their time effectively, and to complete the assigned tasks proficiently and on time. They learn to work in teams to achieve answers from small group participation, and then to share this with other small group participants through effective delegation of work. Some of the material they must access demands that they use information technology effectively to access information that will help to facilitate the delineation of adequately broad differential diagnoses, as well as rational and cost effective management plans.

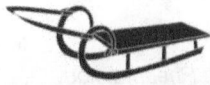

Health advocate

In the answering of the questions and case discussions, the participants are required to consider the risks, benefits, and costs and impacts of investigations and therapeutic alliances upon the patient and their loved ones.

Scholar

By committing to the pre- and post-study requirements, plus the intense three day active learning Practice Review with colleagues is a demonstration of commitment to personal education. Through the interactive nature of the discussions and the use of the "green consult card", they reinforce their previous learning of the importance of collaborating and helping one another to learn.

Professional

The participants are coached how to interact verbally in a professional setting, being straightforward, clear and helpful. They learn to be honest when they cannot answer questions, make a diagnosis, or advance a management plan. They learn how to deal with aggressive or demotivated colleagues, how to deal with knowledge deficits, how to speculate on a missing knowledge byte by using first principals and deductive reasoning. In a safe and supportive setting they learn to seek and accept advice, to acknowledge awareness of personal limitations, and to give and take 360° feedback.

Knowledge

The basic science aspects of gastroenterology are considered in adequate detail to understand the mechanisms of disease, and the basis of investigations and treatment. In this way, the participants respect the importance of an adequate foundation in basic sciences, the basics of the design of clinical research studies to provide an evidence-based approach, the designing of clinical research studies to provide an evidence-based approach, the relevance of their management plans being patient-focused, and the need to add "compassionate" to the Three C's of Medical Practice: competent, caring and compassionate.

"They may forget what you said, but they will never forget how you made them feel."

Carl W. Buechner, on teaching

"With competence, care for the patient. With compassion, care about the person."

Alan B. R. Thomson, on being a physician.

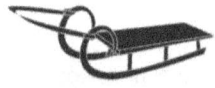

PROLOGUE

HREs, better known as, High Risk Examinations. After what is often two decades of study, sacrifice, long hours, dedication, ambition and drive, we who have chosen Internal Medicine, and possibly through this a subspecialty, have a HRE, the [Boards] Royal College Examinations. We have been evaluated almost daily by the sadly subjective preceptor based assessments, and now we face the fierce, competitive, winner-take-all objective testing through multiple choice questions (MCQs), and for some the equally challenging OSCE, the objective standardized clinical examination. Well we know that in the real life of providing competent, caring and compassionate care as physicians, as internists, that a patient is neither a MCQ or an OSCE. These examinations are to be passed, a process with which we may not necessarily agree. Yet this is the game in which we have thus far invested over half of our youthful lives. So let us know the rules, follow the rules, work with the rules, and succeed. So that we may move on to do what we have been trained to do, do what we may long to do, care for our patients.

The process by which we study for clinical examinations is so is different than for the MCQs: not trivia, but an approach to the big picture, with thoughtful and reasoned deduction towards a diagnosis. Not looking for the answer before us, but understanding the subtle aspects of the directed history and focused physical examination, yielding an informed series of hypotheses, a differential diagnosis to direct investigations of the highly sophisticated laboratory and imaging procedures now available to those who can wait, or pay.

This book provides clinically relevant questions of the process of taking a history and performing a physical examination, with sections on Useful background, and where available, evidence-based performance characteristics of the rendering of our clinical skills. Just for fun are included "So you want to be a such-and-such specialist!" to remind us that one if the greatest strengths we can possess to survive in these times, is to smile and even to laugh at ourselves.

Sincerely,

Alan Thomson

Emeritus Distinguished University Professor, University of Alberta

Adjunct Professor, Western University

 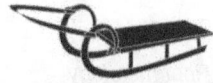

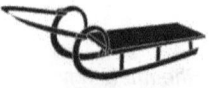

DEDICATION

In the memory of Jim and Dorothy

Whom we will never know.

 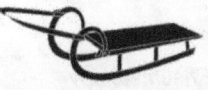

ACKNOWLEDGEMENTS

Patience and patients go hand in hand. So also does the interlocking of young and old, love and justice, equality and fairness. No author can have thoughts transformed into words, no teacher can make ideas become behaviour and wisdom and art, without those special people who turn our minds to the practical - of getting the job done!

Thank you, Naiyana and Duen for translating those terrible scribbles, called my handwriting, into the still magical legibility of the electronic age. Thank you, Sarah, for your creativity and hard work.

My most sincere and heartfelt thanks go to the excellent persons at JP Consulting, and CapStone Academic Publishers. Jessica, you are brilliant, dedicated and caring. Thank you.

When Rebecca, Maxwell, Megan Grace, Henry, Felix, Toby and Grady ask about their Grandad, I will depend on James and Anne, Matthew and Allison, Jessica and Matt, and Benjamin to be understanding and kind. For what I was trying to say and to do was to make my professional life focused on the three C's - competence, caring, and compassion - and to make my very private personal life dedicated to family - to you all.

 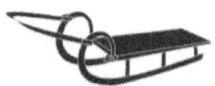

ARE YOU PREPARING FOR EXAMS IN GASTROENTEROLOGY AND HEPATOLOGY?

See the full range of examination preparation and review publications from CAPstone on Amazon.com

Gastroenterology and Hepatology

First Principles of Gastroenterology and Hepatology in Adults and Children - Volume I – Gastroenterology (ISBN: 978-1494345624)

First Principles of Gastroenterology and Hepatology in Adults and Children - Volume II - Hepatology and Paediatrics (ISBN: 978-1494345501)

Medical Mini Review Series in Gastroenterology and Hepatology: Efficient Refresher for the Busy Clinical Gastroenterologist (ISBN: 978-1502472199)

Medical Mini Review Series in Gastroenterology and Hepatology: Efficient Refresher for the Busy Clinical Gastroenterologist (ISBN: 978-1502472199)

Guideline-Based Management in Gastroenterology (ISBN: 978-1515078623)

Guideline-Based Management in Hepatology (ISBN: 978-1502928078)

Endoscopy and Diagnostic Imaging - Part I: Skin, Nail and Mouth Changes in GI Disease; Esophagus; Stomach; Small intestine; Pancreas (ISBN: 978-1477400579)

Endoscopy and Diagnostic Imaging - Part II: Colon and Hepatobiliary (ISBN: 978-1477400654)

Scientific Basis for Clinical Practice in Gastroenterology and Hepatology (ISBN: 978-1475226645)

The Physiology and Pathophysiology of Gastrointestinal and Hepatopancreaticobiliary Disorders: Preparing for Professional Competence. (ISBN: 978-1500298265)

General Internal Medicine

Achieving Excellence in the OSCE - Part One: Cardiology to Nephrology (ISBN: 978-1475283037)

Achieving Excellence in the OSCE - Part Two: Neurology to Rheumatolgy (ISBN: 978-1475276978)

Mastering the Boards and Clinical Examinations in Internal Medicine, Part I: Cardiology, Endocrinology, Gastroenterology, Hepatology and Nephrology (ISBN: 978-1461024842)

Mastering The Boards and Clinical Examinations In Internal Medicine, part II: Neurology, Respirology and Rheumatology (ISBN: 978-1478392736)

Bits and Bytes: Surviving Morning Rounds (ISBN: 978-1478295365)

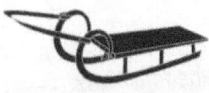

DISCLAIMER

The primary purpose of this publication is education. The author, editor and publisher acknowledge that the development of new material opens to way for possible errors – what is correct today might not be the standard of care tomorrow. Readers are advised to ensure that the doses of drugs which they use are in compliance with their country's product information, and that the use of any therapeutic agent, be it a pharmaceutical or a technology, should be guided by local guidelines. There is often a wide diversity of professional opinion, and guidelines from one country are not always congruent with another.

The author, editor and publisher do not guarantee the safety, reliability, accuracy, completeness or usefulness of this material.

They disclaim any and all liability for damage and claims that may result from the use of information, publications, technologies, products, and for series provided in this publication.

I have made every attempt to trace the holders of copyright for material reproduced in this book. If by some oversight I have omitted a copyright holder, please contact me to correct this. Thank you.

Alan Thomson

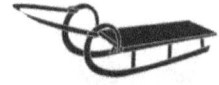

RHEUMATOLOGY

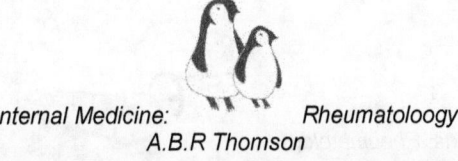

Internal Medicine: *Rheumatoloogy*
A.B.R Thomson

INTRODUCTION

- Take a directed history for a musculoskeletal (MSK) disorder.
  - Joints
    - Pain and stiffness
    - Weight-bearing, activity, time of day
    - Swelling and deformityMotor
      - Weakness, instability, falls
    - Sensation
      - Functional assessment
    - Gait
  - Extra-articular
    - Dry mouth
    - Dry, red eyes
    - Ulcers
    - Raynaud phenomenon
    - Rash
    - Fatigue, weight loss, fever
    - Diarrhea

*hip pain may be referred to knee or lower thigh

Adapted from: Talley NJ, et al. *Maclennan & Petty Pty Limited* 2003, page 252.

- Give the definition of abnormal physical findings in the MSK system.

Physical finding	Definition of Abnormal Finding
• MOTOR EXAMINATION	
○ Weak thumb abduction	- Weakness of resisted abduction, i.e., movement of the thumb at right angles to the palm[a]
○ Thenar atrophy	- A concavity of the thenar muscles when observed from the side
• SENSORY EXAMINATION	
○ Hypalgesia	- Diminished ability to perceive painful stimuli applied along the palmar aspect of the index finger when compared with the ipsilateral little finger
○ Diminished 2-point discrimination	- Diminished ability to identify correctly the number of points using callipers whose points are set 4-6 mm apart, comparing the index with little finger

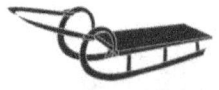

Mastering the Boards: Rheumatology   A.B.R. Thomson

Physical finding	Definition of Abnormal Finding
o Abnormal vibratory sensation	- Diminished ability to perceive vibratory sensations using a standard vibrating tuning fork (128 of 256 Hz), comparing the distal interphalangeal joint of the index finger to the ipsilateral fifth finger
o Abnormal monofilament testing	- Using a Semmes Weinstein monofilament applied to the pulp of the index finger, the patients threshold is greater than the 2.83 monofilament
	• Other Tests
o Square wrist sign	- The anteroposterior dimension of the wrist divided by the mediolateral dimension equals a ratio of greater than 0.70 when measured with calipers at the distal wrist crease
o Closed fist sign	- Paresthesias in the distribution of the median nerve when the patient actively flexes the fingers into a closed fist for 60 s
o Flick sign	- When asking the patient, "what do you actually do with your hand(s) when the symptoms are at their worst?" the patient demonstrates a flicking movement of the wrist and hand, similar to that used in shaking down a thermometer
o Tinel sign	- Paresthesias in the distribution of the median nerve when the clinician taps on the distal wrist crease over the median nerve
o Phalen sign	- Paresthesias in the distribution of the median nerve when the patient flexes both wrists 90° for 60 seconds
o Pressure provocation test	- Paresthesias in the distribution of the median nerve when the examiner presses with his/her thumb on the palmar aspect of the patients wrist at the level of the carpal tunnel for 60 s
o Tourniquet test	- Paresthesias in the distribution of the median nerve when a blood pressure cuff around the patients arm is inflated above systolic pressure for 60 seconds

[a] Most clinicians define weakness as muscle power less than that of the companion muscle in contralateral hand (which has the disadvantage of assuming that the opposite hand has normal strength), or that of a standard of normal strength based on the experience of examining many normal individuals.

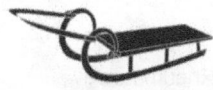

Adapted from: Simel DL, et al. *JAMA* 2009 Table 10-1, page 112; RCE, Table 10.1, page 112.

- Perform a focused physical examination to determine the causes of a patient's motor or sensory neuropathy

    o Motor
      - Immune
        - Guillian-Barre Syndrome
      - Idiopathic
        - Perineal muscular atrophy
      - Metabolic
        - Porphyria
      - Drugs
        - Lead toxicity
        - Dapsone toxicity
        - Organophosphorous poisoning

    o Sensory
      - Metabolic
        - Diabetes mellitus
      - Drugs
        - Alcoholism
      - Infection
        - Leprosy
      - Nutrition
        - Deficiency of B_{12} and B_1
      - Renal
        - Chronic renal failure

Adapted from: Baliga RR. *Saunders/Elsevier* 2007, page165.

"What is not started today is never finished tomorrow"

Johann Wolfgang von Goethe

 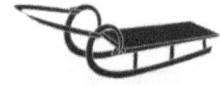

- Perform a focused physical examination of the joints of the upper and lower body and from the abnormal articular findings, give the most likely diagnosis.

Finding	Diagnosis
o Shoulder	
– Inspection	
▪ Flattening of rounded lateral aspect of shoulder	- Anterior dislocation
o Elbow	
– Inspection	
▪ Swelling over anterior elbow	- Glenohumeral synovitis; synovial cyst
▪ Localized cystic swelling over olecranon	- Olecranon bursitis
▪ Swelling obscures paraolecranon grooves	- Elbow synovitis
▪ Nodules over extensor surface of ulna	- Gouty tophi; rheumatoid nodules
o Palpation	
- Elbow pain and tenderness over lateral epicondyle	- Lateral epicondylitis ('tennis elbow')
- Elbow pain and tenderness over medial epicondyle	- Medial epicondylitis ('golfers elbow')
o Wrists and carpal joints	
– Inspection	
▪ Firm, painless cystic swelling, often located over volar or dorsal wrist	- Ganglion (synovial cyst)
▪ Thickening of palmar aponeurosis, causing flexion deformity of MCP joints (4th finger >5th finger > 3rd finger	- Dupuytren contracture
▪ Abnormal prominence of distal ulna	- Subluxation of ulna (from chronic inflammatory arthritis, especially rheumatoid arthritis)
▪ Non-pitting swelling proximal to wrist joint, sparing joint itself; associated clubbing of digits	- Hypertrophic osteoarthropathy

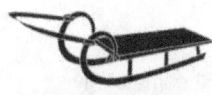

Finding	Diagnosis

- o Fingers
  - – Inspection
    - ▪ Loss of normal knuckle wrinkles — PIP or DIP synovitis
    - ▪ Loss of 'hills and valleys' between metacarpal heads — MCP synovitis
    - ▪ Ulnar deviation at metacarpophalangeal joints — Chronic inflammatory arthritis
    - ▪ Swan neck deformity (flexion contracture at MCP joint, hyperextension of PIP joint, flexion of DIP joint) — Chronic inflammatory arthritis, especially rheumatoid arthritis
    - ▪ Boutonniere deformity (flexion of PIP, hyperextension of DIP) — Detachment of central slip of extensor tendon to PIP, common in rheumatoid arthritis
    - ▪ Osteophytes: Heberden's nodes at DIP, Bouchards nodes at PIP — Osteoarthritis
    - ▪ Mallet finger: flexion deformity of DIP — Detachment of extensor tendon from base of distal phalanx or fracture
    - ▪ 'Telescoping' or 'opera glass hand'; shortening of digits and destruction of IP joints — 'Arthritis mutilans' in rheumatoid or psoriatic arthritis
  - – Palpation
    - ▪ Flexion and extension of digits causes snapping or catching sensation in palm — Trigger finger (flexor tenosynovitis)
    - ▪ Finkelstein test: pain when patients makes fist with fingers over thumb and bends the wrist in an ulnar direction — Tenosynovitis of long abductor and short extensor of thumb ('De Quervain stenosing tenosynovitis')

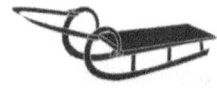

Finding	Diagnosis
o Hip	
– Inspection	
▪ Trauma, hip externally rotated	- Femoral neck fracture; anterior dislocation
▪ Trauma, hip internally rotated	- Posterior dislocation
▪ Pelvic tilt (imaginary line through the anterior iliac spines is not horizontal)	- Scoliosis; anatomic leg length discrepancy; hip disease
o Palpation	
▪ Hip pain, tenderness localized over greater trochanter	- Trochanteric bursitis
▪ Hip pain, tenderness localized over middle third of inguinal ligament, lateral to femoral pulse	- Iliopsoas bursitis
▪ Hip pain and tenderness localized over ischial tuberosity	- Ischiogluteal bursitis ('Weaver bottom')
o Knee	
– Inspection	
▪ Localized tenderness and swelling over patella	- Prepatellar bursitis ('Housemaid's knees')
▪ Generalized swelling of popliteal space	- Baker cyst (enlarged semimembranosus bursa, which communicates with knee joint)
▪ Genu varum and genu valgum	
– Palpation	
▪ Knee pain and tenderness localized over medical aspect of upper tibia	- Anserine bursitis
▪ Distressed reaction if patella moved laterally ('apprehension test')	- Recurrent patellar dislocation

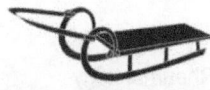

Finding	Diagnosis
o Ankle and feet	
– Inspection	
▪ Flattening of longitudinal arch	- Pes planus
▪ Abnormal elevation of medical longitudinal arch	- Pes cavus
▪ Outward angulation of great toe with prominence over medial 1st MTP joint (bunion)	- Hallux valgus
▪ Hyperextension of MTP joints and flexion of PIP joints	- Hammer toes
– Palpation	
▪ Nodules with Achilles tendon	- Tendon xanthoma
▪ Foot pain, localized tenderness over calcaneal origin of plantar fascia	- Plantar fasciaitis
▪ Foot pain, localized tenderness over plantar surface of MT heads	- Metatarsalgia
▪ Forefoot pain, tenderness between 2nd or 3rd toes or between 3rd and 4th toes	- Morton's interdigital neuroma
▪ Ankle pain, dysesthesias of sole, aggravated by forced dorsiflexion and eversion of foot	- Tarsal tunnel syndrome

Abbreviations: DIP, distal interphalangeal; MCP, metacarpophalangeal; MT, metatarsal; MTP, metatarsophalangeal; PIP, proximal interphalangeal

Permission granted: McGee SR. *Saunders/Elsevier* 2007, Table 53-2, page 627.

- Take a directed history for the common **side effects of non-steroidal anti-inflammatory drugs**.

  - o CNS
    - Delirium/ confusion
    - Headache
    - Dizziness
    - Blurred vision
    - Mood swings
    - Aseptic meningitis

  - o Pulmonary
    - Pulmonary infiltrates
    - Non-cardiac pulmonary edema (aspirin toxicity)
    - Anaphylaxis
    - Bronchospasm
    - Nasal polyps

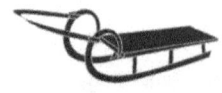

- o GI
  - Nausea, vomiting
  - Abdominal pain
  - ↑/↓ Bowel movement
  - Iron deficiency anemia
  - Peptic ulcer disease
  - Colitis
  - Hemorrhage from diverticulae

- o Kidney
  - ↓ renal blood flow
  - ↓ glomerular filtration rate
  - ↑creatinine clearance
  - Purpura
  - Interstitial nephritis
  - Papillary necrosis
  - Nephrotic syndrome
  - Hyperkalemia
  - Type IV renal tubular acidosis
  - Fluid retention

- o Blood
  - Bone marrow suppression
    - Agranulocytposis
    - Aplastic anemia
  - Platelet-aggregating defect

- o Skin
  - Dermatitis
  - Urticaria
  - Erythema multiforme
  - Exfoliative syndromes (toxic epidermal necrolysis)
  - Oral ulcers

- o Drug interactions
  - ↑ hemostatic effect of warfarin
  - ↑ antihypertensive effect of diuretics, beta -blockers, angiotensin-converting enzyme inhibitors
  - Influence drug metabolism
    - Methotrexate (high doses only)
    - Lithium
    - Oral hypoglycemic agents

Source: Ghosh AK. *Mayo Clinic Scientific Press* 2008, Table 24-21, page 999.

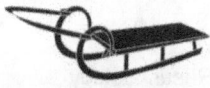

Useful background: Activities of daily living (ADL) and instrumental activities of daily living (IADL)

ADL	IADL
o Bathing	o Use of telephone
o Dressing	o Shopping
o Use of toilet	o Meal preparation
o Mobility	o Housekeeping
o Continence	o Laundry
o Feeding self	o Transportation
	o Taking medicine
	o Money management

Source: Ghosh AK. *Mayo Clinic Scientific Press* 2008, Table 13-8, page 571.

- Give the **abnormal articular findings** of 5 joints and the implied diagnosis.

Finding	Diagnosis
o Fingers	
– Inspection	
▪ Loss of normal knuckle wrinkles	- PIP or DIP synovitis, MCP synovitis
▪ Loss of "hills and valleys" between metacarpal heads	
▪ Ulnar deviation at metacarpophalangeal joints	- Chronic inflammatory arthritis
▪ Swan neck deformity (flexion contracture at MCP joint, hyperextension of PIP joint, flexion at DIP joint)	- Chronic inflammatory arthritis, especially rheumatoid arthritis
▪ Boutenniere deformity (flexion of PIP, hyperextension of DIP)	- Detachment of central slip of extension tendon to PIP, common in rheumatoid arthritis
▪ Osteophytes: Heberden nodes at DIP, Bouchard's nodes at PIP	- Osteoarthritis
▪ Mallet fingers: flexion deformity of DIP	- Detachment of extensor tendon from base of distal phalanx or fracture

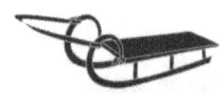

Finding	Diagnosis
▪ "Telescoping" or "opera glass hand"; shortening of digits and destruction of IP joint	- Arthritis mutilans, in rheumatoid or psoriatic arthritis

o Wrists

- Inspection

▪ Firm, painless cystic swelling, often located over volar or dorsal wrist	- Ganglion (synovial cyst)
▪ Thickening of palmar aponeurosis, causing flexion deformity of MCP joints (4th finger > 5th finger > 3rd finger)	- Dupuytren contracture
▪ Abnormal prominence of distal ulna	- Subluxation of ulna (from chronic inflammatory arthritis, especially rheumatoid arthritis)
▪ Non-pitting swelling proximal to wrist joint sparing joint itself, associated clubbing of digits	- Hypertrophic osteoarthropathy

- Special tests

▪ Flexion and extension of digits causes snapping or catching sensation in palm	- Trigger finger (flexor tenosynovitis)
▪ Finkelstein test: pain when patient makes fist with fingers over thumb and bends the wrist in an ulnar direction	- Tenosynovitis of long abductor and short extensor of thumb, or "De Quervain stenosing tenosynovitis")

o Elbows

- Inspection

▪ Localized cystic swelling over olecranon	- Olecranon bursitis
▪ Swelling obscures pata-olecranon grooves	- Elbow synovitis
▪ Nodules over extensor surface of ulna	- Gouty tophi: rheumatoid nodules

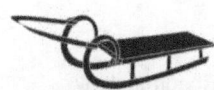

Finding	Diagnosis

- Palpation
  - Elbow pain and tenderness over lateral epicondyle — Lateral epicondylitis ("tennis elbow")
  - Elbow pain and tenderness over medial epicondyle — Medial epicondylitis ("golfer's elbow")

o Shoulder
  - Inspection
    - Flattening of rounded lateral aspects of shoulder — Anterior dislocation
    - Swelling over anterior aspect — Glenohumeral synovitis; synovial cyst

o Hip
  - Inspection
    - Trauma, hip externally rotated — Femoral neck fracture; anterior dislocation
    - Trauma, hip internally rotated — Posterior dislocation
    - Pelvic tilt (imaginary line through the anterior iliac spine is not horizontal) — Scoliosis; anatomic leg-length discrepancy; hip disease
  - Palpation
    - Hip pain, tenderness localized over greater trochanter — Trochanteric bursitis
    - Hip pain, tenderness localized over middle third of inguinal ligament, lateral to femoral pulse — Iliopsoas bursitis
    - Hip pain and tenderness localized over ischial tuberosity — Ischiogluteal bursitis ("Weaver bottom")

o Knee
  - Inspection
    - Localized tenderness and swelling over patella — Prepatellar bursitis ("housemaid's knees")
    - Generalized swelling of popliteal space — Baker's cyst (enlarged semimembranosus bursa, which communicates with knee joint)

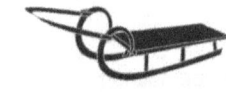

Finding	Diagnosis
▪ Genu varum and genu valgum	- Anserine bursitis

– Palpation
  ▪ Knee pain and tenderness localized over medial aspect of upper tibia
  ▪ Distressed reaction if patella moved laterally ("apprehension test")
	- Recurrent patellar dislocation

○ Ankle and feet
  – Inspection
    ▪ Flattening of longitudinal arch
	- Pes planus

▪ Abnormal elevation of medial longitudinal arch	- Pes cavus
▪ Outward angulation of great toe with prominence over medial 1st MTP joints (bunion)	- Hallux valgus
▪ Hyperextension of MTP joints and flexion of PIP joints	- Hammer toes
– Palpation ▪ Nodules within Achilles tendon	- Tendon xanthoma
▪ Foot pain, localized tenderness over calcaneal origin if plantar fascia	- Plantar fasciitis
▪ Foot pain, localized tenderness over plantar surface of MT heads	- Metatarsalgia

Permission granted: McGee SR. *Saunders/Elsevier* 2007, Table 53-2, pages 625 to 627.

"Let's change the interactions between alerting, orienting and executive functions, and control in a standard curing paradigm."
Grandad

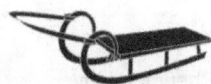

UPPER LIMB

Fingers, Hands and Wrist

- Give the upper limb **movements** and their respective **myotomes**.

Movement	Myotome
o Neck	
– Flexion	C1-C2
– Side flexion	C3
o Shoulder	
– Elevation	C4
– Abduction	C5
o Elbow	
– Elbow flexion and/or wrist extension	C5
– Elbow extension and/or wrist flexion	C7
o Fingers	
– Thumb extension and/or ulnar deviation	C8
– Abduction and/or adduction of hand intrinsic	T1

Source: Filate W, et al. *The Medical Society, Faculty of Medicine, University of Toronto* 2005, Table 12, page 138.

- Give the normal **range of motion** of 5 joints.

Joint	Flexion/ extension (degrees)	Abduction/ adduction (degrees)	Rotation (degrees)
o Shoulder	– 180	▪ 180 (abduction) ▪ 45 (adduction across body)	– 90 (internal rotation) – 90 (external rotation)
o Elbow	– 150 (humero-ulnar)		– 180 (radiohumeral)
o Wrist and carpal joints	– 70 (wrist extension) – 80-90 (palmar flexion)	▪ 50 (ulnar deviation) ▪ 20-30 (radial deviation)	
o Fingers (MCP, PIP and DIP joints)	– 90 (MCP) – 120 (PIP) – 80 (DIP)	▪ 30-40 (MCP combined abduction/ adduction)	

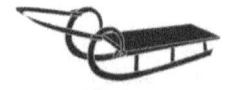

Joint	Flexion/ extension (degrees)	Abduction/ adduction (degrees)	Rotation (degrees)
o Hip	– 10-20 (extension) – 120 (flexion, knee flexed)	▪ 40 (abduction) ▪ 25 (adduction)	– 40 (internal rotation) – 45 (external rotation)
o Knee	– 130		
o Ankle and feet	– 45 (plantar flexion) – 20 (dorsiflexion)		– 30 (inversion) – 20 (eversion)

Permission granted: McGee SR. *Saunders/Elsevier* 2007, Table 53-1, page 624.

- Give the causes of **wasting of small muscles of hand.**

  o CNS/ PNS
    - Cord (C8, T1)
      ▪ Motor neuron disease
      ▪ Tumour
      ▪ Syringomyelia
      ▪ Meningovascular disease
      ▪ Cord compression
    - Roots
      ▪ Cervical spondylosis
      ▪ Neurofibroma etc
    - Brachial plexus
      ▪ Klumpke paralysis
      ▪ Cervical rib
    - Ulnar or median nerve lesions

  o MSK
    - Arthritis of hand or wrist
    - Disuse atrophy
    - Muscle diseases

Adapted from: Burton JL. *Churchill Livingstone* 1971, page 86.

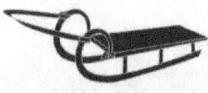

- Give the common deformities of the hand, and their associated conditions.

Name of deformity		Associations
o Mallet finger/thumb	– Flexed DIP caused by damage to the extensor tendon	▪ Trauma or RA
o Swan neck deformity	– Flexed DIP and hyperextended PIP	▪ RA, but has many other causes
o Boutonniere deformity	– Hyperextended DIP and flexed PIP – Occurs when the central slip of the extensor tendon detaches from the middle phalanx	▪ Trauma or RA
o Dupuytren contracture	– Flexion deformity of the fingers at the MCP and IPs associated with nodular thickening in the palm and fingers	▪ Diabetes, epilepsy, alcoholism ,and hereditary
o Heberden nodes	– Hard dorsolateral nodules of DIPs, often associated with a deviation of the distal phalanx	▪ OA
o Bouchard nodes	– Similar to Heberden nodes, but affects the PIPs	▪ OA

Abbreviations: OA, osteoarthritis; RA, rheumatoid arthritis

Adapted from: Filate W, et al. *The Medical Society, Faculty of Medicine, University of Toronto* 2005, page 135.

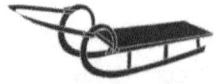

- Perform a focused physical examination of the hand to distinguish between rheumatoid arthritis (RA) and osteoarthritis (OA).

Sign	RA	OA
o PIP	+	+
o DIP		+
o Swan-neck deformity*	+	
o Deviation		
– Ulnar ***	+	
– Lateral		+
o Boutonniere deformity**	+	

*Swan-neck deformity extension at PIP and DIP
** Boutonniere deformity PIP joint, fixed flexion; DIP joint, extension
*** ulnar deviation at the metacarpal phalangeal joints

Source: Mangione S. *Hanley & Belfus* 2000, page 20.

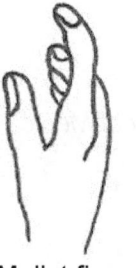   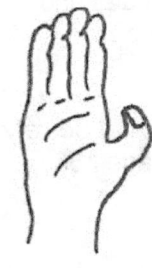

Mallet finger   Mallet thumb

- o A flexed DIP caused by damage to the extensor tendon
- o Interpretation of trauma or RA

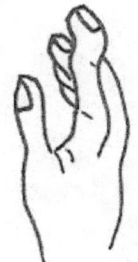

Swan – neck deformity

- o A flexed DIP and hyperextended PIP
- o Interpretation of RA, but has many other causes

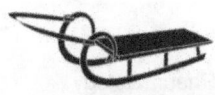

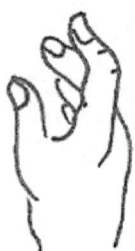

Boutonniere deformity

- Hyperextended DIP and flexed PIP
- Occurs when the central slip of the extensor tendon detaches from the middle phalanx
- Trauma or RA
- Ulnar deviation
- Deformity

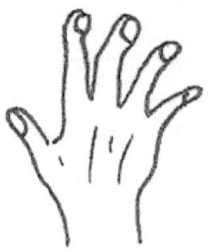

Dupuytren contracture

Heberden nodes and Bouchard nodes

Adapted from : Filate W, et al. *The Medical Society, Faculty of Medicine, University of Toronto* 2005, Figure 2, page 135.

"The real voyage of discovery consists not in seeking new lands but seeing with new eyes"

Marcel Proust

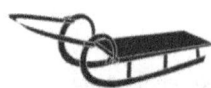

Useful background: More deformities

Site	Location of MSK disorder
➢ Finger	
○ Loss of normal knuckle wrinkles	- PIP or DIP synovitis
○ Loss of "hills and valleys" between metacarpal heads	- MCP synovitis
○ Ulnar deviation at metacarpophalangeal joints	- Chronic inflammatory arthritis
○ Swan-neck deformity (flexion contracture at MCP joint, hyperextension of PIP joint, flexion of DIP joint)	- Chronic inflammatory arthritis, especially rheumatoid arthritis
○ Boutonniere deformity (flexion of PIP, hyperextension of DIP)	- Detachment of central slip of extensor tendon to PIP, common in rheumatoid arthritis
○ Mallet finger: flexion deformity of DIP	- Detachment of extensor tendon from base of distal phalanx or fracture
○ "Telescoping" or "opera glass hand": shortening of digits and destruction of IP joints	- "Arthritis mutilans", in rheumatoid or psoriatic arthritis

➢ Proximal and distal interphalangeal joints

- ○ Spindle-shaped deformity of finger (tensynovites, especially in psoriatric arthritis)
- ○ Tophi (gout)
- ○ Wasting of small muscles of the hand
- ○ Heberden nodes – bony nodules at DIP joints (OA)
- ○ Bouchard nodes – long nodules at PIP joints(OA)
- ○ Deformity of thumb
- ○ Ulnar deviation of thumb

➢ Wrists and carpal joints

Site	Location of MSK disorder
○ Ganglion (synovial cyst):	- Firm, painless cystic swelling, often located over volar or dorsal wrist

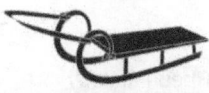

Site	Location of MSK disorder
o Dupuytren contracture:	- Thickening of palmar aponeurosis, causing flexion deformity of MCP joints (4th finger > 5th finger > 3rd finger)
o Subluxation of ulna (from chronic inflammatory rthritis, especially rheumatoid arthritis):	- Abnormal prominence of distal ulna
o Hypertrophic osteoarthropathy:	- Non-pitting swelling proximal to wrist joint, sparing joint itself; associated clubbing of digits

> Special tests
- o Trigger finger (flexor tenosynovitis):   - Flexion and extension of digits causes snapping or catching sensation in palm
- o Tenosynovitis of long abductor and - Finkelstein's test: pain when short extensor of thumb, or "De Quervain's stenosing tenosynovitis": patient makes fist with fingers over thumb and bends the wrist in an ulnar direction

> Elbows
- o Subcutaneous nodules
- o Psoriatric rash

> Palpation – (Feel and move passively and actively)

> Hands
- o Tenderness or pain
- o Synovitis
- o Effusions
- o Range of movement
- o Crepitus
- o Subluxation
- Hand function
  - Grip strength
  - Key grip (abduction of thumb)
  - Opposition strength
  - Practical ability
    - Button and unbutton clothes
    - Pincer movement
    - Writing

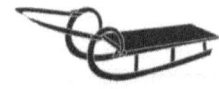

➢ Palms
  ○ Scars, palmar erythema, pale palmar creases (anemia
  ○ Wasting of thenar and hypothenar eminence
  ○ Palmar tendon crepitus
  ○ Erythema
  ○ Thickening of palmar fascia (Dupuytren's contracture)

➢ Wrists
  ○ Synovitis
    - Effusions
    - Range of movement
    - Crepitus
  ○ Carpal tunnel syndrome tests

Useful background: Thumb movements

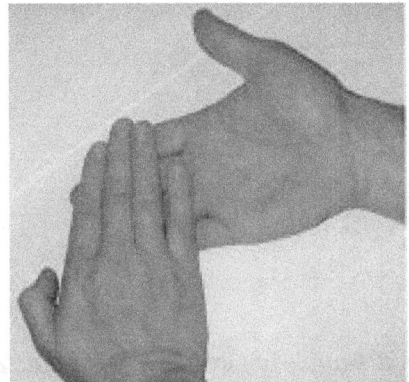 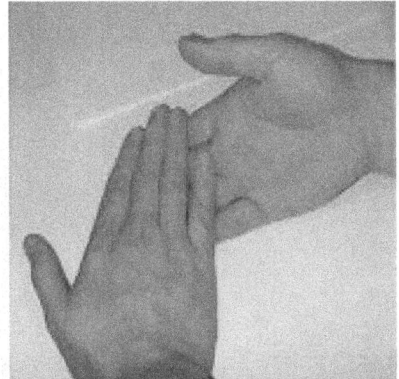

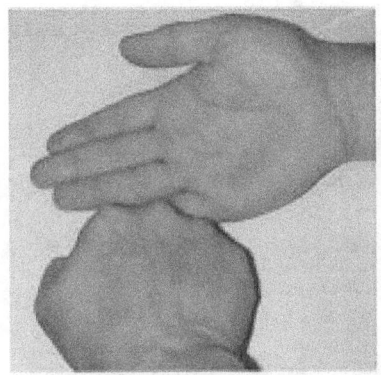 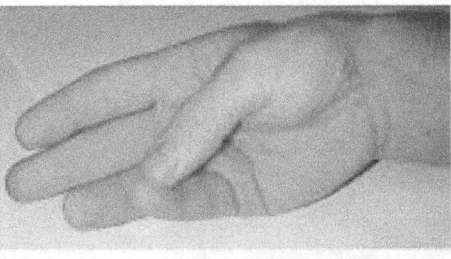

Adapted from: Talley NJ, et al. *Maclennan & Petty Pty Limited* 2003, Figure 8.10, page 267.

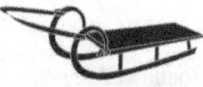

Useful background: Testing the superficial and profundus flexor tendons

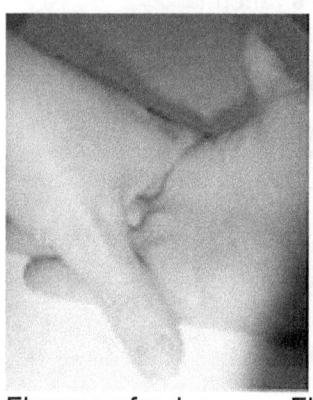 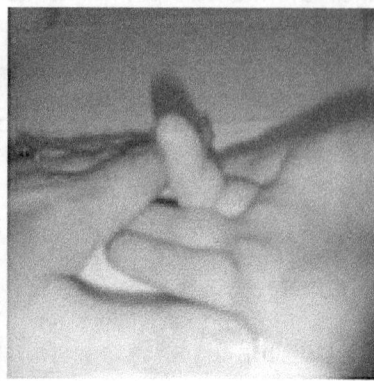

Flexor profundus   Flexor superficialis

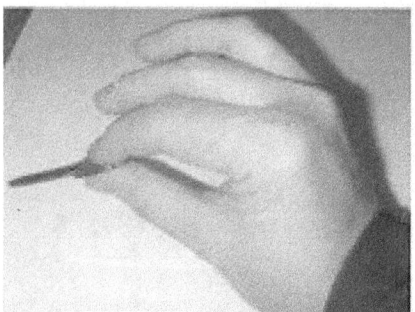

The key grip

Adapted from: Talley N. J., et al. *Maclennan & Petty Pty Limited* 2003, page 268.

Useful background: MCP and IP joint movements

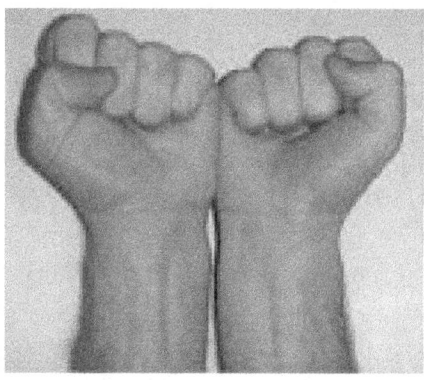 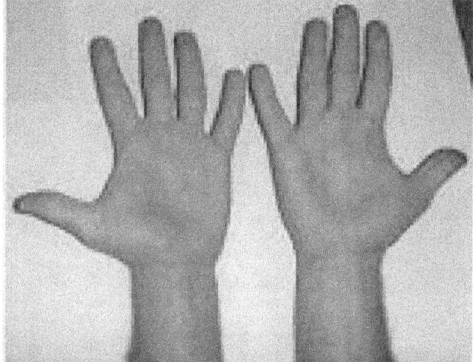

Flexion   Extension

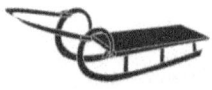

Abbreviations: DIP, distal interphalangeal joint; IP, interpharangeal joint; MCP, metacarpopharyngeal joint; MT, metatarsal; OA, osteoarthritis; PIP, proximal interphalangeal joint; RA, rheumatoid arthritis.

Adapted from: Talley NJ, et al *Maclennan & Petty Pty Limited* 2003, Figure 8.1, page 269; Filate W, et al. *Medical Society, Faculty of Medicine* 2005, Table 7, page 135, pages 124 and125; and McGee SR. *Saunders/Elsevier* 2007, Table 53-2, pages 626 and 627.

- Give the normal **ranges of wrist motion.**

Movement	Normal range of motion
o Flexion	75°
o Extension	75°
o Radial deviation	20°
o Ulnar deviation	35°
o Supination	80° from vertical (with pencil grasped in hand)
o Pronation	75° from vertical (with pencil grasped in hand)

Source: Filate W, et al. *The Medical Society, Faculty of Medicine, University of Toronto* 2005, page133.

- Give the normal **ranges of hand motion**

Movement	Normal range of motion
o Flexion	145°
o Extension	0°
o Supination	80° from vertical (with pencil grasped in hand)
o Pronation	75° from vertical (with pencil grasped in hand)

Source: Filate W, et al. *The Medical Society, Faculty of Medicine, University of Toronto* 2005, page 132.

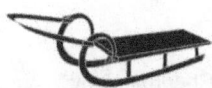

- Give the normal ranges of motion of the **joints in the hand**.

Digit	Joint	Range of motion
o Fingers	MCPs	0-90°
	PIPs	0-100°
	DIPs	0-80°
o Thumb	MCP	5° extension; 55° flexion
	IP	20° extension; 80° flexion
o Wrist and carpal joints		70˚ (wrist extension)
		80˚-90˚ (palmar flexion)
		50˚ (ulnar deviation)
		20˚-30˚ (radical deviation)
o Fingers (MCP, PIP, and DIP joints)		90˚ (MCP)
		120˚ (PIP)
		80˚ (DIP)
		30˚-40˚ (MCP, combined abduction/adduction)

Abbreviations: DIP, distal interphalangeal joint; IP, interpharangeal joint; MCP, metacarpopharyngeal joint; MT, metatarsal; OA, osteoarthritis; PIP, proximal interphalangeal joint; RA, rheumatoid arthritis.

- Give the **nerve supply** of the hand.

Nerve	Sensory	Motor
• Motor and sensory		
o Radial	- Dorsum of first webspace	▪ Extension of fingers, thumb, and wrist
o Ulnar	- Dorsal tip of small finger - Pulmar surface of small finger/ medial ring finger	▪ Finger abduction and adduction of ring and small finger ▪ DIP flexion of fingers ▪ Opposition of small finger ▪ Wrist flexion
o Median	- Dorsal tip of index/ middle/ lateral half of ring finger - Palmar surface of index/ middle/ lateral half of ring finger	▪ Thumb IP flexion ▪ Index/ middle finger flexion ▪ Wrist flexion

Nerve	Sensory	Motor
• Motor		
o Posterior interosseous branch		▪ Extension of thumb
o Anterior interosseous branch		▪ Flexion of index/ middle finger
o Lateral terminal branch		▪ Opposition of thumb

Adapted from: Filate W, et al. *The Medical Society, Faculty of Medicine, University of Toronto* 2005, Table 9, page 136.

- Give the **distribution of arthritis** in the hand and wrist in osteoarthritis and in rheumatoid arthritis.

Joint	Osteoarthritis	Rheumatoid arthritis
o DIP	– Very common	▪ Rare
o PIP	– Common	▪ Very common
o MCP	– Rare	▪ Very common
o Wrist	– Rare	▪ Very common

*Osteoarthritis will sometimes affect only the carpometacarpal joint of the thumb

Abbreviations: MCP, metacarpophalangeal; PIP, proximal interphalangeal; DIP, distal interphalangeal

Source: Filate W., et al. *The Medical Society, Faculty of Medicine, University of Toronto* 2005, Table 10, page 136.

- o Special tests
    - – For intact flexor digitorum superficialis: restrict motion of 3 out of 4 fingers by holding down distal phalanges with the dorsum of the patients hand (palm up) rested on a table; ask the patient to flex the free finger and look for PIP flexion
    - – For intact flexor digitorum profundus; hold down both the proximal and middle phalanges and ask the patient to flex fingers; look for DIP flexion

Adapted from: Filate W, et al. *The Medical Society, Faculty of Medicine, University of Toronto* 2005, pages 133, and 136.

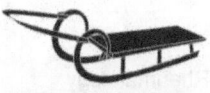

Wrist movements

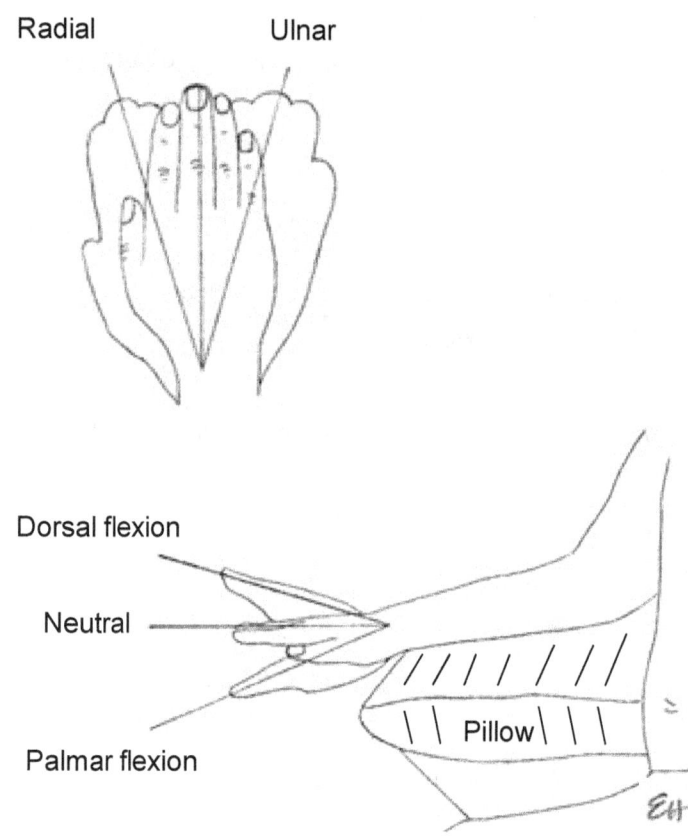

Adapted from: Talley NJ, et al. *Maclennan & Petty Pty Limited* 2003, Table 8.7, page 264.

- Perform a focused physical examination for **carpal tunnel syndrome**. (actually, Tinel sign is the reproduction of symptoms any nerve; eg, Tinel sign may be positive over ulnar nerve at the medial side of the elbow)

  o Tinel sign – symptoms reproduced by pressure on median nerve at wrist.

  o Phalen sign – symptoms reproduced by flexing wrists and holding dorsal sides together for 1 minute.

  o Sensory loss on thenar half of palm.

Adapted from: Mangione S. *Hanley & Belfus* 2000, page 463.
Useful background: Tinel sign (left) and Phalen sign (right)

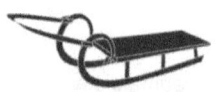

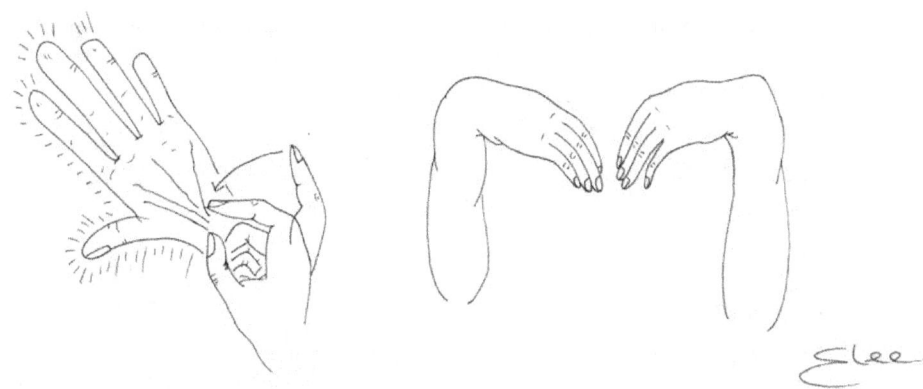

Adapted from: Mangione S. *Hanley & Belfus* 2000, page 465.

What is "the best"? There are no "best" clinical tests of physical examination for carpal tunnel syndrome, since the likelihood of each of the previous tests is < 2.

Carpal Tunnel Syndrome

- Give the systemic conditions which are associated with the **carpal tunnel syndrome**.

  o Rheumatoid arthritis

  o Diabetes

  o Thyroid disease

  o Pregnancy

  o Katz hand diagram
    - Classic or probable hand diagram has a sensitivity of 64% and a specificity of 73%

  o Hypalgesia in the median nerve territory
    - Pooled studies yielded PLR, 3.1; NLR, 0.7

  o Weak thumb abduction
    - Pooled studies yielded PLR, 1.8; NLR, 0.5

Note: Several traditional findings of Carpal Tunnel Syndrome have little or no diagnostic value including: nocturnal paresthesia; Phalen and Tinel signs; thenar

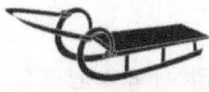

- Give the performance characteristics of clinical examination for Carpal Tunnel Syndrome (CTS). Note that the PLR for all of these are < 2.0, making each of the physical signs of limited value.

Physical sign	PLR	NLR
o Tinel sign	1.5	0.82
o Phalen test	1.3	0.74
o Provocation tests	1.1	0.89
o Mulivariate model	1.7	0.39
o Flick or Tinel	1.5	0.79
o Phalen or Tinel	1.5	0.81
o Flick	1.4	0.85
o Flick or Phalen	1.3	0.82
o Abnormal monofilament in digits	1.2	0.11

Abbreviations: CI, confidence interval, PLR, positive likelihood ratio; NLR, negative likelihood ratio.

Adapted from: Simel DL, et al. *JAMA* 2009, Table 10-5, page 123; Filate W, et al. *The Medical Society, Faculty of Medicine, University of Toronto* 2005, page 134.

- Give a systematic approach to localized areas of **translucent bone** seen on diagnostic imaging.
    - o Cysts
        - – Fluid
        - – Fibrous tissue
    - o Tumor
        - – Multiple bones, fibrous tissue in cyst; "poly ostotic fibrous dysplasia"
    - o Leukemia
    - o Metastases
        - – Thyroid
        - – Bronchus
        - – Breast
        - – Kidney
        - – Myeloma
    - o Sarcoidosis
    - o Histiocytosis X

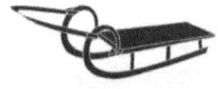

- Give a systematic approach to localized areas of calcified bone (periostitis).

    o Subperiosteal bleeding
      - Trauma
      - Hemophilia
      - Leukemia

    o Associated with fracture

    o Bone infections

    o Tumors – primary, secondary

    o Pulmonary osteo-arthropathy

- Perform a focused physical examination of the wrist for rheumatoid arthritis.

    o Tendon of extensor carpi ulnaris – swelling
    o Radial ulnar ligaments – protrusion and instability of distal ulna from lax ligaments.
    o Carpal rows
      - Subluxation to dorsal side
      - Bayonet deformity

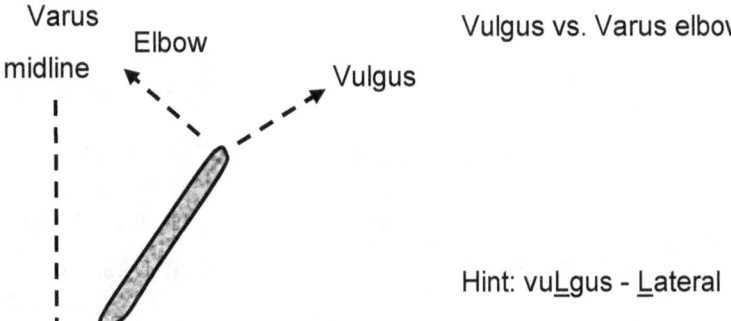

Vulgus vs. Varus elbow

Hint: vuLgus - Lateral

Adapted from: Mangione S. *Hanley & Belfus* 2000, pages 463, 468 and 472.

- Perform a directed physical examination of the hands for **acromegaly, Marfan syndrome, and Turner syndrome**.

    o Acromegaly – enlarged distal portion of body, with hands shaped like shovels (spades).

    o Marfan syndrome
      - Arachnodactyly: long, thin, "spider-like" fingers
      - Marfan's thumb sign is positive normally, when the thumb is extended into the palm and the remaining 4 fingers are curled over the thumb, the fist covers the thumb; in Marfan's , the end of the thumb sticks out beyond the fifth finger (ulnar) end of the fist, Marfan's thumb sign is also positive with the hypermobile joints in Ehlers-Danlos syndrome.

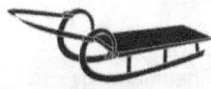

- o Turner syndrome
  - A short, inwardly dimpled fourth knuckle
  - Also seen in pseudohypoparathyroidism, and in 10% of otherwise normal persons.

SO YOU WANT TO IMPRESS YOUR STAFF!

When a person's fingers are exposed to the cold, they may become pale, then blue from the arterial vasospasm and ischemia, then with redness from reperfusion. This latter phase from a decline in the spasm and therefore ischemia may be associated with pain and paresthesia as well as the redness. In some persons (20%) no cause/association may be found, and this progression of white-blue-red is called Reynaud's disease (i.e., Reynaud's phenomenon, with no known underlying disorder. However, the Raynaud's phenomenon may proceed a number of conditions.

- Perform a focused physical examination for the causes of the **Raynaud phenomenon**.

  - o MSK
    - Rheumatoid arthritis
    - Scleroderma
    - Systemic lupus erythematosis
    - Mixed connective disease
    - Dermatomyositis
    - Polymyositis

  - o Hematological disorders
    - Cryoglobulinemia
    - Polycythemia
    - Monoclonal gammopathy

  - o Arterial
    - Compression
      - Thoracic outlet syndrome
      - Carpal tunnel syndrome
    - Artherosclerosis
    - Vasculitis
    - Prinznetal angina

  - o Drugs and toxins
  - o Endocrine disorders
    - Hypothyroidism
    - Acromegaly
    - Addison's disease

  - o Pulmonary disorders
    - Idiopathic pulmonary hypertension

  - o Neurological
    - Reflex sympathetic dystrophy

  - o Life style
    - Occupational use of percussion or vibratory tools (e.g. a jack hammer)

ELBOWS

- Give the normal **ranges of motion**.

Movement	Normal range of motion
o Forward flexion	– 165°
o Backward extension	– 60°
o Abduction	– 170°
o Adduction	– 50°
o External rotation (with elbows at sides)	– 70°
o Internal rotation (with shoulder abducted to 90° & elbow flexed)	– 70°

Source: Filate W, et al. *The Medical Society, Faculty of Medicine, University of Toronto* 2005, page 129.

- Perform a **focused physical examination** of the elbow.

- o Inspection
  - – Olecranon bursitis:
    - ▪ Localized cystic swelling over olecranon
    - ▪ Swelling obscures para-olecranon grooves
  - – Elbow synovitis:
  - – Gouty tophi; rheumatoid nodules:
    - ▪ Nodules over extensor surface of ulna

- o Palpation
  - – Lateral epicondylitis ("tennis elbow"):
    - ▪ Elbow pain and tenderness over lateral epicondyle
  - – Medial epicondylitis ("golfer elbow"):
    - ▪ Elbow pain and tenderness over medial epicondyle

- o Active Movement   Normal range of movement (ROM)
  - – Flexion
    - ▪ 145°
  - – Extension
    - ▪ 0°
  - – Supination
    - ▪ 80° from vertical (with pencil grasped in hand)
  - – Pronation
    - ▪ 75° from vertical (with pencil grasped in hand)
  - – Rotation
    - ▪ 180° (radio humeral)

Adapted from: Filate W, et al. *The Medical Society, Faculty of Medicine, University of Toronto* 2005, Table 3, page 132; McGee SR. *Saunders/Elsevier* 2007, Table 53-2, page 627.

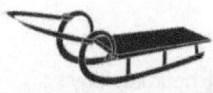

- Take a directed history and a focused physical examination for features **differentiating diseases** affecting the elbow.

Clinical feature	Rheumatoid arthritis	Psoriatic arthritis	Acute gout	Osteo-arthritis	Lateral epicondylitis
o Age	3-80	10-60	30-80	50-80	20-60
o Pain onset	Gradual	Gradual	Abrupt	Gradual	Gradual
o Stiffness	Very common	Common	Absent	Common	Occasional
o Swelling	Common	Common	Common	Common	Absent
o Redness	Absent	Uncommon	Common	Common	Absent
o Deformity	Flexion contrac-tures, usually bilaterally	Flexion contractures, usually bilaterally	Flexion contractures, only in chronic state	Flexion contrac-tures	None
	Subcutaneous nodules	Psoriatric nails	Gout tophi		

Permission granted: Filate W, et al. *The Medical Society, Faculty of Medicine, University of Toronto* 2005, Table 4, page 132.

Pain in the elbow may be caused by infection (Staphylococcus aureus), gout or trauma. In this context, give the meaning of "**tennis elbow**".

- o "tennis elbow", aka lateral epicondylitis

- o Lateral epicondylitis does not involve the elbow joint, but instead affects the soft tissue around the joint

- Perform a focused physical examination of the elbow to distinguish between **"tennis" and "golfer" elbow**.

	Tennis (lateral epicondylitis)	Golf (lateral epicondylitis)
o Site of injury	- Proximal attachment of the extensor muscles of the forearm	- Flexor attachment of muscles of forearm
o Pain, tenderness	- Lateral epicondyle	- Medial epicondyle
o Examination technique		

Midline   Midline

Resisted wrist flexion

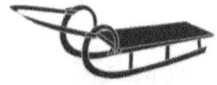

SHOULDERS

Useful background: Anatomy of the shoulder

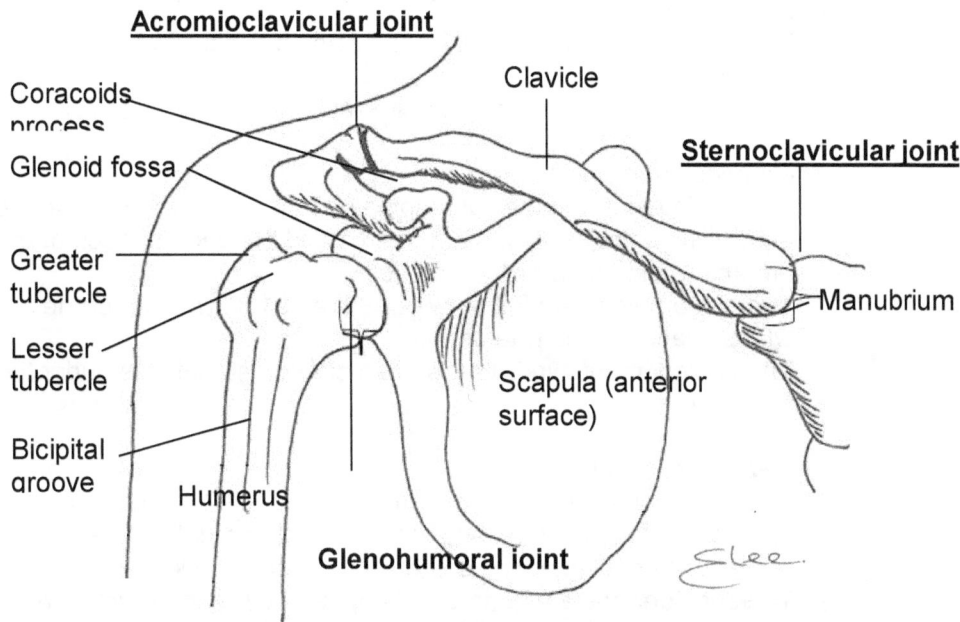

Adapted from: Filate W, et al. *The Medical Society, Faculty of Medicine, University of Toronto* 2005, Figure 1, page 129.

- In the context of a painful shoulder, give the meaning of the following

    o The painful arc sign
    o Tears of
       - Supraspinatus
       - (partial) rotator cuff

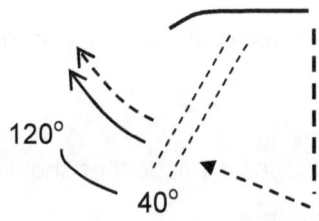

    o Glenohumeral arthritis
    o No active abduction from midline (0°): complete rotator cuff tear

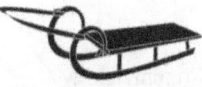

- o Instability
  - The relocation test and the anterior release test are the most useful in diagnosing anterior instability (labrum lesion)
  - Relocation test: PLR, 6.5
  - Anterior release test: PLR, 8.3.
  - The sulcus sign for inferior instability has a sensitivity of 31% and a specificity 89%
  - The apprehension test is of limited value due to low specificity.

- o The impingement syndrome is
  - The impingement of the supraspinatus tendon between the greater tuberosity of the head of the humerus and the undersurface of the acromion and acromioclavicular joint.
  - There is a painful arc felt between 90° and 130°, and tenderness with palpation of the rotator cuff.
  - The impingement syndrome is often due to osteophytes under the acromion

- o The apprehension test
  - Used to identify anterior shoulder dislocations. The patient's affected arm is abducted and externally rotated until a look of apprehension is noted if the shoulder is dislocatable.
  - The shoulder has a "squared off" appearance, with reduction of internal rotation and possible loss of sensation and contraction over the lateral deltoid muscle.
  - The causes of posterior shoulder dislocation include:
    - Epileptic seizures
    - Ethanol intoxication,
    - Electrolution/electroshock therapy
    - Encephalitis.

- Perform a focused **physical examination** of the shoulder.

  - o Inspection
    - Swelling
      - Flattening aspect of shoulder; anterior dislocation
    - Erythema
      - Swelling over anterior aspect; glenohumeral synovitis; synovial cyst
    - Assymetry/atrophy
    - Deformity
    - Skin changes

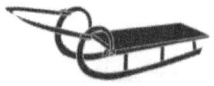

- o Palpation
    - Tenderness
    - Temperature
    - Edema
    - Crepitus
    - Biceps groove
    - Subdeltoid bursa
- o Passive and active movement
- o Normal ranges of motion (ROM)

Movement	Normal ROM
o Forward flexion	165°
o Backward flexion	60°
o Abduction	170°
o Adduction	50°
o External rotation (with elbows at sides)	70°
o Internal rotation (with shoulder abducted to 90° & elbow flexed)	70°

- o Note
    - One way to test for limitations of passive motion is to ask the patient to bend over and try to touch his or her toes. In those with normal shoulder passive motion, the arms dangle toward the floor.

Abbreviation: ACJ, acromioclavicular joint; ROM, ranges of motion

Adapted from: McGee SR. *Saunders/Elsevier*, 2007, Table 53-3, page 629; Filate W, et al. *The Medical Society, Faculty of Medicine, University of Toronto*, 2005, Table 1, page 129.

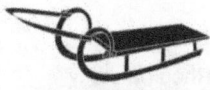

➢ Active movements of Shoulder

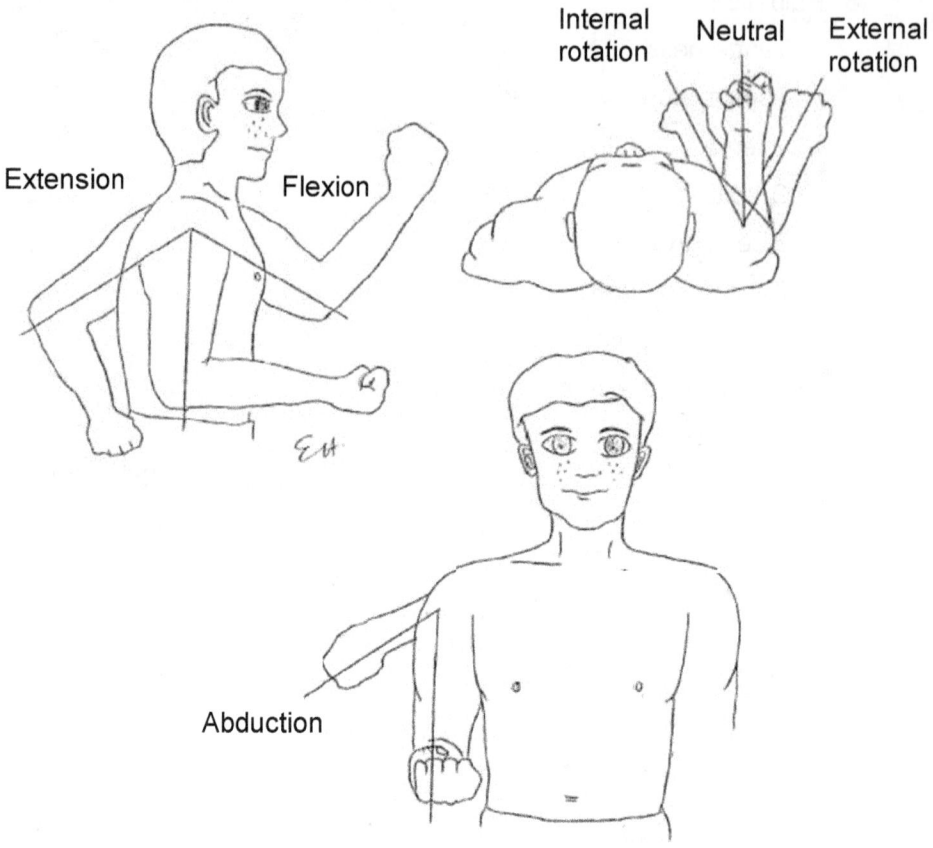

Adapted from: Talley NJ, et al. *Maclennan & Petty Pty Limited* 2003, page 271.

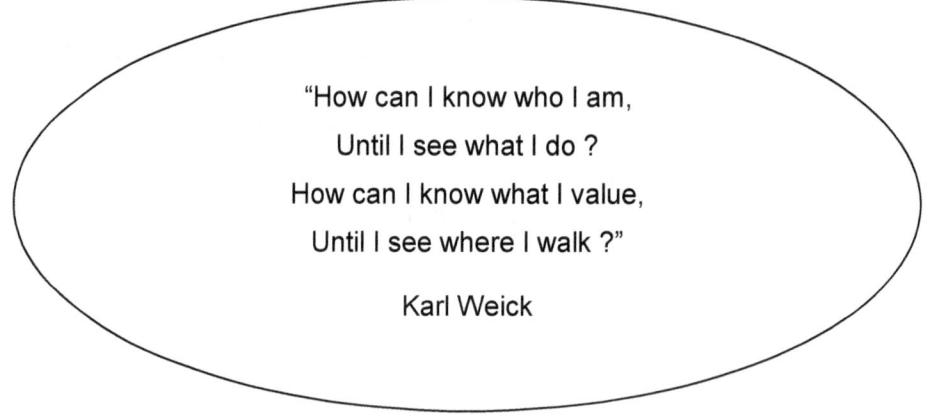

"How can I know who I am,

Until I see what I do ?

How can I know what I value,

Until I see where I walk ?"

Karl Weick

➢ Passive movements

Neer impingement sign   Hawkins impingement sign

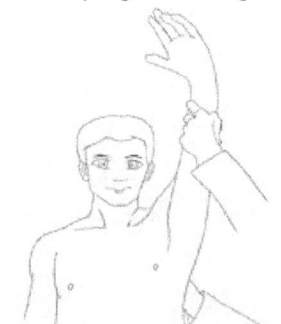 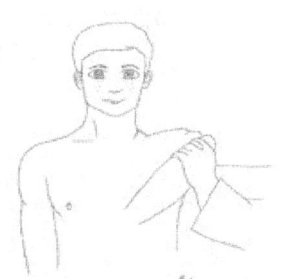

Adapted from: McGee SR. *Saunders/Elsevier* 2007, Figures 53-1 and 53-2, pages 630 and 631.

Yergason sign   Suprasinatus test

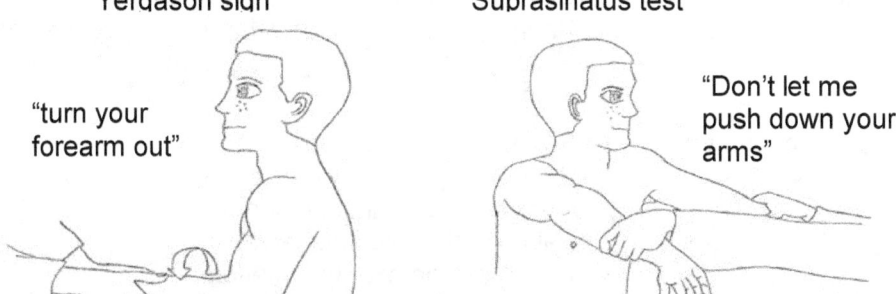

"turn your forearm out"   "Don't let me push down your arms"

The "supraspinatus test" is also known as the "empty can" or "Jobe" test.

Adapted from: McGee SR. *Saunders/Elsevier* 2007, pages 631 to 633.

➢ Special tests

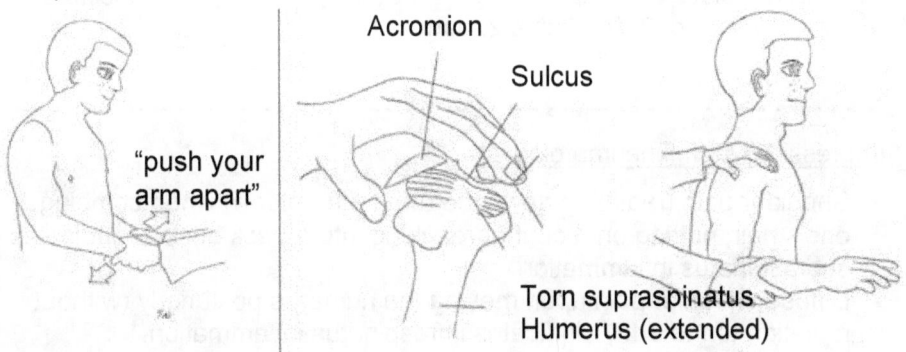

"push your arm apart"   Acromion   Sulcus

Torn supraspinatus Humerus (extended)

Adapted from: McGee SR. Evidence *Saunders/Elsevier* 2007, pages 634 and 635.

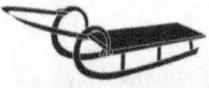

> Range of motion
  o Active and passive ROM for
    - Flexion/extension
    - Abduction/adduction
    - Internal/external rotation

> Special maneuvers
  o Apprehension test

Source: Filate W., et al. *The Medical Society, Faculty of Medicine, University of Toronto* 2005, Table 1, page 129.

Useful background: **Common clinical conditions** of the shoulder

Condition	Clinical features
o Rotator cuff tendinitis	– Shoulder pain on activity – Sharp pain on elevation of arm into overhead position – History of chronic usage (e.g. throwing, swimming) or trauma
o Rotator cuff tear/ rupture	– Sharp pain after trauma – Pain over greater tuberosity – Characteristic shoulder shrug – Pain on attempted abduction – Weakness on external rotation
o Bicipital tendinitis	– Generalized anterior tenderness over long head of biceps – Pain, especially at night – Reproduction of anterior shoulder pain during resistance to forearm supination

Adapted from: Filate W, et al. *The Medical Society, Faculty of Medicine, University of Toronto*, 2005, Table 2, page 131.

Impress the staff Rheumatologist!

> Shoulder pain (radiating down the arm to the elbow) when combing one's hair, putting on a coat or reaching into a back pocket - indicates supraspinatus inflammation.
> Diffuse shoulder pain upon moving the humerus posteriorly (without radiation to the arm) - indicates infraspinatus inflammation.

Source: Filate W, et al. *The Medical Society, Faculty of Medicine, University of Toronto* 2005, page 130.

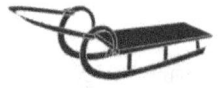

- Give the common MSK conditions that affect the shoulder.
  - o Acromioclavicular strain
  - o Biceps tendinitis
  - o Frozen shoulder
  - o Glenohumeral osteoarthritis
  - o Impingement syndrome
  - o Rotator cuff tenditinitis
  - o Rotator cuff tendon tear
  - o Subscapular bursitis

Source: Jugovic PJ, et al. *Saunders/ Elsevier* 2004, page 184.

- Perform a focused physical examination for **causes of shoulder pain**.

o Referred pain

   1. Cervical spine

     - Up to neck

     - +/- down into forearm + hand

   2. Myocardial infarction

   3. Diaphragmatic irritation

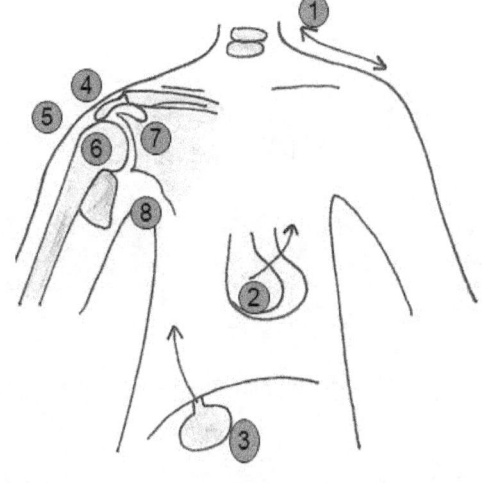

o Local causes

   4. Points of shoulder: ACJ joint arthritis

   5. Supraspinatus tendinitis (painful mid-arc)

     – Capsular syndromes

     – Acute bursitis

     – Subacromial syndromes

   6. Subacromial bursitis

   7. Glenohumeral arthritis

   8. Bicipital tendinitis

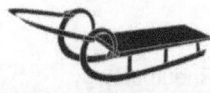

Palpation diagnosis	Finding/ Range of passive motion

o Capsular syndromes
  – Adhesive capsulitis
  – Glenohumeral arthritis
	▪ All motions limited (especially external rotation and abduction)

o Acute bursitis	▪ Abduction limited
o Acromioclavicular joint (ACJ) pain	▪ Normal ▪ Tenderness of ACJ, especially ▪ Tenderness with compression of ACJ ▪ Pain worse during adduction of arm across body
o Subacromial syndromes – Rotator cuff tendonitis	▪ Shoulder pain on activity ▪ Sharp pain on elevation of arm into overhead position ▪ History of chronic usage (e.g. throwing, swimming) or trauma ▪ Sharp pain after trauma ▪ Pain over greater tuberosity ▪ Characteristic shoulder shrug and pain on attempted abduction
– Rotator cuff tear	▪ Painful arc ▪ Weakness on external rotation ▪ Hawkin's impingement sign ▪ Neer's impingement sign ▪ Supraspinatus test ▪ Atrophy ▪ Weakness ▪ Infraspinatus weakness, atrophy ▪ Dropped arm test ▪ Palpable tear
– Bicipital tendinitis	▪ Generalized anterior tenderness over long head of biceps ▪ Associated with pain, especially at night ▪ Hallmark is reproduction of anterior shoulder pain during resistance to forearm supination

Abbreviation: ACJ, acromioclavicular joint

Adapted from: Jugovic PJ, et al. *Saunders/ Elsevier* 2004, page 183; McGee SR. *Saunders/Elsevier* 2007, Table 53-3, page 629.

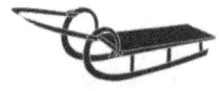

➤ Special tests

    o Tests for anterior shoulder instability

        – Anterior apprehension test – limited valve due to low specificity

        – Relocation test

            – With patient supine, patient's arm is passively abducted to 90°, elbow is flexed to 90° and arm is externally rotated 90°.

            – Examiner applies downward (posterior) pressure to humeral head.

            – Relief of symptoms of apprehension or pain is a positive result.

            – PLR, 6.5

        - Anterior release test

            – The relocation test is performed, and the examiner's hand is suddenly removed from the proximal humerus. Expression of apprehension or pain is a positive result.

            – PLR, 8.3

    o Test for inferior shoulder instability (Sulcus sign)

        - The patient stands or sits with the arm by the side and shoulder muscles relaxed

        - The arm is pulled vertically downward.

        - The presence of a sulcus sign (indentation between acromion and humeral head) is suggestive of interior should instability

        - Sensitivity, 31%; specificity, 89%

    o Tests for anterior shoulder instability

        - With the patient supine, the arm is abducted to 90° and the humerus is maximally internally rotated.

        - Examiner applies downward (posterior) pressure to humeral head

        - Apprehension by the patient is a positive result and indicates posterior instability

    o Labrum lesion: sensitivities of ≥ 83%, specificities of ≥ 90%

        - The biceps load I and II tests

        - The pain provocation test

        - The internal rotation resistance strength test

Adapted from: Filate W, et al. *The Medical Society, Faculty of Medicine, University of Toronto* 2005, pages 129 and 130.

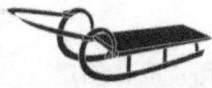

- Give the performance characteristics for detecting **rotator cuff tendonitis and tear**.
  - o Neither the Neer nor the Hawkin impingement sign, the supraspinatus test causing pain, infraspinatus weakness, or the painful arc sign are clinically significant to diagnose rotator cuff tendonitis or rotator cuff tear, or have a positive likelihood ratio (PLR) > 2.0.

Finding	PLR
➢ Detecting rotator cuff tendonitis	
o Yergason sign	2.8
➢ Detecting rotator cuff tear-individual findings	
o Age ≥ 60 years	3.2
o Supraspinatus atrophy	2.0
o Infraspinatus atrophy	2.0
o Supraspinatus weakness	2.0
o Dropped arm test	5.0
o Palpable tear	10.2
➢ Detecting rotator cuff tear – Combined findings	
o 3 findings	48.0 ...
o 2 findings	4.9 ...

*Note: findings with PLR< 2 are outlined, include
- o Neer impingement sign
- o Hawkin impingement sign
- o Supraspinatus testing causes pain
- o Infraspinatus weakness
- o Painful arc sign

Adapted from: McGee SR. *Saunders/Elsevier* 2007, Box 53-1, pages 636-637.

What's "the best"?

- o The "best" clinical test for the presence of rotator cuff tendonitis is
  - a positive Yergason sign

- o The "best" clinical tests for the presence of a rotator cuff tear are
  - a palpable tear
  - a positive dropped arm test, and
  - age ≥ 60 years.

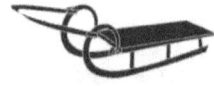

SO YOU WANT TO BE A RHEUMATOLOGIST!

- Examination of the shoulder demonstrates a painful arc, suggesting a subarcomial syndrome. Perform a focused physical examination to distinguish rotator cuff tear from tendonitis.
  - o Tear – weak cuff muscle strength
  - o Tendonitis – normal cuff muscle strength

- Perform a focused physical examination for shoulder syndromes

Syndrome	Location of pain	Range of passive motion	Other findings
o Capsular syndromes – Adhesive capsulitis – Glenohumeral arthritis	- Outer arm	- Limited (all motions limited, especially external rotation and abduction)	
o Acute bursitis	- Outer arm	- Limited (Abduction especially limited)	
o Acromioclavicular pain	- Point of shoulder	- Normal	- Tenderness of acromioclavicular joint

SO YOU WANT TO BE A RHEUMATOLOGIST!

- Fluid is palpated over the anterior surface of the joint. In this context, give what is the shoulder pad sign, and what is its usual cause?
  - o The shoulder pad syndrome is bilateral shoulder effusions.
  - o The usual cause of bilateral shoulder effusions is amyloidosis.

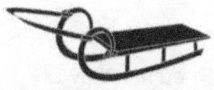

- Take a directed history and perform a focused physical examination to diagnosed the types of **tendon damage** to the shoulder and rotator cuff tear.

Clinical finding	Tendon			Frozen shoulder	Rotator cuff tear
	Tendinitis	Tear	Rupture		
o Pain	+	+	+++	+	+
o Weakness		+	+++		+
o Stiffness				+	
o External rotation abduction					
– Active				+	+
– Passive				+	-

"Knowledge speaks, but wisdom listens"

Jimi Hendrix

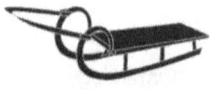

SPINE

➤ Cervicle

- Give the **cervical spine movements** and their respective myotomes

Movement	Myotome
o Neck flexion	C1-C2
o Neck side flexion	C3
o Shoulder elevation	C4
o Shoulder abduction	C5
o Elbow flexion and/ or wrist extension	C5
o Elbow extension and/ or wrist flexion	C7
o Thumb extension and/ or ulnar deviation	C8
o Blood vessels	T1

Abduction and/ or adduction of hand intrinsics

Source: Filate W, et al. *The Medical Society, Faculty of Medicine, University of Toronto* 2005, page 138.

- Give the active movements of the cervical spine and their normal range of motion.

Maneuver	Normal ROM
o Flexion ("touch your chin to your chest")	80-90°
o Extension ("put your head back")	70°
o Side flexion* ("touch each shoulder with your ear without raising your shoulders)	20-45°
o Rotation* ("turn your head to the left and right"; Look for symmetrical movements)	70-90°

Abbreviation: ROM, range of motion.

Source: Filate W, et al. *The Medical Society, Faculty of Medicine, University of Toronto* 2005, Table 11, page 138.

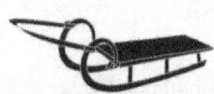

➤ Thoracolumbar

• Give the causes of lower back symptoms.

   o Degenerative
     - Disk herniation

   o Infiltrative
     - Primary, metastatic

   o Inflammatory
     - Seronegative/spondyloarthropathies
     - Prostatitis, endometriosis, pyelonephritis, pancreatitis

   o Infectious
     - Osteomyelitis, TB

   o Metabolic
     - Osteoporosis with fractures
     - Osteomalacia
     - Paget's disease

   o Compression
     - Cauda equine syndrome
     - Abdominal aortic aneurysm

   o Neurological deficits of cauda equine syndrome
     - Saddle anesthesia
     - Decreased anal tone or perianal sensory loss
     - Fecal incontinence
     - Urinary retention
     - Severe or progressive neurological deficit

Adapted from: Filate W, et al. *The Medical Society, Faculty of Medicine, University of Toronto* 2005, page 137; Jugovic PJ, et al. *Saunders/ Elsevier* 2004, page 110.

Clinical Pearl

Acute onset of L2-L3 lumbar plexopathy plus a "psoas sign" after trauma suggests an ilio psoas hematoma, which can be diagnosed early by CT of the abdomen, and weeks later by EMG showing degeneration some 3 weeks after the trauma

---

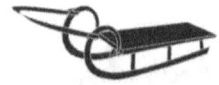

➤ Clinical

• Take a directed history and perfom a focused physical examination of back pain.

➤ History
  o Case – pain
    - How, when, where, why, what is quality of life
  o Complications
    - Fever, chills, night sweats
    - Anorexia, weight loss
    - Fatigue
    - Bowel bladder symptoms (retention, incontinence)
    - Nerve compression (sensory, motor, erectile dysfunction)
    - Cauda equina syndrome

➤ Causes
  o Joint
    - Inflammation, seropositive, seronegative
  o Bone
    - Infection, osteomyelitis, TB, immunosuppression
  o Inflammation
    - Pancreatitis, prostatitis, endometriosis, pyelonephritis
  o Malignancy
    - 1°, 2° (pancreas, prostate)
  o Metabolic
    - Osteoporosis, Paget's, fracture
  o Blood vessels
    - AAA rupture

Abbreviation: AAA, abdominal aortic aneurysm

Adapted from: Jugovic PJ, et al. *Saunders/ Elsevier*, 2004, page 110.

"Science, like good diagnosis, represents
incremental progress
of small steps taken slowly on solid ground."

Grandad

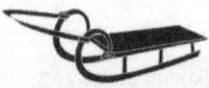

➢ Physical

- Perform a focused physical examination of thoracolumbar back pain.

o Inspection	– Symmetry; deformity
	  ▪ Lordosis
	  ▪ Kyphosis
	  ▪ Scoliosis
	– Trauma, scars
	– Inflammation
	– Edema

o Palpation	– Tenderness
	  ▪ Spinous processes
	  ▪ Paraspinal
	– Range of motion
	  ▪ Flexion, extension, lateral flexion, rotation
	  ▪ Chest expansion

o Nerve compression	– Straight leg raising – (L4,5; S1,2,3) – L4 medial calf, knee jerk, squat and rise – L5 first web space, heel walk – S1 lateral foot, ankle jerk, toe walk
o Pulses/bruits	– Femoral, papliteal, dorsalis pedis

Source: Jugovic PJ, et al. *Saunders/ Elsevier* 2004, pages 111 and 112.

o Active movements

Maneuver Thoracic and lumbar	Normal range of motion	
	Thoracic spine	Lumbar spine
– Forward flexion: ('Bend forward and touch your toes')*	20-45°	40-60°
– Extension: ('Arch your back')	25-45°	20-35°
– Side flexion: ('slide your hand down your leg')**	20-40°	15-20°
– Rotation: ('rotate toward each side')	35-50°	3-18°
– Chest expansion: (difference between rest and full inspiration	Normal is > 5cm	N/A

*With forward flexion
  o The distance from the fingers to the ground is measured; the majority of patients can reach the ground within 7cm.

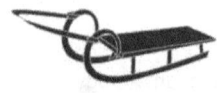

o Other methods are:
- The examiner first measures the length of the spine from the C7 spinous process to the T12 spinous process with the patient standing.
- The patient is then asked to bend forward, and the spine is measured again- a 2-7 cm difference in tape measure length is considered normal.

**With side flexion, distance from fingertips to floor is measured and compared with the other side- should be same

Adapted from: Filate W, et al. *The Medical Society, Faculty of Medicine, University of Toronto* 2005, page 140.

Useful background

➢ Active movements of the thoracolumbar spine

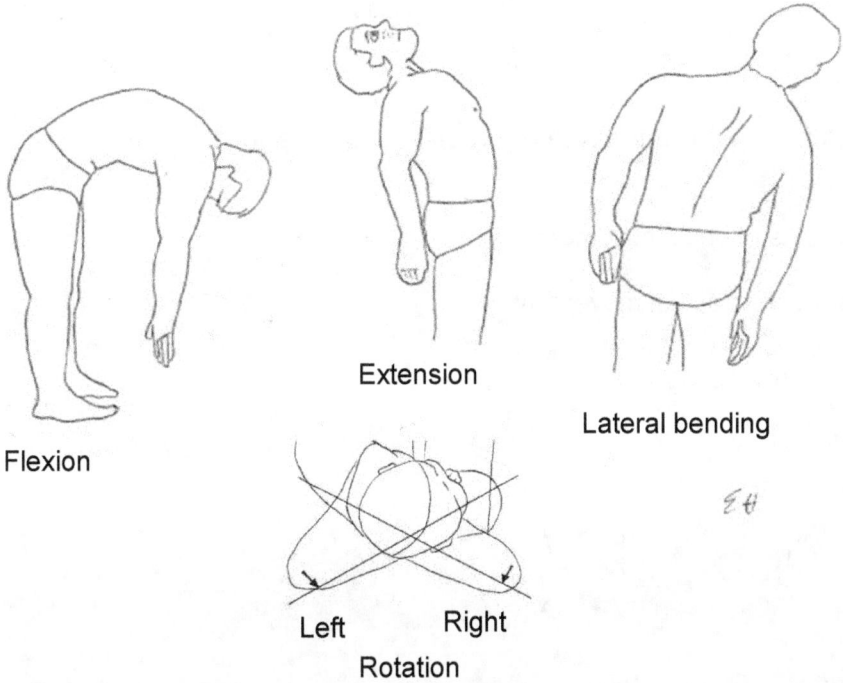

Extension

Lateral bending

Flexion

Left   Right
Rotation

Adapted from: Talley NJ, et al. *Maclennan & Petty Pty Limited* 2003, Figure 8.22, page 277.

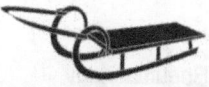

➢ Common causes of **kyphoscoliosis**

- o Idiopathic

- o Rib cage   – Thoracoplasty
  -       – Empyema

- o Connective   – Marfan syndrome
  tissue   – Ehlers-Danlos syndrome
  -       – Morquio syndrome

- o Spine   – Osteoporosis
  -       – Osteomalacia
  -       – Vitmain D-resistant rickets
  -       – Tuberculous spondylitis
  -       – Neurofibromatosis

- o Neuromuscular   – Muscular dystrophy
  -       – Poliomyelitis
  -       – Cerebral palsy
  -       – Friedreich ataxia

Adapted from: Mangione S. *Hanley & Belfus* 2000, page 283.

Special tests of back movement

➢ Restriction of spinal movement

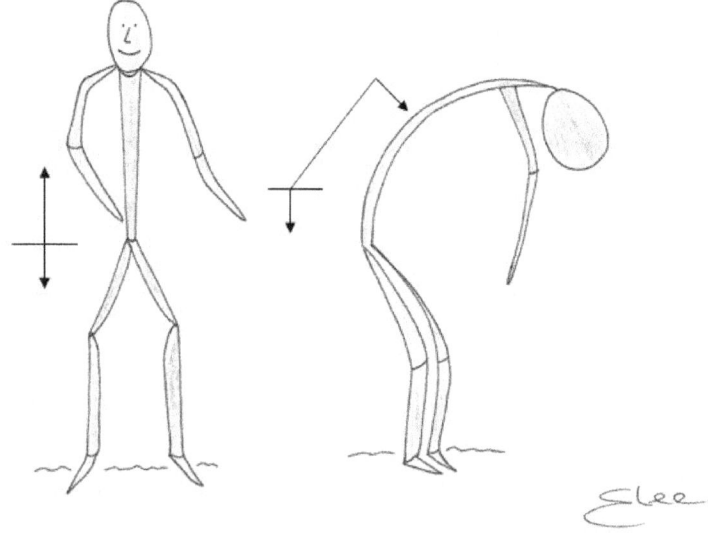

 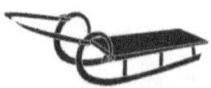

Movement and instructions	ROM	
	Thorax	Lumbar
– Forward flexion: ("Bend forward and touch your toes")	20-45°	40-60°
– Extension: (Arch your back")	25-45°	20-35°
– Side flexion: ("Slide your hand down your leg")	20-40°	15-20°
– Rotation: (twist toward each side")	35-50°	3-18°
– Chest expansion: (with a tape measure)	> 5 cm	N/A

- Schober test
    - In health an increase from 15 to 22 cm is seen on forward flexion measured above (10 cm standing) and below (5 cm) a line drawn between the dimples of Venus.
    - In those with decreased spinal flexibility the distance measured increases to < 22 cm.

o Lumbar vertebral fractures

o A rib-pelvis distance value < 2 fingerbreadths had a good sensitivity (87%) and moderate specificity (47%) for lumbar vertebral fracture

o Straight leg raising test for lumbar disc herniation

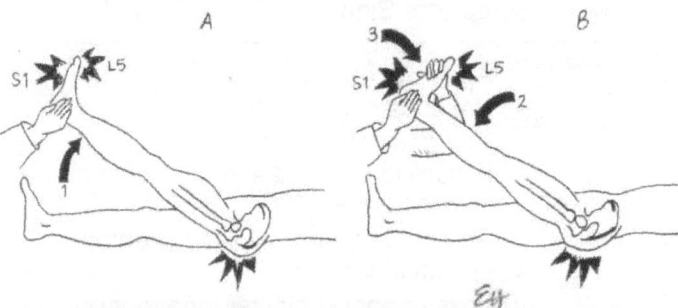

- Diagnostic value of this straight-leg raising test in detecting lumbar disc herniation may lie primarily in ruling out its presence, because sensitivity (0.8) is far greater than specificity (0.4).
- However, the crossed **straight** leg raise test (positive result = reproduction of contralateral pain with elevation and abduction of unaffected leg) identified lumbar disc herniation with a sensitivity of 25% and a specificity of 90% in patients with sciatica.

Adapted from: Filate W, et al. *The Medical Society, Faculty of Medicine, University of Toronto* 2005, Table 13, page 140; Figure 3, page 142 and 143.

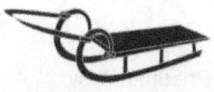

➢ "Red Flags"

- Give the "Red flags" that may indicate potential serious etiology of low back pain.

  o Age > 50 years

  o History of recent bacterial infections, malignancies, trauma, or inflammatory disease

  o Bowel or bladder dysfunction

  o Saddle anesthesia

  o IV drug use

  o Chronic disease

  o Neurological deficits

Source: Jugovic PJ., et al. *Saunders/ Elsevier* 2004, page 113.

Another Approach

- Give the "Red Flag" symptoms/signs in the assessment of low back pain.

Condition	Symptoms/Signs
o Cancer	– Age >50 – Previous cancer history – Unexplained weight loss – Failure to improve after 1 month therapy
o Cauda Equina Syndrome	– Acute urinary retention or overflow incontinence – Loss of anal sphincter tone/fecal incontinence – Perineal numbness – Change in sexual function – Weakness of legs
o Epidural abscess	– Intravenous drug abuse or sources of infection – Local or radicular pain unrelieved by position change – Fever – Sensory loss – Paraparesis or quadriparesis – Bowel/bladder impairment

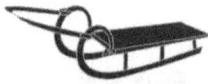

Condition	Symptoms/Signs
o Herniated Nucleus Pulposus	– Positive SLR (leg pain at <60°) – Weak dorsiflexion of ankle (L4-5) or great toe (L5-S1 or L4-5) – Reduced ankle reflex (L5-S1) – Reduced light touch in L4, L5 or S1 dermatomes of foot/leg
o Spinal Fracture/Compression Fracture	– Age >50 – Female gender – Major trauma – Pain and tenderness – Distracting painful injury – Also consider a history of osteoporosis or corticosteroid use
o Spinal Osteomyelitis	– Intravenous drug abuse – Sources of infection (e.g., skin, teeth, urinary tract or indwelling catheter) – Fever – Vertebral tenderness

Abbreviations: MRI = magnetic resonance imaging; SLR = straight leg raising

Reproduced with permission: Therapeutics Choices. Sixth Edition. Ottawa, Canada: *Canadian Pharmacist Association* 2012, Table 1, page 1095.

- Give performance characteristics of the Clinical Examination for Herniated Disk or Cancer among patients with Back Pain

Test	PLR	NLR
o Sit-to-stand test for upper lumbar herniation	26 (1.7-41.3)	0.35 (0.22-0.56)
o Nocturnal pain for cancer-induced back pain	1.7 (1.2-1.19)	0.17 (0.03-0.73)
o Crossed straight-lef raise for disk herniation	1.6-5.8	0.59-0.90
o Ipsilateral straight-leg raise for disk herniation	0.99-2.0	0.04-0.5

Abbreviation: NLR, negative likelihood ratio; PLR, positive likelihood ratio

Source: Simel DL, et al. *JAMA* 2009, Table 7-8, page 86

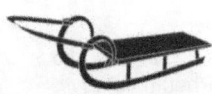

HIPS

➢ Clinical

   o Pain in the hip

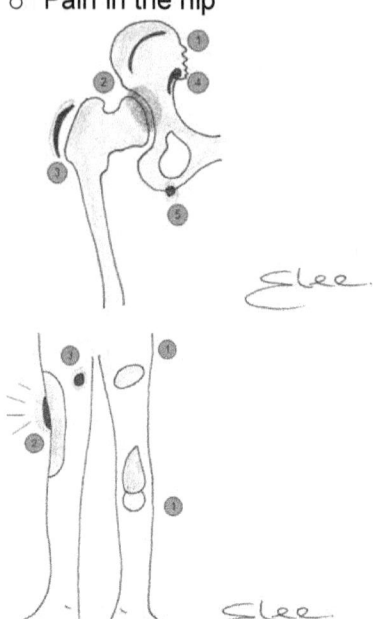

- Structures giving rise to pain around the hip and buttocks
  1. Sacro-iliac joint
  2. Hip joint (OA, RA, sepsis)
  3. Trochanteric bursa (overuse, mechanical imbalance)
  4. Ischiogluteal bursa (posterior)
  5. Insertion of adductor tendon

- Patterns of pain around the hip
  1. Intrinsic hip or knee joint pain
  2. Trochanteric bursitis
  3. Adductor tendinitis

   o Compensatory postures that might be seen in an examination of the hip if there is:
- A scoliotic deformity - flexion of the longer leg
- An abduction deformity - flexion of ipsilateral knee
- An adduction deformity - flexion of contralateral knee
- A flexion deformity - exaggerated lordosis.

Source: Jugovic PJ, et al. *Saunders/ Elsevier* 2004, page 171.

   o Radiation of pain (Where is the pain felt in the following conditions?)
- Osteoarthritis → to groin
- Bursitis → superior margin of the greater trochanter
- Sacroiliitis → sacroiliac joint

   o Compensatory postures of the lower leg, knee or spine if there are associated deformities
- A scoliotic deformity - flexion of the longer leg
- An abduction deformity - flexion of ipsilateral knee
- An adduction deformity - flexion of contralateral knee
- A flexion deformity - exaggerated lordosis.

Adapted from: Jugovic PJ, et al. *Saunders/ Elsevier* 2004, page 171.

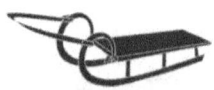

o Maneuvers for the hip and normal range of motion (ROM).

Maneuver	Normal ROM
– Flexion – with patient lying supine, have patient pull knee to chest; knee is also flexed	120°
– Extension – with patient lying on side, palpate the ASIS and PSIS and have patient fully extend the leg until pelvis shifts	15°
– Abduction – place one hand on the contralateral ASIS and with the other hand, grasp the heel and abduct the patient's leg until the pelvis shifts	40°
– Adduction – place one hand on the ipsilateral ASIS and with the other hand, grasp the heel and adduct the patient's leg until the pelvis shifts	25°
– Rotation – flex knee and hip to 90°, grasp the lower leg and move medially (external rotation) and laterally (internal rotation)	▪ External rotation in ext -35° ▪ External rotation at 90° ▪ Flex -45°
– Or with patient lying supine with the leg fully extended, roll the leg medially and laterally	▪ Internal rotation in ext: -45° ▪ Internal rotation at 90° ▪ Flex -45°

Abbreviation: ROM; range of motion

Source: Filate W, et al. *The Medical Society, Faculty of Medicine, University of Toronto* 2005, page 145.

➢ Normal ROM of hip

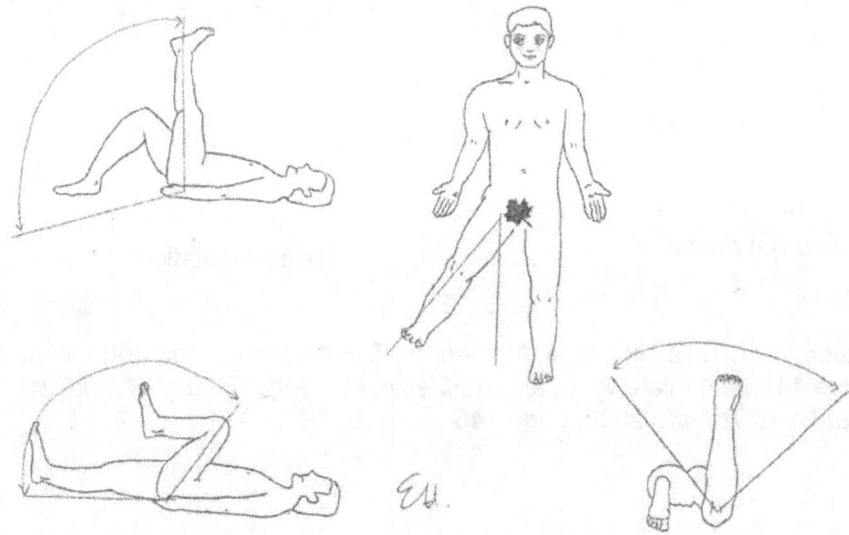

Adapted from: Talley NJ, et al. *Maclennan & Petty Pty Limited* 2003, page 279.

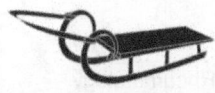

- Give the **lower limb movements** and their respective **myotomes**.

Lower limb movement	Myotome
○ Hip flexion	○ L2
○ Knee extension	○ L3
○ Ankle dorsiflexion	○ L4
○ Great toe extension	○ L5
○ Ankle plantar flexion, ankle eversion, hip extension	○ S1
○ Knee flexion	○ S2

Source: Filate W, et al. *The Medical Society, Faculty of Medicine, University of Toronto* 2005, Table 14, page 141.

Useful background: Internal and external rotation of the hip

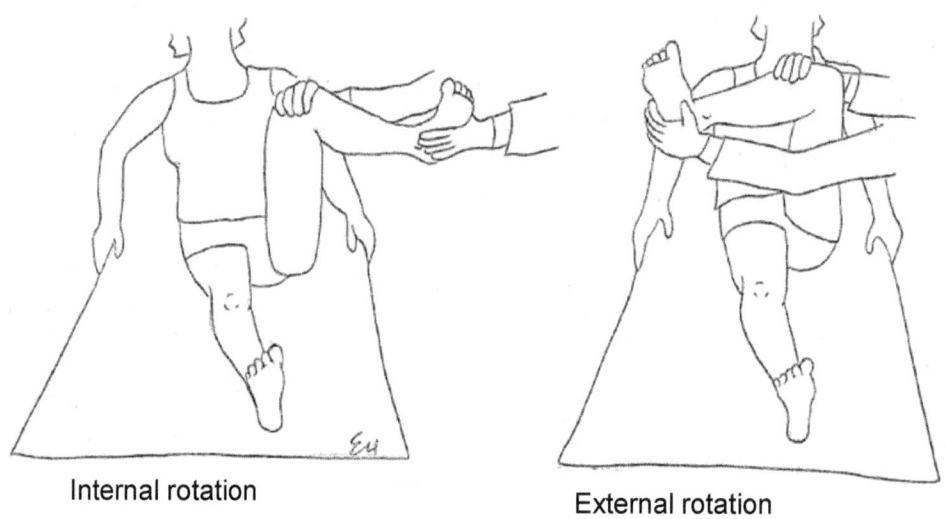

Internal rotation

External rotation

Adapted from: Talley NJ, et al. *Maclennan & Petty Pty Limited* 2003, Figure 4, page 145; and Filate W, et al. *The Medical Society, Faculty of Medicine, University of Toronto* 2005, page 145.

SO YOU WANT TO BE A RHEUMATOLOGIST!

- In the context of a screening physical examination for hip disease, what is the FABER maneuver?

    o   The FABER maneuver is the movement of the hip so that it is Flexed, ABducted, and Externally Rotated.

- In the context of redness and swelling of the calf of one leg, give is the meaning of the "crescent sign", and give what diagnosis does it suggest.

    o   If there is crescent-shaped bruising of the calf from the medial to the lateral malleolus, they likely have pseudothrombophlebitis from a ruptured cyst.

- While on a camping trip in Europe, a gentleman develops an annular rash. He returns home to North Overshoe, and six weeks later he develops a painful knee joint and a unilateral facial nerve (CN VII) palsy. Give the likely etiology.

    o   Lyme disease, and the confirmatory test is an antibody titre against *Borrelia burgdorferi*.

"The impossible is often the untried"
Jim Goodwin

 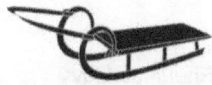

GLUTEAL MUSCLES

- Perform a focused physical examination for **gluteal muscle weakness**.

  o Trendelenburg sign (TS)
    - Stand on one leg, the pelvis on the other side normally becomes elevated
    - TS is positive with lack of elevation or sagging of buttock.

  o Trendelenburg gait
    - Weakness/ paralysis of gluteal muscles causing awaddling gait (common in progressive muscular dystrophy)

Adapted from: Mangione S. *Hanley & Belfus* 2000, page 472.
A patient with IBD (inflammatory bowel disease presents with pain in the groin, which is considered to arise from the hip.

- Give the causes of **hip pain** in the person with inflammatory bowel disease (IBD), ulcerative colitis and Crohn disease..

  o ON (osteonecrosis, aka avascular necrosis)

  o OP (osteoporosis)

  o IBD-associated arthritis

  o Trochanteric bursitis
    - Lateral joint tenderness
    - ↓ abduction

- Give the differential diagnosis for **lateral hip pain**.

o Trochanteric bursitis	– ↑ pain on active hip abduction
o Iliotibial band syndrome	– Pain radiated down lateral surface of leg – Tenderness along band – ↑ pain on adduction of knee
o Lumbar radiculopathy	– Positive straight-leg-raising test
o Osteoarthritis / synovitis of hip	– ↑ pain on passive motion – ↓ ROM (range of movement) due to ↑ pain

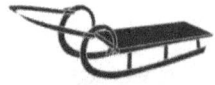

KNEES

- Give the common causes of a **painful knee joint**.

    o Musculoskeletal
      - Rheumatoid arthritis
      - Osteoarthritis
      - Gout
      - Pseudogout

    o Infection
      - Viral infection
      - Septic arthritis
      - Borrelia burgdorferi

    o Metabolic
      - Gout
      - Pseudogout

    o Hematology
      - Hemophilia

    o Trauma

Adapted from: Baliga RR. *Saunders/Elsevier* 2007, pages 344 and 345.

```
SO YOU WANT TO BE A RHEUMATOLOGIST!

• In the context of a painful knee joint, give what Lyme disease is.

    o Lyme disease causes painful knee, skin rash and unilateral CN
      VII (facial nerve) paralysis due to an infection with Borrelia
      burgdorferi
```

- Perform a directed physical examination of the knee.

    o Inspection
      - For symmetry, deformity, genu valgum or varum, rubor, swelling,
        quadriceps, atrophy (assess with tape)
      - Skin bruising and any abnormal movements used to compensate
        for pain/stiffness in knee joint
      - Assess gait
      - Assess standing, feet together (hip, knee, ankle in straight line)

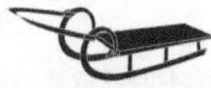

- o Palpation – Flex knee for best assessment
  - - Joint line and along course of medial and lateral collateral ligaments, tibial tubercle and intrapatellar tendon, bursal areas including anserine, prepatellar and infrapatellar popliteal fossa (for cyst, etc)
    - Tenderness at 90°, 180°
    - Flexion, 135°; extension, 0°
    - Warmth
    - Popliteal fossa Baker cyst
    - Swelling of patella
    - Crepitation

  - - Knee should be flexed for best assessment

  - - Effusions
    - Temperature
    - Wipe test
    - Ballotment
    - Fluid displacement sign
    - Patellar tap

  - - Bulge sign/fluid displacement sign
  - - Balloon sign.fluctuation test

- o Active and passive ROM: flexion/extension
- o Stability (ligaments)
  - - Anterior and posterior cruciate draw test
  - - Collateral and medial collateral ligament stability

  - - Provocative tests
    - Meniscal tests
      - - McMurray /Apley tests)
      - - Apprehension test
      - - Femoral-patelar grind test
      - - Crouch compression test
    - Anterior drawer test (anterior cruciate ligament)
    - Pivot shift test
    - Posterior drawer test (posterior cruciate ligament)
    - Stability of lateral and medial collateral ligaments

Adapted from: Filate W, et al. *The Medical Society, Faculty of Medicine, University of Toronto* 2005, page 147; Jugovic PJ, et al. *Saunders/ Elsevier* 2004, page 175; McGee SR. *Saunders/Elsevier* 2007, Table 53.2, pages 626-7.

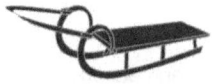

> What is "the best"? The three "best" clinical tests for osteoarthritis of the knee in a person with chronic pain are bony enlargement, varus (not valgus)

- o Anterior drawer sign

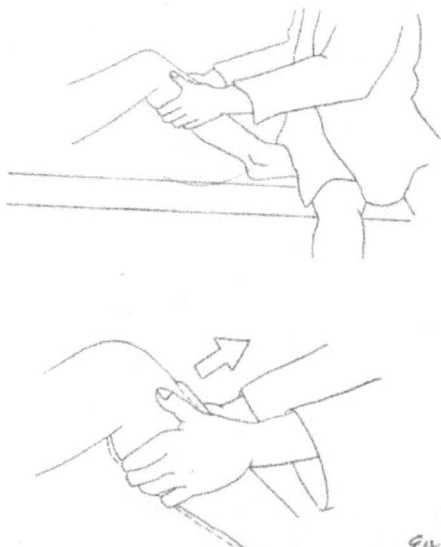

Adapted from: McGee SR. *Saunders/Elsevier* 2007, Figure 53.7, page 641.

- o Posterior anterior drawer sign

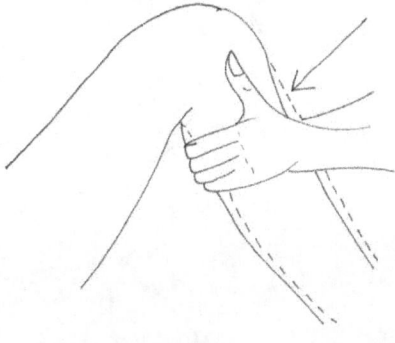

- With the patient positioned as for the anterior drawer sign, the clinician pushes posteriorly on the patient's upper calf.
- In the PCL-deficient knee, this force reveals an abnormal posterior tibial movement (arrow) with a soft endpoint

Adapted from: McGee SR. *Saunders/Elsevier* 2007, Figure 53.11, page 646.

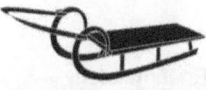

o   Pivot shift sign

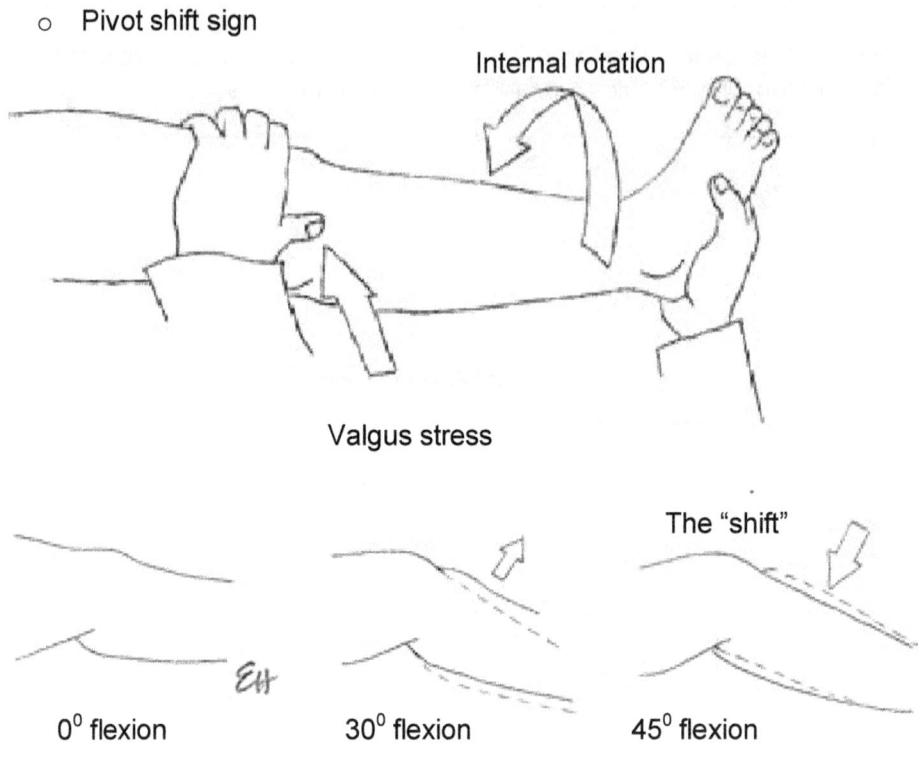

Internal rotation

Valgus stress

The "shift"

0⁰ flexion   30⁰ flexion   45⁰ flexion

Adapted from: McGee SR. *Saunders/Elsevier* 2007, Figure 53.9, page 643.

Lachman sign

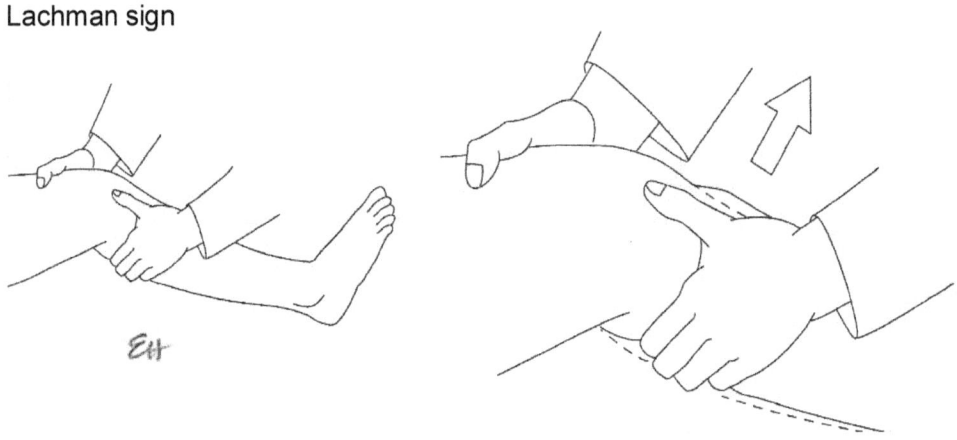

Adapted from: McGee SR. *Saunders/Elsevier* 2007, Figure 53.8, page 642.

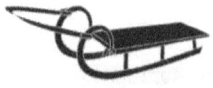

o The McMurray test

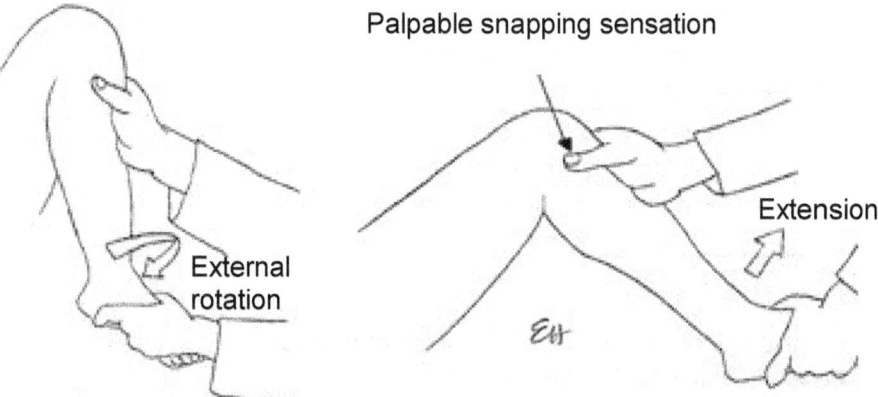

Palpable snapping sensation

External rotation

Extension

Adapted from: McGee SR. *Saunders/Elsevier* 2007, Figure 53.2, page 647.

- Give the performance characteristics of physical examination for detecting **anterior cruciate ligament** rupture or tear

Finding	PLR
o Detecting anterior cruciate ligament ruptureor tear	
– Lachman sign	17.0
– Anterior drawer sign	11.5
– Pivot shift sign	8.0
o Detecting meniscal injury	
– McMurray sign	8.2
– Block to full extension	3.2

o Note that joint line tenderness does not have significant values for PLR/ NLR.

Abbreviation: PLR, positive likelihood ratio

Adapted from: McGee SR. *Saunders/Elsevier* 2007, Box 53-4, page 651.

What is "the best"?

  o The three "best" clinical tests for the presence of an anterior cruciate ligament tear are
    - Positive Lachman sign
    - Anterior drawing sign
    - Pivot shift sign.

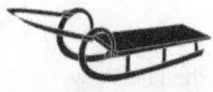

What is "the best"?
- o The three "best" tests of physical examination for clinically significant knee fracture are
  - Inability to flex the knee beyond 90°
  - Inability to bear weight
  - Tenderness at the head of the fibula.

- Give the performance characteristics of physical examination for clinically significant **knee fracture**.

Finding	LR+
o Age ≥ 55 years	3.0
o Joint effusion	2.5
- Limitation of knee flexion;	
▪ Not able to flex beyond 90 degrees	2.9
▪ Not able to flex beyond 60 degrees	4.7
o Isolated tenderness of patella	2.2
o Tenderness at head of fibula	3.4
o Inability to bear weight, immediately and in emergency department	3.6

➢ Combined findings
- o Ottawa knee rule* positive   1.7

* Ottawa rule for knee fracture: A knee radiograph is indicated (and the rule is positive) if any of the following are present:

- o Age ≥ 55 years
- o Tenderness at head of fibula
- o Isolated tenderness of patella (no bone tenderness of knee other than patella)
- o Inability to flex to 90 degrees

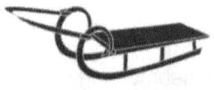

- o Inability to bear weight both immediately and in the emergency department (4 steps); unable to transfer weight twice onto each lower limb regardless of limping

- o Ecchymosis does not have significant values for PLR/-

Abbreviation: PLR, positive likelihood ratio

Adapted from: McGee SR. *Saunders/Elsevier* 2007, page 649, and page 639.

- Give the performance characteristics of tests for **osteoarthritis of knee** in patients with chronic pain

Finding	PLR
o Individual findings	
– Morning stiffness <30 minutes	3.0
– Bony enlargement	11.8
– Varus deformity	3.4
o Combined findings	
– At least 3 out of 6:	3.1
– Age > 50 years	
– Stiffness < 30 minutes	
– Crepitus	
– Bony tenderness along margins of joint	
– Bone enlargement	
– No palpable warmth	
– Note:	

- Valgus deformity does not have a significant PLR values for osteoarthritis of the knee, nor does crepitus on passive movement (PLR, 2.1) or a palpable increase in the temperature of the knee.

Adapted from: McGee SR. *Saunders/Elsevier* 2007, Box 53-2, page 648.

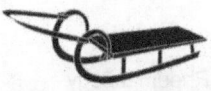

ANKLES

- Perform a focused physical examination of the ankle.

Finding	Diagnosis
o Inspection	
– Flattening of longitudinal arch	▪ Pes planus
– Abnormal elevation of medial longitudinal arch	▪ Pes cavus
	▪ Hallux valgus
– Outward angulation of great toe with prominence over medial 1st MTP joint (bunion)	▪ Hammer toes
– Hyperextension of MTP joints and flexion of PIP joints	
o Palpation	
– Nodules within Achilles tendon	▪ Tendon xanthoma
– Foot pain, localized tenderness over calcaneal origin of plantar fascia	▪ Plantar fasciitis
– Foot pain, localized tenderness over plantar surface of MT heads	▪ Metarsalgia
– Forefoot pain, tenderness between 2nd or 3rd toes or between 3rd and 4th toes	▪ Morton's interdigital neuroma
– Ankle pain, dysesthesias of sole, aggravated by forced dorsiflexion and eversion of foot	▪ Tarsal tunnel syndrome

Printed with permission: McGee SR. *Saunders/Elsevier* 2007, Table 53-2, page 627.

➤ Active Movement: Normal ROM

Joint	Flexion/extension	Rotation
o Ankle and feet	– 45° (plantar flexion)	▪ 30° (inversion)
	– 20° (dorsiflexion)	▪ 20° (eversion)

Abbreviations: DIP, distal interphalangeal; MCP, metacarpophalangeal; MT, metatarsal; PIP, proximal interphalangeal

Source: McGee SR. *Saunders/Elsevier* 2007, Table 53-1, page 624.

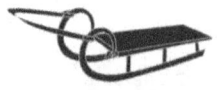

- Give performance characteristics for ankle and midfoot fracture*

Finding	PLR	NLR
o Detecting ankle fracture		
– Tenderness over posterior lateral malleolus	2.4	0.4
– Tenderness over posterior medial malleolus	4.8	0.6
– Inability to bear weight immediately after injury	2.6	0.5
– Inability to bear weight 4 steps in the emergency room	2.5	0.3
o Detecting midfoot fracture		
– Tenderness at the base of the 5th metatarsal	2.9	0.1
– Ottawa foot rule	2.1	0.1

- Note: Some clinical findings are deleted because their PLR is < 2. These include:
  - Ottawa ankle rule
  - Tenderness of navicular bone
  - Inability to bear weight immediately, and
  - Inability to bear weight 4 steps in the emergency room.

Adapted from: McGee SR. *Saunders/Elsevier* 2007, Box 53-5, page 654.

SO YOU WANT TO BE A RHEUMATOLOGIST!

- Give the difference between Trousseau syndrome, Trousseau sign and Chevostek sign?

  o Trousseau syndrome
    - Migratory, superficial or deep thomboplebitis
    - Associated with carcinoma of the lung, breast, stomach, pancreas or prostate

  o Trousseau sign
    - Carpopedal spasm, extension of the body, and spisthotonos finger extensors and wrist flewors (aka obstertrocoam's hand, or main d'accoucheur).
    - Due to due low Ca^{2+}, Mg^{2+}, PO_4^{2-}; alkalemia

  o Chvostek sign
    - For muscle hyperexicitability; (from low Ca^{2+}, Mg^{2+}, PO_4^{2-}; alkalemia)
    - Sensitivity of 27%; false positive rate of 4-29% in adult (i.e. sign is "worthless")

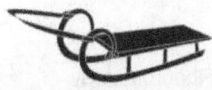

FEET

- Perform a focused physical examination of the feet.

  o Inspection
     - For skin rash, scars
     - At the nails for changes of psoriasis
     - At the forefoot for hallux valgus, clawing and crowding of the toes (rheumatoid arthritis)
     - At the callus over the metatarsal heads which may occur in subluxation
     - At both the arches of the foot, in particular medial and longitudinal (flat foot, pes cavus)

  o Palpate
     - Ankles for synovitis, effusion, passive movements at the subtalar joints (inversion and eversion) and talar joint (dorsiflexion and plantar flexion); remember that tenderness on movement is more important that the range of movement
     - Metatarsophalangeal joints for tenderness
     - Individual digits, for synovial thickening
     - Bottom of heel, for tenderness (plantar fasciitis), and Achilles tendon for nodules.

Adapted from: Baliga RR. *Saunders/ Elsevier* 2007, page 334-335; Filate W, et al. *The Medical Society, Faculty of Medicine, University of Toronto* 2005, page 151.

Gem, Pearl, Tid-Bit and Non-sense

  o Notwithstanding that "there are never 'nevers'" in medicine, RA never involves the DIP joints.

Foot pain: Plantar Fasciitis, Morton Neuroma

- Take a directed history and perform a focused physical examination to distinguish plantar fasciitis from a (Morton) neuroma.

Clinical Feature	Plantar Fasciitis	Morton Neuroma
o ↑ pain with walking	+	+
o ↑ pain by wearing tight or high-heeled shoes	-	+
o ↑ pain after nighttime sleep or after resting	+	-
o Tenderness along plantar fascia or calcaneal insertion site	+	-
o Tenderness when squeezing forefoot	-	+

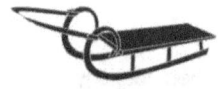

INFECTIOUS ARTHRITIS

- ➢ Common causes
  - ○ Bacterial
  - ○ Fungal
  - ○ Viral

- ➢ Diagnosis
  - ○ Joint aspiration
    - − Synovial fluid analysis
      - − PMN > 50 x 10^9 /L (50,000 mL) suggest
        - − Infection
        - − Gout
        - − RA (rheumatoid arthritis)
    - − Culture of synovial fluid

Clinical Pearl

- ○ Synovial fluid > 50 x 10^9 PMN may occur in infectious arthritis as well as in gout or RA (rheumatoid arthritis), but these other conditions may become infected with a secondary infectious arthritis.

- ○ Bacterial infectious arthritis can occur in the absence of a positive culture.

Gems and Pearls in Septic Arthritis

- ○ Common causes
  - − In young persons: Gonococcal arthritis
    - ▪ Systemic symptoms or skin papules / macules / pustules are uncommon
    - ▪ Blood cultures positive in only 50%

  - − Old, immune suppressed, post-operative, IV catheters
    - ▪ Think gram-negative organisms

  - − Persons with systemic fungal infection
    - ▪ Develops subacute monoarthritis
    - ▪ Think fungal arthritis

  - − Person for TB endemic area, previous exposure, on immunosuppressants / anti-TNF drugs
    - ▪ Think tuberculous arthritis, even if TB skin test is negative

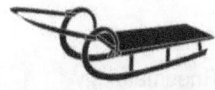

Clinical Caution

- o The cause of septic arthritis must be diagnosed from **aspiration** of synovial fluid, measurement of WBC / PMNs, and culture.

- o Non-inflammatory: synovial fluid WBC 200-2000 / μL, PMN < 25%
    - OA (osteoarthritis)
    - ON (osteoarthritis)
    - HH (hereditary hemochromatosis)
    - SCD (sickle cell disease)

- o Inflammatory: synovial fluid WBC > 2000, PMN > 50%

    - MSK
        - RA (rheumatoid arthritis)
        - SAP (spondyloarthropathy)
        - SLE (systemic lupus erythematosis)

    - Crystalline arthropathy

    - Infectious
        - GC gonococcal
        - Staphylococcal
        - TB

Helpful Clues:

- o In crystalline arthropathy synovial fluid, WBC is > 50,000 / μL
    - Watch out for secondary infection

- o For infectious arthropathy, WBC is usually > 100,000 / μL
    - 40% have no fever
    - May complicate OA (osteoarthritis)

"Use diagnostic imaging to guide your clinical impression, not to make the diagnosis."

Dr. Joel Hurwitz

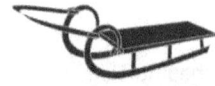

BACTERIAL ARTHRITIS

- Give the **microorganisms** which commonly cause bacterial arthritis

    o Gram-positive

    - Staphylococcus
        - Aureus
            - Common
        - Epidermidis
            - Prosthetic joints

    - Streptococcus species
        - Diabetes

    - Escherichia coli (common)

    - Pseudomonas aerugenosa

    o Gram-negative

    - Neisseria gonorrhea
        - Monoarticular
            - Knee
            - Wrist
            - Ankle
        - Migratory associated
            - Fever, chills
            - Rash, vesiculopustular (disseminated GC disease)
            - Tenosynovitis (dorsa of hands, feet)

    - Salmonella
        - Sickle cell disease

    - Pseudomonas
        - IVDU (intravenous drug users)

➤ Treatment

- Give the treatment of bacterial arthritis.

    o No gram stain
    - If Neisserria gonorrhea suspected
        - Ceftriaxome
    - If N. gonorrhea not suspected
        - Ceftriaxone or cefotaxime

    o Gram-positive cocci
    - Oxacillin / nafcillin or cefazoline
    - If MRSA a possibility
        - Vancomycin or linezolid

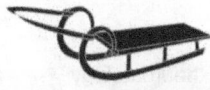

- o Gram-negative bacilli
  - – Ceftriaxone or
  - – Cefotaxime
- o Pseudomonas aeruginosa
  - – Cefazidine plus gentamicin or carbapenems
- o Chlamydia
  - – Doxycycline or azithromycin

- o Note:
  - – Repeated needle or arthroscopic drainage, or surgical debridement if refractory
  - – Remove infected joint, and replace after antibiotic clearance of all infection

Tuberculosis

- o Only < 2% of M. tuberculosis infections affect the joints
- o With / without pulmonary TB
- o Usually monoarticular
- o Pott disease
  - – TB of an intervertebral disk
  - – Associated osteomyelitis

- o Diagnostic imaging   – CT or MRI more sensitive than radiography
- o Diagnosis   – Synovial-fluid aspiration
   – Biopsy

A fisher accidently pricks himself with a hook, and develops nodular papules at the site. The lesion ulcerates, and the adjacent joints become painful. Cellulitis is suspected, but appropriate antibiotics for this diagnosis fail.

- • In the context of infectious arthritis, give the name of the likely organism, and give the methods to confirm the diagnosis.

  - o The puncture of the skin allowed infection with the marine organism Mycobacterium marinum

  - o The diagnosis is made by examination of a synovial fluid aspiration or biopsy of the synovium

  - o Treat with minocycline, clarithromycin, or trimethoprim sulfamethoxazole

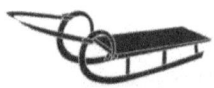

Lyme Disease

➤ Phases
- o Early infection with Borrelia burgdorferi
- o Early
  - Polyarthritis
- o Late
  - Chronic arthritis
  - Monoarthicular
    - Knee
    - Hip
    - Ankle

➤ Diagnosis

- o Joint fluid aspiration
  - PMN
    - 10 to 20 x 10^9 (10,000 to 20,000 / μL)
  - Culture negative
  - PCR (polymerase chain reaction)
    - Positive

- o Biopsy of synovium
  - Direct microscopy → B. burgdorferi
- o Serological testing not reliable

Fungal Arthritis

➤ Causes

Fungal infections of the joints occur in endemic areas, and are also likely to occur in persons who are immunocompromised.

- Give the common fungal causes of arthritis, and the clinical features.

  - o Causative Organisms
    - Coccidoides
    - Cryptococcus
    - Histoplasma
    - Aspergillus
    - Blastomyces
    - Candida

  - o Clinical
    - Monoarticular
    - Medium / large joints
    - Diagnosis made from examination of synovial fluid aspirate or biopsy of synovium

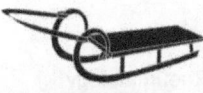

Viral Arthritis of Joints

Case Scenario

A mother of two toddlers attending a daycare facility develops a fever, arthralgias and myalgias. She then develops a large red mark on her face that appears as if she had been physically abused. She consulted her physician, who recognized that the patient was likely suffering from a viral infection, which included the joints, rather than being a victim of abuse by her spouse.

- Give the name of the likely virus, and the specific diagnostic test.
  - o The "slapped cheek" of the facial rash plus the symptoms of a flu-like illness suggest a parvovirus B19 infection.
  - o The clinical suspicion as confined with the finding of IgM anti-parvovirus antibodies

---

Buzz Words

- o Fever, cough, lymphadenopathy, morbilliform rash, plus symmetric or migratory arthralgia: name the likely causes of viral arthritis.
- o Morbilliform rash → think rubella, and you're correct, rubella arthritis

---

Useful recollections
- o Patients with HBV or HCV infections may develop arthralgias / arthritis
- o HBV
  - – Symmetric
  - – Polyarticular
- o HCV
  - – Chronic polyarthralgia, or
  - – Polyarthritis, from essential mixed cryoglobulinemia

Watch Out – Clinical Alert

- o Inflammatory or crystalline arthropathies injure joints and increase the risk of bacterial infection.

- o Prosthetic joints may become infected < 3 mon after implantation or > 3 mon from hematogenous spread: look for erosion or loosing around the implant.

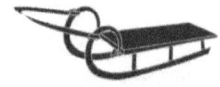

INFLAMMATORY CRYSTAL INDUCED ARTHROPATHIES

➢ Causes/Associations

- Give the causes of inflammatory crystal-induced arthropathies.
  - Gout
  - Pseudogout (calcium pyrophosphate deposition disease [CPPDA])
  - Basic calcium phosphate (BCP) deposition
  - Infection
  - Trauma
    - R/O
      - Fracture
      - Hamarthrosis
    - May precipitate attacks of
      - Gout
      - Pseudogout
  - Degeneration
  - Reactive arthritis

➢ Diagnosis
  - Aspiration of synovial fluid from acutely inflamed joint
    - PMN > 3.0×10^9 / L (> 3000 / mL)
    - Phagocytosed needle-shaped, negatively birefringent urate crystal on polarized light microscopy
  - X-ray
    - Acute
      - Soft tissue swelling
    - Chronic
      - "punched out" lesion (urate deposit)
      - Tophi, destroying joint

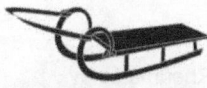

Gouty Arthritis

➢ Definition: "Gout is a disease in which monosodium urate monohydrate (MSU) crystals deposit in joints, soft tissue such as cartilage, tendons and bursa, or in renal tissues such as glomeruli, the interstitium and tubules".

   o The deposition of MSU crystals "….can result in gouty arthritis, tophi, nephropathy or uric acid nephrolithiasis" (Kapur S and Kraag G, et al. Chapter 44. In: Therapeutic Choices. Grey J, Ed. 6th Edition, *Canadian Pharmacists Association*: Otttawa, ON, 2011, page 1011).

   o MSU tophi may cause joint deformities and destruction, and tophi in the cardiac conduction system may lead to dysarrythmias.

➢ Pathophysiology

• Give the pathophysiology of gout.

   o ↑ intake
   - High purine foods
   - ↑ fructose intake
   - Obesity
   - ↑ intake of beer

   o ↑ synthesis
   - Hereditary
   - ↑ activity of PRPP (phosphoribosyl pyrophosphate) → ↑ production of purine → ↑ uric acid
   - ↓ activity of HPRT (hypoxanthine guanine phosphoribosyl transferase) synthase → ↓ purine → ↓ xanthine / hypoxanthine → ↓ purine salvage → purine deficiency → ↓ feedback inhibition on PRPP synthase → synthesis of uric acid

   o ↑ cell turnover
   - Blood disorders
     ▪ Erythropoietin
     ▪ Granulocyte colony-stimulating factor)
     ▪ Granulocyte-macrophage colony-stimulating factor
   - Treatment of blood disorders
     ▪ Hemolytic anemia
     ▪ Polycythemia vera
     ▪ Leukemia
     ▪ Lymphoma
     ▪ Ineffective erythroparesis
   - Psoriasis
   - Tumor lysis (usually treatment for acute leukemia or lymphoma)

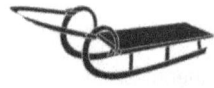

- o ↓ renal excretion (underexcreters of urate)

  - Primary
    - GFR (glomerular filtration ratio) is normal, but urate secretes in proximal renal tubule may be defective

  - Secondary
    - ↓ GFR-related disorders (↑ retention of urate)
    - Drugs
      - ↓ urate
    - Excreting transporters in proximal renal tubule → hyperuricemia
    - Examples
      - Competitive blocking
      - Weak acids diuretics
      - ASA (low-dose aspirin)
      - Nicotinic acid
      - Diuretics
      - Ethambulol
      - Pyrazinamide
      - Non-competitive blocking
    - Dehydration, alkalosis → ↑ retention of Na^+, H^+, urate

- ➢ Causes

  - o Associations
    - Hypertension
    - Diabetes
    - Cardiovascular disease

  - o Hyperuricemia

- Give 15 causes of **hyperuricemia**.

  - o Primary gout

  - o Chronic renal failure

  - o ↑ Production of uric acid

  - o ↓ Excretion of uric acid
    - Chronic renal failure
    - Hyperparathyroidism
    - Ketosis and lactic acidosis

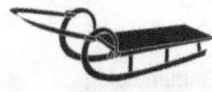

- o Increased cell turnover
  - Polycythemia
  - Leukemia
  - Reticulosis
  - Myelosclerosis
  - Psoriasis

- o Drugs
  - Salicylates (in low doses)
  - Thiazides and furosemide
  - Pyrazinamide

- o High purine diet and alcohol

- o Down syndrome
- o Metabolic
  - Obese
  - Hypertensive patients

- o Congenital
  - Lesch-Nyhan syndrome (congenital mental deficiency, choreo-athetosis and lip chewing)

Adapted from: Burton JL. *Churchill Livingstone* 1971, page 116.

➢ Clinical
- o Early in disease course
  - Sudden onset at night time
  - First metarsophalangeal joint
  - Monoarticular

- o Late
  - May have chronic arthritis, against a background of
  - ↑ frequency of acute gouty arthritis

- o Tophi
  - Urate (needle-shaped, negatively birefringent)
    - Bursae
    - Skin
    - Cartilage
    - Subchondral bone
    - Infected tophaceous gouty tophi

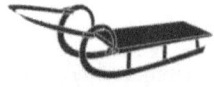

In the patient with painful arthritis, the examination of synovial fluid by birefringent microscopy may show needle-shaped, negatively birefringent crystals which are diagnostic of gouty arthritis.

- Give clinical features suggestive of gouty arthritis which do **not prove** the diagnosis of gout.
  - o Uric acid tophi
    - – Yellow nodules of monosodium urate found on
      - Extensor surface of extremities
      - Finger pads
      - Tendons
  - o Monoarticular arthritis of first MTP (metatarsophalangeal) joint ("podagra") or tarsal joints
  - o Hyperuricemia

➤ Laboratory

Pearls and Gems

- o If synovial fluid aspirate shows monosodium urate crystals as well as WBC > 50,000 / μL – beware: there may be an associated bacterial infection
- o Indicate which medications must **not** be used in persons with gout plus renal disease
  - – NSAIDs
  - – Probenecid
  - – Colchicine
  - – Allopurinol

- Give the **precautions** which must be followed when starting allopurinol.
  - o Give low-dose colchicine when starting allopurinol;
  - o Once the uric acid level is stable, stop the colchicine;
  - o If the allopurinol cannot be taken (poor tolerance, renal disease, use febuxostat).
- In the patient being treated with allopurinol, give the reason for discontinuing use of hydrochlorothiazide, if at all possible.
  - o The combination of allopurinol plus hydrochlorothiazide may cause fatal
    - – Hypersensitivity syndrome
      - Fever
      - Eosinophilia
      - Dermatitis, sever
      - Hepatic necrosis
      - Acute nephritis

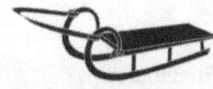

- Give the ways to distinguishing between gout and pseudo-gout (CPPDD).

Crystalline arthritis	Sex distribution	Joint involvement	Crystal	Crystal characteristics
o Gout*	Male > female	Asymmetrical distal joints, especially great toe	Uric acid	Long, needle-shaped Negative birefringence
o Calcium pyrophosphate deposition disease (pseudo-gout)	Female > male	Proximal joints, especially knee and wrist	Calcium pyrophos -phate	Rectangular, positive birefringence

Examine ears, olecranon bursae and Achilles tendons for tophi.

Source: Ghosh AK. *Mayo Clinic Scientific Press* 2008, Table 10-3, page 385.

➢ Diagnostic imaging

- Give the radiological features of **gout**
  - o Punched out erosions of joint margins
  - o Erosions occur beyond joint capsule
  - o Spotted appearance of carpals
  - o Cartilage loss
  - o No osteoporosis or new bone formation

Source: Burton JL. *Churchill Livingstone* 1971, page 113.

➢ Causes of radiological erosions in hands
  - o Musculoskeletal
    - Gout
    - Rheumatoid arthritis
    - Chondromata
  - o Infection
    - Sarcoidosis
  - o Trauma
    - Traumatic cysts
  - o Ideopathic
    - Localized osteitis fibrosa cystica

Adapted from: Burton JL. *Churchill Livingstone* 1971, page 116.

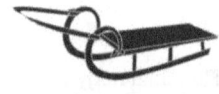

SO YOU WANT TO BE RHEUMATOLOGIST!

- A nodule is palpated at the extensor surface of the elbow. How can you differentiate between a rheumatoid nodule and a gouty tophus on physical examination?

    o You can't! usually aspiration or biopsy is needed, unless the gouty tophus drains to the surface.

SO YOU WANT TO BE RHEUMATOLOGIST!

- Give the radiological changes of gouty arthropathy.

    o Periarticular   - Punched-out, circular erosions
                           - Inflammation
                           - Tophi
                           - Deformity

➢ Treatment

- Give the treatment of gouty arthritis

    o Acute   - Increasing serum concentrations of urate will precipitate an attack, but curiously, so also will decrease urate concentrations
                      - Treat the acute episodes
                      - Colchicine 1.2 mg, with 0.6 mg given one hour later
                      - NSAIDs, Coxibs
                          ▪ po, IV, IA (intra-articularily)

    o Maintenance (for ≥ 2 attacks per year)
        - Pharmacological
            ▪ For 6-mon use 0.6 mg colchicine while serum urate levels are being reduced, to prevent an acute attack
            ▪ Allopurinol or febuxostat, in doses to reduce and maintain serum urate at ≤ 0.35 mmol/mL (≤ 6.0 mg/dL)
            ▪ Acts by ↓ activity of xanthine oxidase, so will ↑ concentration of serum azathioprine

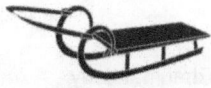

- For gouty tophi, use longterm xanthine oxidase inhibitors to achieve target serum urate concentration of ≤ 0.29 mmol/L (≤ 5.0 mg/dL)
- Probenecid – use only when
  - GFR is normal
  - Urine urate is ↑ ("primary under excreters from defects in reabsorption of urinary urate by PCT (proximal convoluted tubular) URAT-1 transporter

Note: Probenecide ↑ urinary urate → ↑ risk of urate renal calculi

- Non-pharmacological
  - Life style issue re diet, ↑ BMI

For persons with hyperuricemia, but no previous attack of gouty arthritis, use life-style treatment to ↓ serum urate concentration.

Calcium Pyrophosphate Deposition Disease (CPPD)

➤ Definition:
  o CPPDD (calcium pyrophosphate deposition disease) results from the deposition of calcium pyrophosphate into cartilage (chondrocalcinosis) or into the joint, resulting in acute crystal-induced arthritis (pseudogout), degenerate cartilage disease (osteoarthritis-like, or chronic inflammatory arthritis)

  o "CPP arthropathy is a clinical diagnosis made by observing typical osteoarthritis features, along with chondrocalcinosis in locations atypical for osteoarthritis (e.g. write, 2nd / 3rd metacarpophalangeal joint." MKSAP 16, Rheumatology 2012, page 53.

➤ Pathophysiology

• Give the pathophysiology of pseudogout.

  o Chondrocytes → ↑ production of pyrophosphate plus extracellular Ca^{2+} form crystal → CPP crystals deposited in cartilage and joint space → acute inflammatory reaction CPP crystals may cause osteoarthritis.

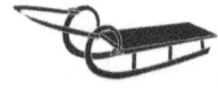

➢ Causes / associations

- Give the disease associations of pseudogout (acute arthritis from CPPDD).

  o Familial   - Hypocalciuria hypercalcemia

  o Endocrine   - Hyperparathyroidism
                          - Hypothypoidism
                          - Hemochromatosis

  o Electrolyte   - Hypophosphatasia
    disturbances   - Hypomagnesia

➢ Clinical

- Give the typical sites for asymptomatic **chondrocalcinosis**, and 3 metabolic conditions for which screening for CPPDD must be performed in the patient < 50 yr.

  o Sites of chondrocalcinosis
    - Wrist
      ▪ Triangular fibrocartilage between distal ulna and carpal bones
    - Symphysis pubis joint
    - Menisci of the knee joint

  o Metabolic disorders associated with CPDD
    - Hyperparathyroidism
    - Hypothyroidism
    - Hemochromatosis, hereditary (HH)
    - Gout

➢ Diagnosis
  o Imaging
    - CPP deposits seen as a liver calcified dependent below and parallel to the cartilage surface, typically of the knee.
    - Joint aspiration
      - Birefringent, rhomboid-shaped crystals
  o CPPDD is partially diagnosed from positive birefringence of rhomboid-shaped crystals in the aspirate of synovial fluid.

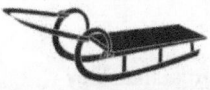

- o The full diagnosis rests on the demonstration of both positive birefringence calcification of cartilage or joint capsule.
- o These linear calcifications of the meniscus and articular cartilage are characteristic for chondrocalcinosis.

- Give the distinction between gouty arthritis and CPPDD on birefringent microscopy of an aspirate of synovial fluid.

Condition	Birefringent crystals	Shape of crystals
o Gout	– Negative	– Needle-like
o CPPDD	– Positive	– Rhomboid

Basic Calcium Pyrophosphate (BCP) **Disease**

In the context of should pain and effusion which develops after trauma, give the characteristics of the Milwaukee shoulder syndrome.

- o Destructive inflammatory effusion
- o Bloody, non-inflammatory effusion
- o ↓ active movement destruction of cartilage of joints associated tendons
- o Radiographs calcification articular and periarticular
- o Joint aspirate
  - BCP (basic calcium pyrophosphate) crystals
  - Seen as aggregates after alizarin red attaining

Clinical Pearl

- o Before performing an upper endoscopy (EGD, esophagogastroduodenostomy) in a patient with long-term RA
  - Obtain a radiogram of the cervical neck to ensure there is no atlantoaxial subluxation, and therefore possible instability of the neck.

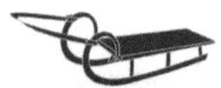

CARDIAC DISEASE AND SYSTEMIC INFLAMMATORY DISORDERS

- Give the rheumatological disorders with the following cardiac conditions.

  o Pericarditis disease
  - SLE (25%-50%)
  - RA (~30%)
  - SSC
  - BS

  o Myocardial disease
  - SSC
  - BS
  - PN
  - SAR

  o Aortitis, arteritis
  - AS (25%-60%)
  - TA

  o Endocarditis
  - SLE (~20%-60%)

  o Premature CAD
  - SLE (↑ risk 50x!)
  - RA
  - KD

  o Valve disease
  - AR SLE (~20%), AS (~40%), BS
  - Leaflet fibrosis
  - RA (~15%)

  o LV diastolic dysfunction
  - AS

  o Conduction defects, arrhythmias
  - AS (~10%)
  - BS
  - SAR

  o Systemic hypertension
  - SSC
  - SSC renal crisis
  - TA

  o Pulmonary artery hypertension
  - SSC

  o Peripheral artery disease
  - GCA

Note: All of these systemic inflammation disorders are MSK (musculoskeletal) disorders, also considered in the Chapter on Rheumatological disorders

Abbreviations: AR, aortic regurgitation; AS, ankylosing spondylitis; BS, Behcet syndrome; GCA, giant cell arthritis; KD, Kawasaki disease; PAN, polyarteritis nodosa; RA, rheumatoid arthritis; SAR, sarcoidosis; SLE, systemic lupus erythematosus; SSC, systemic sclerosis; TA, Takayasu arteritis

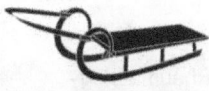

A.B.R. Thomson

- Give the cardiac conditions associated with AS, BS, GCA, KD, RA, SAR, SLE, SSC, and TA.

  o AS
    - Aortic arteritis
    - LV diastolic dysfunction
    - Conduction defects
    - Arrhythmias
    - Valve disease

  o BS
    - Pericarditis
    - Myocardial disease
    - Arrythmias
    - Conduction defects
    - Valve disease

  o GCA
    - Peripheral artery

  o KD
    - Premature CAD

  o RA
    - Pericarditis
    - Premature CAD
    - Valve disease

  o SAR
    - Myocardial disease
    - Conduction defects
    - Arrhythmias

  o SLE
    - Pericarditis
    - Endocarditis
    - Valve disease

  o SSC
    - Aortitis arteritis
    - Systemic hypertension

  o TA
    - Pericarditis
    - Myocardial disease
    - Systemic hypertension
    - Pulmonary hypertension

Abbreviations: AS, ankylosing spondylitis; BS, Behcet syndrome; GCA, giant cell arthritis; KD, Kawasaki disease; PAN, polyarteritis nodosa; RA, rheumatoid arthritis; SAR, sarcoidosis; SLE, systemic lupus erythematosus; SSC, systemic sclerosis; TA, Takayasu arteritis

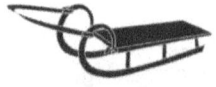

OLIGOARTHRITIS AND POLYARTHRITIS

➤ Causes

- Give the most common causes of oligoarthritis and polyarthritis.

- Oligoarthritis
  - Inflammatory
    - Acute
      - GC (gonorrhea)
      - RF (rheumatic fever)
    - Chronic
      - Spondyloarthritis
      - Connective tissue disease
  - Non-inflammatory
    - Chronic
      - Osteoarthritis
- Polyarthritis
  - Acute
    - Viral infection
      - HBV
      - HIV
      - Rubella
      - Paravirus B19
  - Chronic
    - RA (rheumatoid arthritis)
    - SLE (systemic lupus erythematosis)
    - Sponyloarthritis
      - AS (ankylosing spondylitis)
      - Psoriatric arthritis
      - Reactive arthritis
        - Salmonella
        - Shigella
        - Yerinia
        - Campylobacter
        - Clostridium

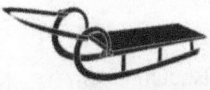

- Perform a focused physical examination for patterns of arthropathy.

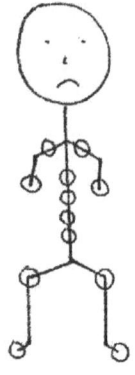

Primary osteoarthritis

Symmetrical, affecting many joints

- Great toes and thumbs: MP joints
- Fingers: terminal IP joints
- Acromio-clavicular joints

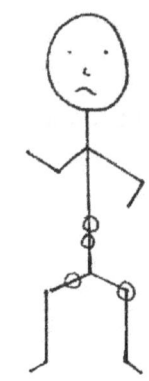

Secondary osteoarthritis

Asymmetrical, affecting weight bearing joints:

- Knees
- Hips
- Intervertebral discs

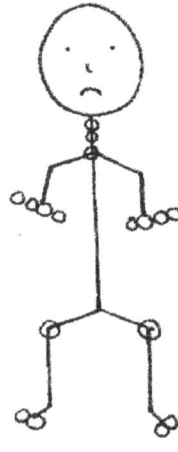

Rheumatoid arthritis

- Hands: intercarpal joints, MP joints and proximal IP joints
- Feet: tarsal and lateral MP joints
- Knees
- Small joints of cervical spine and subacromial bursae

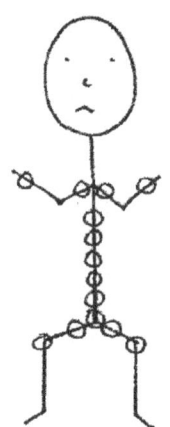

Ankylosing spondylitis

- Spine and both sacro-iliac joints
- Knees, shoulders, wrists

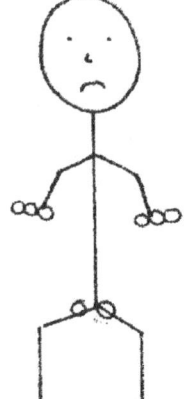

Psoriasis

- Hands, terminal IP joints
- Sacro-iliac joints
- 'Rheumatoid' pattern

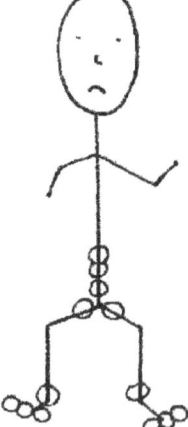

Reactive (Reiter) arthritis

- Ankles and all joints of feet
- Knees
- Hips, sacro-iliac joint and spine

Source: Burton JL. *Churchill Livingstone* 1971, page 112.

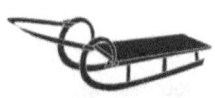

RHEUMATOID ARTHRITIS

➤ Definition: Rheumatoid arthritis (RA) is a systemic autoimmune disease manifesting primarily as a symmetric and erosive poly arthritis" (Hazlewood G and Bykerk VP. In: Therapeutic Choices. Grey J, Ed. 6th Edition, *Canadian Pharmacists Association*: Otttawa, ON, 2011, page 1040).

- o Rheumatoid arthritis is a systemic disorder of unknown cause in which chronic inflammation may lead to joint destruction and disability

- o "most patients have systemic polyarthritis involving small and large joints [MCP, metacarb, phalangeal joints; PIP, proximal interphalangeal joints; wrist; MTP, metaphalangal pints] that is associated in the prolonged morning stiffness

- o Specificity for RA of 80%

➤ Demography

- o Incidence $30/10^5$ per year

- o Prevalence $1000/10^5$ in Caucasian females

➤ Points of interest

- o Persons with RA have an increased risk of
  - Cardiovascular disease and cardiovascular mortality
  - Infections
  - Lymphoma
  - Osteoporosis

- o Only 30% of patients diagnosed with RA have a positive serum RF (rheumatoid factor) at the time of their initial presentation with symptoms.

- o A negative RF "....does not exclude the possibility of rheumatoid arthritis

➤ Causes/Associations

• Give the factors which contribute to the causation of rheumatoid arthritis (RA).

- o Environmental
  - Exposure to
    ▪ Smoking
    ▪ Asbestos
    ▪ Silica
  - Low socioeconomic status
- o Hormone
  - More common in women

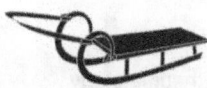

- o Antibiotics
  - RF (rheumatoid factor)
  - CCP (anti-cyclic citrullinated peptide in 60% of RA patients; specificity of RA 95%
  - Neither are necessary or sufficient to cause RA
- o Genetics
  - Shared epitope of several HLA-DR B chains polymorphisms
    - STAT4 (a transcription factor which responds to cytokines)

➤ Clinical

o Key symptoms of inflammation

- Stiffness: worst in the early morning, or after prolonged inactivity, progressively easing as the day goes on
- Pain: inflammatory pain is usually present at rest as well as on movement
- Both are greatly relieved by non-steroidal anti-inflammatory drugs (NSAIDs)

Source: Davey P. *Wiley-Blackwell* 2006, page 114.

- Give the American Rheumatism Association (ARA) criteria for the diagnosis of rheumatoid arthritis (RA).

  - o Morning stiffness for at least 1 hour for duration of 6 weeks or more

  - o Swelling of at least three joints for 6 weeks or more

  - o Swelling of wrist, metacarpophalangeal or proximal interphalang 6 weeks or more

  - o Symmetry of swollen joint areas for 6 weeks or more

  - o Subcutaneous nodules

  - o Positive rheumatoid factor

  - o Radiographic features typical of rheumatoid arthritis, i.e. erosions periarticular osteopenia.

When <u>four or more</u> of the above criteria are met, there is 93% sensitivity and 90% specificity for the diagnosis of rheumatoid arthritis.

Adapted from: Baliga RR. *Saunders/Elsevier* 2007, page 339.

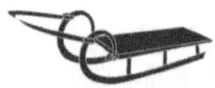

- Perform a focused physical examination for rheumatoid arthritis (RA), and its complications.

  o Poor general health
    - Weight loss
    - Pale
    - Depression and social problems

  o Joints
    - Metacarpophalangeal (MCP) joints
      - Synovitis
      - Effusions
      - Low range of movement
      - Crepitus
      - Subluxation, deformity
      - Boutonniere deformity (fixed flexion of PIP and extension of DIP, due to protrusion of the PIJ through ruptured extensor tendon)
      - Z deformity (thumb IPJ hypertension and fixed flexion and of subluxation of MCJ)
      - Tendon rupture
    - Arms
      - Entrapment neuropathy (e.g. carpal tunnel)
      - Subcutaneous nodules
    - Elbow, shoulder joint
      - Axillary nodes
      - Baker synovial cyst
    - Back, hips, knees

  o Lower limbs
    - Ulceration (vasculitis)
    - Calf swelling (ruptured synovial cyst)
    - Peripheral neuropathy
    - Mononeuritis multiplex
    - Pressure sores
    - Infected ulcers (from nodules)
    - Cord compression

  o Joint complications
    - Deformity, subluxation
    - Pyoarthrosis
    - Tendon rupture (due to attrition or nodules)
    - Nerve compression (due to tenosynovial swelling)
    - Cord or root compression (due to cervical subluxation)
    - Baker synovial cyst
    - Acute rupture of synovial sac (especially in knee)

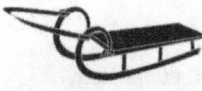

- Hoarseness, due to crico-artenoid arthritis
- Deafness, due to arthritis of auditory ossicles

o MSK
   - Osteoporosis
   - Muscle atrophy

o Eye
   - Episcleritis
   - Scleritis
   - Scleromalacia perforans, scleromalacia
   - Uveitis
   - Sjogren syndrome
   - Pyoderma gangresnosa

o Face
   - Eyes – dry eyes (Sjögren sndrome), scleritis, episcleritis, scleromalacia perforans, uveitis, Sjogren's syndrome, anemia, cataracts (corticosteroids, chloroquine)
   - Fundi – hyperviscosity
   - Face – parotid enlargement (Sjögren syndrome),
   - Mouth – dryness, ulcers, dental caries
   - Temporomandibular joint (crepitus)
   - Hoarseness (crico-arytenoid arthritis)
   - Ears – deafness (arthritis of auditory ossicles)

o Neck
   - Cervical nodes
   - Swan neck (hyperextension at PIJ [subluxation], and fixed flexion deformity of DIJ [tendon shortening]
   - Thyroiditis

o Skin
   - Pressure sores and infected ulcers (due to nodules)
   - Pyoderma gangrenosum

o Heart/CVS
   - Pericardial effusion
   - Pericarditis
   - Arteritis
   - Aortic regurgitation
   - Rheumatoid granuloma of heart
   - Murmurs from rheumatic heart disease

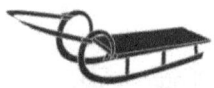

A.B.R. Thomson

- o Lung
  - Pleuritis, pleural effusion
  - Nodules in lung or pleura
  - Fibrosing alveolitis
  - Caplan syndrome (in pneumoconiosis)
  - Fibrosis
  - Infarction
  - Infection
  - Arteritis

- o Arteritis
  - Digital ischemia
  - Raynaud syndrome
  - Leg ulcers
  - Mesenteric ischemia
  - Arteritis of lungs, kidneys, liver
  - Peripheral and autonomic neuropathy
  - Amyloidosis
  - May develop renal vein thrombosis

- o Abdomen
  - Mesenteric ischemia
  - Arteritis of kidneys, liver
  - Splenomegaly
  - Pernicious anemia
  - Subfertility
  - Urine: protein, blood (drugs, vasculitis, amyloidosis)
  - Rectal examination (blood)
  - Complications of therapy
  - Renal/ vein thrombosis
  - Splenomegaly (e.g. Felty syndrome: RA, splenomegaly, leucopenia)
  - Inguinal nodes
  - Felty syndrome (splenomegaly, RA and leucopenia)
  - Character and distribution of deformities
    - Contractures, hyperextension, ulnar deviation (late finding), abnormal posture, nodules, muscular atrophy
    - Bony swelling
    - Soft tissue swelling, redness or rash, palmar erythema, fingernail or finger tuft abnormalities, Dupuytren's contractures
    - Range of motion (ROM)

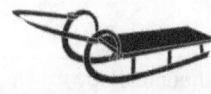

- Active
- Passive, to include:
  - Wrist flexion/extension
  - Making fist
  - Grip strength
  - Finger flexion/extension
  - Opposition of thumb and 5th finger/thumb and index finger

- Functional assessment in rheumatoid arthritis
  - Class 1: Normal functional ability
  - Class 2: Ability to carry out normal activities, despite discomfort or limited mobility of one or more joints
  - Class 3: Ability to perform only a few of the tasks of the normal occupation or of self-care
  - Complete or almost complete incapacity with the patient confined to wheelchair or to bed

- Complications of therapy

- Associated autoimmune disease
  - Pernicious anemia (PA)
  - Thyroiditis
  - Hemolytic anemia

- ↓ fertility (prior to development of arthritis)
  - Chronic brucellosis
  - CNS
    - Posterior and anterior neuropathy
    - Nerve entrapment
  - Eye-keratoconjunctivitis sicca
    - Uveitis
    - Corneal ulceration
    - Cystoid bodies
  - Endocrine
    - Thyroiditis
  - Skin-infection
    - Ulcers
  - Bone marrow
    - Normochromic normocytic anemia
    - Pernicious anemia
    - Hemolytic anemia
    - Lymphadenopathy
    - Splenomegaly

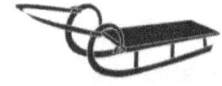

- Lung
  - Fibrosis
  - Pleural effusion
  - Nodules
  - Caplan syndrome
- Kidney
  - Proteinuria
  - Amyloid

Adapted from: Burton JL. *Churchill Livingstone* 1971, page 115; Baliga RR. *Saunders/Elsevier* 2007, page 338; Talley NJ, et al. *Maclennan & Petty Pty Limited* 2003, Table, 8.31, page 286; Jugovic PJ, et al. *Saunders/ Elsevier* 2004, pages 146 and 147.

- Give clinical conditions suggesting **periarticular involvement** in RA.

  o Bursa   - Bursitis

  o Tendon   - Tendinopathy
                   - Teno synovitis

  o Neck   - Swan neck

  o Hands   - Boutonniere deformities

  o Flexion contractures

  o Cysts   - Popliteal
                   - Ganglion

- In the context of RA (rheumatoid arthritis), give the components of the **Felty syndrome**.

  o Skin   - Ulcers (rheumatoid vasculitis)
                   - Nodules

  o Eye   - Scleral ulceration
                   - Scleritis

  o Lung   - Interstitial lung disease

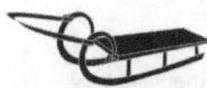

- Give the classic sites of symmetric joint involvement in RA.

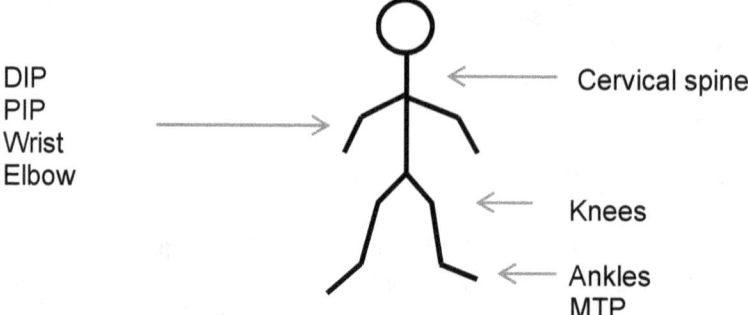

DIP
PIP
Wrist
Elbow

Cervical spine

Knees

Ankles
MTP

Abbreviations: MCP, metacarpophalangeal; MTP, metatarsophalangeal; PIP, proximal interphalangeal

From: Baliga RR. *Saunders/Elsevier* 2007, page 336.

- Give **extra-articular** clinical components of RA, and their cause.

o Eye	– Red, painful	▪ Scleritis ▪ Sjogren syndrome ▪ Keratoconjunctivitis sicca ▪ Uveitis ▪ Corneal ulceration ▪ Cystoids bodies ▪ Scleromalacia perforans	
o Voice	– Hoarseness	▪ RA of cricoarytenoid	
o Skin	– Ulcers	▪ RA vasculitis ▪ Infection ▪ Ulcers ▪ Raynaud phenomenon	
o Heart	– CAD (coronary heart disease) – Heart failure (HF)	▪ Use of anti-TNF treatment	
o CNS / PNS	– Neuropathy – Mononeuritis multiplex – Wrist or foot drop – Paresthesias / ↑ DTR in arms	▪ RA vasculitis ▪ Vasculitis ▪ Peripheral neuropathy ▪ Nerve entrapment ▪ Sublaxation of C1-C2	

- o Lung
  - – BOOP (bronchiolitis obliterans organizing pneumonia
  - – Multiple basilar nodules
  - – Effusion
  - – Rheumatoid pleuritic
  - – Interstitial lung disease
  - – Fibrosis
  - – Pulmonary hypertension
  - ▪ Caplan syndrome

- o Bone
  - – Osteoporosis
  - ▪ Use of corticosteroids
  - ▪ Deficiency of Calcium, vitamin D

- o Blood
  - – Splenomegaly
  - – Granulocytopenia
  - ▪ Felty syndrome

- o Endocrine
  - – Thyroiditis
  - – Infertility

- o Renal
  - – Proteinuria
  - – Amyloid

SO YOU WANT TO BE A "RHEUM –WITH- A -VIEW" (Rheumatologist)!

- Give the meaning of palindromic rheumatoid arthritis.
  - o Acute recurrent arthritis, usually affecting one joint, with symptom-free intervals of days to months between attacks

Source: Baliga RR. *Saunders/Elsevier* 2007, page 345.

SO YOU WANT TO BE A RHEUMATOLOGIST!

- A patient with rheumatoid arthritis (RA) is found to have **splenomegaly**. Give the causes of splenomegaly in this patient which are related to the RA.
  - o Adult – Felty syndrome
  - o Child – Still disease
  - o Amyloidosis
  - o Associated SLE
  - o Beucellosis

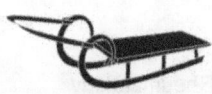

SO YOU WANT TO BE A RHEUMATOLOGIST!

- Give causes **arthritis plus nodules**.

  o Rheumatoid arthritis
  o Systemic lupus erythematosus (rare)
  o Rheumatic fever (Jaccoud arthritis) (very rare)
  o Granulomas- e.g. sarcoid (very rare)

Source: Talley NJ, et al. *Maclennan & Petty Pty Limited* 2003, page 269.

- Perform a focused examination for the rheumatoid foot.

  o Pes planus – inward rotation of the medial malleolus
  o Loss of anterior arch – wide front part of foot
  o Hallux valgus – bending of the big toe towards the second toe
  o Cock-up deformities of the toes – flexion of the IP joint of the toes
  o Dropped metatarsal leads - subluxation of the metatarsal heads

SO YOU WANT TO BE A RHEUMATOLOGIST!

- Give the poor **prognostic factors** for RA.

  o Systemic features: weight loss, extra-articular manifestations
  o Insidious onset
  o Rheumatoid nodules
  o Presence of rheumatoid factor more than 1 in 512

Source: Baliga RR. *Saunders/Elsevier* 2007, page 339.

➢ Causes of **deforming polyarthopathy**
  o Rheumatoid arthritis
  o Psoriatic arthritis
  o Ankylosing spondylitis
  o Reiter disease
  o Chronic tophaceous gout
  o Osteoarthritis
  o Lyme arthritis

➢ Causes of **arthropathy plus nodules**
  o Rheumatoid arthritis
  o Systemic lupus erythematosus
  o Rheumatic fever
  o Sarcoidosis

Adapted from: Talley NJ, et al. *Maclennan & Petty Pty Limited* 2003, page 261-9.

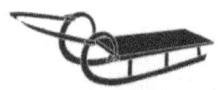

➢ Differential

• Give causes of **symmetric arthritis** other than RA (rheumatoid arthritis), and the clinical findings suggestive that the diagnosis is not RA.

o Infection	– Parvovirus B12	▪	Exposure to infants, young children
	– Rubella	▪	Arthritis after immunization
o MSK	– SLE (systemic lupus erythematosus)	▪	Skin rash
	– SSC (systemic sclerosis)	▪	Sclerodactyly
		▪	Raynaud phenomenon
	– Psoriatic arthritis	▪	Typical skin and nail changes
	– PM / DM (polymyositis / dermatomyositis)	▪	Proximal muscle weakness
		▪	Skin changes
o Metabolic	– HH (hereditary hemochromatosis)	▪	Bronze skin
		▪	Hepatomegaly
		▪	Diabetes

➢ Laboratory

• Give conditions in which the ESR (erythrocyte sedimentation rate) may be **falsely elevated** in the absence of an inflammatory condition).

o Diabetes

o Chronic renal disease

o Pregnancy

The specificity of rheumatoid factors (serology) for (RF) for RA (rheumatoid arthritis) is ~ 80%.

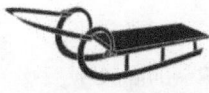

- Give the approximate proportion of persons with other autoimmune disorders who are positive for RF, as well as the prevalence of RF in the healthy population.

Condition	Approximated % positive for RF
o Mixed cryoglobulinemia	100
o Sjogren syndrome	70
o SLE	25
o Healthy normal persons	10

- Give the **performance characteristics of RF** (rheumatoid factor) and anti-CCP antibody assay in RA (rheumatoid arthritis).

Test	Sensitivity	Specificity
RF	80%	87%
Anti-CCP	76%	96%

Serological tests play an important role in the investigation of rheumatologic disorders. There may be overlap between diagnosis due to the varying performance characteristics of these tests.

- Give the usual serological abnormalities in the following disorders.

Rheumatologic Disorder	Serological abnormality
o AIH (autoimmune hepatitis)	Anti-smooth muscle
o CSS (Churg-Straus syndrome)	p-ANCA
o GPA (granulomatosis with polyangiitis)	c-ANCA
o Mixed connective tissue disease)	Anti-RNP
o Microscopic polyangiitis	p-ANCA
o Polymyositis	Anti-Jo-1
o Rheumatoid arthritis	Anti-CCP

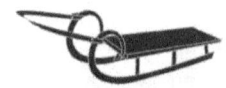

Rheumatologic Disorder	Serological abnormality
o SLE (systemic lupus erythematosus)	Anti-ds DNA
	Anti-La / SSB
– Drug-induced	Anti-histone
– Subacute	Anti-Ro / SSA
o Sjogren syndrome	Anti-La / SSB
	Anti-Ro / SSA
o SSc (systemic sclerosis) type	
– Limited cutaneous, +/- CREST syndrome	Anti-centromere pattern of ANA
– Diffuse cutaneous	Anti-smooth muscle

- In the patient suspected to have RA, but in whom the rheumatoid factor (RF) is negative, measure anti-CCP (cyclic citrullinate peptide), since this is

  o Sensitive, 50%

  o Specific ,95%

➢ Disease Activity

- Give the methods to evaluate disease activity and damage of rheumatoid arthritis.

  o Subjective   – Degree of joint pain (scored /10 on ascending pain scale)
                        – Duration of morning stiffness (in minutes or hours)
                        – Degree of fatigue (scored /10)
                        – Physician and patient global assessment of disease activity
                        – Limitation of function

  o Physical examination
                        – Number of actively inflamed/swollen joints
                        – Mechanical joint problems
    - Loss of motion
    - Crepitus
    - Instability
    - Malalignment and/or deformity
                      – Extra-articular manifestations including
    - Dry eyes
    - Nodules
    - Pulmonary findings
    - Carpal tunnel syndrome

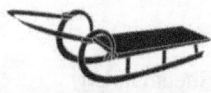

o   Laboratory   – Erythrocyte sedimentation rate/C-reactive protein level: monitor every 1-2 months
- Rheumatoid factor titre/anti-CCP antibody: at baseline
- Complete blood cell count: monitor during most therapies every 1-3 months
- Creatinine level: monitor at least twice per year
- Urinalysis at baseline and during an annual visit
- Synovial fluid analysis if available: at baseline to exclude other conditions or sepsis

o   Imaging   – Radiographs of hands and feet and selected involved joints annually and as indicated

Consider joint ultrasound or, if available, MRI to identify subclinical erosions if radiographs normal in the first year

Reproduced with permission: Therapeutics Choices. Sixth Edition. Ottawa, Canada: Canadian Pharmacist Association 2012, Table 1, page 1041.

➢ Diagnostic imaging

- Give the radiological features of Rheumatoid arthritis.

  o Osteoporosis

  o Cartilage loss

  o Marginal and surface erosions

  o Subluxations, dislocations and carpal ankylosis

  o No sclerosis or new bone formation

Source: Burton JL. *Churchill Livingstone* 1971, page 113.

- Give a justification **periodic radiographic evaluation** of the joints in RA.

  o Joint RA damage may occur even on the absence of symptoms

  o If there is radiological evidence of active RA, therapy may need to be changed

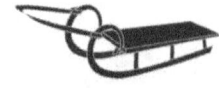

➢ Treatment

- In the context of the patient with rheumatoid arthritis of sufficient severity to fail NSAIDs and acetaminophen, give name 6 **DMARDs** (disease-modifying anti-rheumatic drugs)

  o "Gold standard" DMARDs

  o Stop alcohol in MTX (methotrexate)-treated persons

  o Warn patients to plan their pregnancy and stop MTX 3 mon before conception

- Give the rationale for concurrent therapy of allopurinol with azathioprine / 6-MP (mercaptopurine)

  o Allopurinol is a purine analog which inhibits xanthine oxidase, and there by increases the blood concentrations of azathioprine and 6-MP

  o Non-biologics   – DMARDs
                                    – Methotrexate
                                    – Cyclosporine
                                    – Hydrochloroquine
                                    – Sulfasalazine
                                    – Minocycline
                                    – Leflunomide

  o Biologics   – TNF-α inhibitors (e.g. infliximab, adalimumab, enternacept)
                                    – Anti-CD20 B cell depleting monoclononal antibody (rituximab)
                                    – IL-6 receptor antagonist (tecilizumab)
                                    – CTLA4: Fc (cytotoxic T-lymphocyte antigen 4; e.g. abatacept)
                                    – Anti-IL-12 / IL-23 mAb ustekinumab
                                    – Anti-BLyS mAb (anti-B-lymphocyte stimulator, e.g. belimumab)
                                    – IL-1
                                         ▪ IL-1R antagonist Anakinra
                                         ▪ IL-1B trap Rilonacept
                                         ▪ Anti-IL-1B mAb Canakinumab

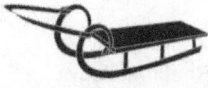

- T cell costimulation may be blocked at two sites. Give the name of two biological agents used to treat RA which act at different sites to block T cells.

  o Abatacept and Rituximab are two different biologicals used to treat RA

    - Their sites of action.

  o Dendritic cells   – Abatacept

  o B cells   – Abatacept
                                       – Rituximab

    - Patients with RA who fail anti-TNF therapy may be switched to periodic infusions of **tocilizumab**. Regular monitoring is required.

Blood test	R/O (rule out)
o CBC	– Leukopenia
	– Thrombocytopenia
o Hepatic enzymes	– Transaminases, ALT, AST
	– AP, alkaline phosphatase
o Lipids	– LDL cholesterol

"The combination of methotrexate with a TNF-α inhibitor is associated with greater efficacy than therapy with methotrexate or a TNF-α inhibitor alone" MKSAP 16, Rheumatology 2012, page 140.

Before beginning the patient with immunosuppressants or before immunomodulating therapies, it is recommended to vaccinate against influenza.

- Give the **influenza vaccine** which is recommended in the setting of using immunomodulating therapy

  o Intramuscularily administered trivalent virus, or

  o Intranasal influenza vaccine

  o The trivalent vaccine is inactivated virus, and is safe to give to the patient on immunosuppression or biologicimmunomodulating therapies.

  o The intranasal influenza vaccine is liver virus, and as such is contraindicated in such a patient for fear of developing disseminated viral infection.

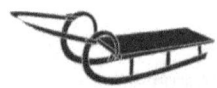

Clinical Alert

- o Your patient with severe and long standing RA is being scheduled for an elective operative procedure requiring a **general anesthetic**.

- • Give the preoperative radiogram which is necessary

  - o Cervical spinal film to ensure there is no risk for atlantoaxial sublaxation and instability of the spine, with damage to the cord.

- • Give the safe timing before and during **pregnancy** of stopping drugs used to treat RA.

  - o 3 mon before conception   – Methrotrexate
    - – Leflunomide
    - – Sulfasalazine (in males)

  - o Before 2 weeks of gestation   – Corticosteroids

  - o Early pregnancy   – NSAIDs (also avoid in T3 to prevent
    - ▪ Premature closure of ductus arteriosis
    - ▪ Interferes with labour
    - – ASA

  - o Before lactation   – Methotrexate

Clinical Tips

o	Methotrexate	– Methotrexate (MTX) is the DMARD (disease-modifying anti-rheumatic drugs) of choice in RA (rheumatoid arthritis)
		– Because of risk of DILI (drug-induced liver injury) in the liver of persons on MTX long-term, there is an alcohol caution ↑ liver damage (hepatitis)
o	Hydroxychloroquine	– In high dose or with long-term use, hydroxychloroquine may be deposited in the retina, causing retinal damage
		– Retinal examinations should be performed regularly in persons on long-term hydroxychloroquine
		– No firm guideline for interval of surveillance; recommendations very from q 6 mon to annual after 5 g of therapy

---

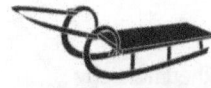

- Perform a focused physical examination of extra – articular complications of rheumatoid arthritis (RA).

RA is usually symmetrical, involving the proximal interphalangeal and metacarpophalangeal (MCP) joints in the hands, the wrist joints, the tarsal and metatarsophalangeal (MTP) joints in the small joints of the upper cervical spine

- o General
  - – Recurrent fevers, with or without infections
  - – Weight loss

- o CNS
  - – Neuropathy

- o Eyes
  - – Keratoconjunctivitis sicca (KS)
  - – Sjogren syndrome (KS, plus xerostomia)
  - – Scleromalacia (including scleromalacia perforans)
  - – Scleritis
  - – Episcleritis

- o Skin
  - – Nodules
    - ▪ Flexor and extensor tendons
    - ▪ Especially of hands, sacrum, heal (Achilles tendon)
  - – Vasculitis
  - – Infarction of nail folds
  - – Skin hyperpigmentation
  - – Lower extremity ulcers

- o Lung
  - – Rheumatoid nodules
  - – Caplan syndrome rheumatoid nodules at periphery of lung fields
  - – Fibrosing alveolitis
  - – Pleural effusion

- o Heart
  - – Pericardial effusions
  - – Arteritis
  - – Nodules
  - – Cardiomyopathy
  - – Aortic regurgitation

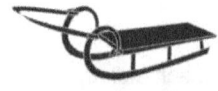

- ○ Spleen
  - – Splenomegaly
  - – Felty syndrome (splenomegaly and hypersplenism, usually in a seropositive RA patient)

- ○ Hematology
  - – Lymphadenopathy
  - – Cytopenias besides leukopenia
  - – Anemia – normochromic – hypochromic – macrocytic (B12, PA)
  - – Felty syndrome (classic triad)
    - ▪ Rheumatoid arthritis
    - ▪ Leukopenia
    - ▪ Splenomegaly

- Give causes of **pyoderma gangrenosum**.

  - ○ MSK
    - – Rheumatoid arthritis (RA)
    - – Seronegative arthritis associated with gastrointestinal symptoms

  - ○ GI
    - – IBD (Ulcerative colitis, Crohn disease)
    - – Chronic active hepatitis

  - ○ Hematology
    - – Acute and chronic myeloid leukemia
    - – Myelocytic leukemia
    - – Hairy cell leukemia
    - – Polycythemia rubra vera
    - – Multiple myeloma
    - – IgA monoclonal gammopathy

Source: Baliga RR. *Saunders/Elsevier* 2007, page 467.

Clinical Gems: No!
- ○ **No** osteoporosis or new bone formation with gout
- ○ **No** ankylosis with osteoarthritis
- ○ **No** sclerosis or new bone formation with rheumatoid arthritis

---

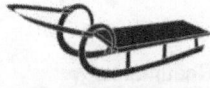

SJÖGREN SYNDROME

➢ Definition: "Sjogren syndrome is a slowly progressive autoimmune disorder which usually causes dry eyes (kerratoconjunctivitis sicca) and dry mouth (xerostomia), as well as numerous multisystem extraglandular association (~ 50%)

➢ Pathophysiology

This syndrome occurs in rheumatoid arthritis, and also with other connective tissue diseases.

- Give the pathoimmunology / physiology of Sjogren syndrome.

  o Lymphocytic invasion of epithelial tissue
  o Immune-complex-mediated inflammation
  o Associations HLA-DR / -DQ alleles
  o Triggers HCV, as well as other viruses

➢ Clinical
  o Classic triad
    - Arthritis, typically episodic polyarthritis
    - Dry eyes
    - Dry mouth

  o Physical examination
    - Dry eyes: conjunctivitis, keratitis, corneal ulcers (rarely vascularisation of the cornea)
    - Dry mouth
    - Arthritis
    - Chest: infection secondary to reduced mucus secretion, pleurisy or interstitial pneumonitis
    - Kidneys; renal tubular acidosis or nephrogenic diabetes insipidus
    - Genital tract: atrophic vaginitis
    - Pseudolymphoma: lymphadenopathy and splenomegaly, which may rarely progress to a true (usually non-Hodgkin's) lymphoma

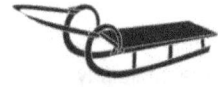

- o Other features
  - - Constitutional features: fatigue, malaise, myalgia
  - - Raynaud phenomenon
  - - Cutaneous vasculitis
  - - CNS abnormalities
    - • Cerebritis, CNS vasculitis
    - • Stroke
    - • Multiple sclerosis-like illness
  - - Peripheral neuropathy
    - • Sensory
    - • Autonomic
    - • Heart aortic regurgitation

Adapted from: Ghosh AK. *Mayo Clinic Scientific Press* 2008, Table 24.5, page 978; Talley NJ, et al. *Maclennan & Petty Pty Limited* 2003, Table 8.7, page 256.

➢ Extraglandular associations

• Give **extraglandular associations** of Sjogren syndrome.

o Constitutional	– Fatigue	
	– Fever	
o CNS / PNS	– Cognitive dysfunction	
	– TIA / CVA	
	– MS-like syndrome	
	– Transverse myelitis	
	– Peripheral neuropathy	
o CVS	– Vasculitis, small vessel	
	– Raunaud phenomenon	
o Lung	– Bronchi	
	▪ COPD	
	▪ Chronic bronchitis	
	▪ Bronchiectasis	
	▪ Bronchiolitis obliterans	
	– Interstitium	
	▪ Interstitial pneumonitis	
	▪ Pneumonia	
	– Lymphoid tissue	
	▪ Pseudolymphoma	

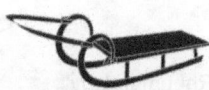

- o GI   – PBC (primary biliary cirrhosis)
- o Kidney   – Glomerulonephritis
  - – Tubular interstitial nephritis
  - – RTA (renal tubular acidosis), type 1

- o Hematology   – Lymphadenopathy
  - – Marginal zone B-cell lymphoma mucosa-associated lymphoid tissue (MALT) (↑↑ risk)

  - – Anemia
  - – Leukopenia
  - – Thrombocytopenia

- o MSK   – Arthralgia
  - – Arthritis
  - – Myositis

➢ Diagnosis: Use the **classification criteria** for Sjogren syndrome of the American-European Consensus Group.

- o Primary
  - – 4 criteria of the 6, which must include
    - ▪ #4 characteristic histopathology of lip biopsy, and
    - ▪ # 6 positive autoantibodies
      - – Anti-Ro / SSA and
      - – Anti-La / SSB
  - – Or 3 criteria of #4 and #6 (i.e. 3 of # 3, 4, 5, 6)
    - ▪ 3 keratoconjunctivitis sicca positive Schirmer test (↓ wetting of tear test strip), or
    - ▪ Positive Rose Bengal staining of cornia
  - – # 5 xerostomia
    - ▪ ↓ unstimulated saliva flow abnormal parotid sialography abnormal salivary scintigraphy

- o Secondary connective tissue disease, plus
  - – # 1 symptoms of dry eye, or
  - – #2 symptoms of dry mouth
  - – Plus #3, 4, 5

- o Autoantibodies
  - – Anti-La / SSB (40%)
  - – Anti-Ro / SSA (~70%)
  - – ANA, speckled pattern (> 80%)
  - – Rheumatoid factor (> 80%)
  - – ↑ globulins (cryoglobulins in 30%

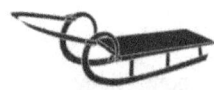

Seronegative Arthritis

➢ Definitions
  o Palindromic – Recurrent acute attacks of periarticular structures
    rheumatism – No permanent joint deformity
          – Seronegative

- Give causes of seronegative (rheumatoid factor [RF] negative; commonly an asymmetrical) arthritis.

  o Ankylosing spondylitis
    – Sacroilliac joints and spine
    – Hips, knees and shoulders
    – Psoriatic arthritis
    – Terminal interphalangeal joints
    – Sacroilliac joints
    – Rheumatoid pattern

  o Reiter syndrome
    – Sacroilliac joints and spine
    – Hips
    – Knees
    – Ankles, and most of the joints of the feet

  o Infections
    – Brucellosis
    – Chronic active hepatitis
    – Filiarisis
    – Infectious mononucleosis
    – Influenza
    – Kala-azar
    – Leprosy
    – Malaria
    – Salmonellosis
    – Sarcoidosis
    – Schistosomiasis
    – Syphilis
    – Trypanosomiasis
    – Tuberculosis
    – Vaccinations

  o Miscellaneous
    – Hypergammaglobulinemic purpura
    – Asbestosis

Adapted from: Ghosh AK. *Mayo Clinic Scientific Press* 2008, page 975; Talley NJ, et al. *Maclennan & Petty Pty Limited* 2003, page 253

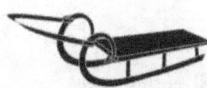

Juvenile Chronic Arthritis: Still Disease

➢ Definition of Still disease

  o Arthritis of unknown cause for 6 weeks or longer

  o Associated with daily temperature spikes to 39.4°C (103°F) for at least 2 weeks

  o With or without maculopapular rash

- Juvenile chronic arthritis (Still disease) may be pauciarticular and polyarticular. Define Still disease and its two major forms. Perform a focused physical examination for juvenile chronic arthritis and its complications.

  o Pauciarticular (~ 75%)
  – ≤ 4 or fewer joints

  o Polyarticular (~25%)
  – ≥ 5 joints involved
  – Usually upper cervical apophyseal, carpometacarpal and terminal interphalangeal joints
  – Fusion of jaw, resulting in a
  – Fusion of cervical spine
    ▪ Micrognathia
    ▪ Receding chin
    ▪ Splenomegaly and lymph adenopathy

"We don't see things the way they are.
We see them the way WE are."

Talmud

 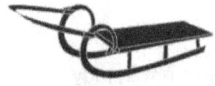

Adult-onset Still Disease (AOSD)

➢ Clinical
- o Daily spiking fever — Peaks in late evening
- o Skin rash — Salmon-skin
  - — Trunk
  - — Proximal extremities
- o Arthralgia / arthritis — Wrist
  - — Knees
  - — Ankles
  - — May progress to ankylosis
- o Hematology — Hemophagocytic syndrome

- Give the complications of juvenile chronic arthritis.

  - o General
    - — Lethargy, anorexia and irritability
    - — Growth failure

  - o MSK
    - — Sacrolitis (more commonly seen in boys)
    - — Joint contractures
    - — Joint failure

  - o Eye
    - — Iritis and anterior uveitis (more commonly seen in girls)
    - — Chronic anterior uveitis

  - o Hematology
    - — Anemia
    - — Amyloidosis
    - — Splenomegaly

Adapted from: Baliga RR. *Saunders/Elsevier* 2007, page 351.

➢ Laboratory
- o ↑ WBC, ↑ ESR, ↑ CRP, ↑ platelets
- o ↑ ferritin (acute phase reactant)
- o ↓ hemoglobin
- o Abnormal LEs
- o No autoantibodies (seronegative) or low complement

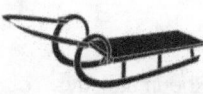

- ➢ Differential
  - o Vasculitis
  - o Autoinflammatory syndrome (e.g. FMF, familial Mediterranean fever)

- ➢ Treatment
  - o NSAIDs
  - o Corticosteroids
  - o Methotrexate
  - o Anti-TNFα drugs
  - o Inhibitors of IL-1, IL-6

Abbreviation: LE, liver enzymes; SLE, systemic lupus erythematosus

---

Clinical Scenario

A 40 yr old man presents with FUO (fever of unknown origin), characterized by daily spikes of fever, non-specific symptoms of malaise, fatigue, myalgia and arthralgia. There is a pink skin rash, and physical findings suggestive an inflammatory arthritis but no signs of chronic liver disease. The hematological and rheumatological blood screens are normal. The serum transaminases and alkaline phosphatase are normal; the serum ferritin is > 250 ng/mL, but genetic testing for hereditary hemochromatosis is negative.

- • Give the likely diagnosis, and treatment of this disorder.
  - o The patient likely has AOSD (adult-onset Still disease)
  - o Treatment includes
    - – NSAIDs, for refractory disease, treatments include
    - – Corticosteroids
    - – Methotrexate
    - – TNF-α inhibitors
    - – Anakinra (IL-1 receptor antagonist)

Psoriatric Arthritis

- ➢ Clinical
  - o Skin and nail changes of psoriasis
    - – Do not correlate with severity / extent of joint disease
    - – Precede joint disease in 85%

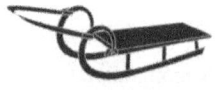

o Joint changes – Large joints ▪ 40% symmetrical oligoarthritis of legs and feet

– Small joints ▪ 25% symmetrical, like RA (rheumatoid arthritis)

– Spine ▪ 50% spinal disease

- Perform a focused physical examination for psoriatic arthritis.

  o Arthritis (in only 5% of persons with psoriasis)
    - Asymmetrical terminal joint involvement
      ▪ Monoarticular and oligoarticular arthritis of the hands and feet.
      ▪ May occur with psoriatic nail changes
    - Symmetrical joint involvement (most common like rheumatoid arthritis, but seronegative)
      ▪ Arthritis mutilans (destructive polyarthritis, with telescoping of digits)

  o Nail changes (nails involved in 80% of persons with associated arthritis)
    - Pitting, onycholysis, ridging, hyperkeratosis, discoloration
    - Distal interphalangeal joints
    - Arthritis matilans (osteolysis with deformity of digits)
    - Spondylitis
    - Onychodystrophy
    - Psoriatic, reddish plaques, with silvery scales and well-defined edges (most prominent on elbows [extensor surfaces], scalp, submammilary and umbilical regions)
  o Skin
    - Scalp
    - Behind ear
    - Entesor surfaces
    - Umbilicus
    - Gluteal cleft

Adapted from: Baliga RR. *Saunders/Elsevier* 2007, page 343; Talley NJ, et al. *Maclennan & Petty Pty Limited* 2003, page 290.

➢ Diagnostic imaging

- Give the radiological features of psoriatic arthritis
  o 'Fluffy' periostitis
  o Destruction of small joints
  o 'Pencil and cup' appearance
  o Osteolysis, ankylosis and telescoping in arthritis mutilans
  o Non marginal syndesmophytes in spondylitis (*Q J Med* 1977;46:411)

Adapted from: Baliga RR. *Saunders/Elsevier* 2007, page 343.

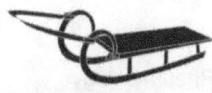

➤ Laboratory	– RF-positive	▪ Psoriasis ~ 15%
		▪ Psoriasis plus arthropathy ~ 15%
	– ↑ uric acid	▪ Do not confuse with gouty arthropathy
➤ Treatment	– Mild disease	▪ NSAIDs
		▪ Methotrexate
		▪ TNF-α inhibitors for failure of methotrexate (do not use in pregnancy)
	– Axial disease	▪ Consider early use of TNF-α inhibitors
	– Dactylitis, enthesitis (painful heels)	▪ Local injected corticosteroids
		▪ TNF-α inhibitors

NSAIDs, hydroxychloroquine and sulfasalazine are used for mild RA.

- Give the **caution** about the use of **NSAIDs and hydroxychloroquine** in psoriatric arthritis.
  - o NSAIDs and hydrochloroquine may worsen the clinical course of psoriasis

"Understand how you apply your medical art."
James Calvin

 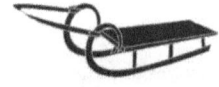

AXIAL SPONDYLITIS / ARTHROPATHY

➢ Types

- Give the inflammatory joint disorders
  - o Psoriatric arthritis
  - o Reactive arthritis
  - o Ankylosing spondylitis
  - o IBD-associated arthritis

  - o Also known as
    - – Sponyloarthropathy
    - – Serronegative spondyloarthropathies
    - – Reactive arthritis (Reiter Syndrome)
  - o Remember:
    - – **The four 'A's of ankylosing spondylitis**: anterior uveitis, pulmonary apical fibrosis, aortic regurgitation, Achilles tendonitis
    - – Psoriasis and Reiter syndrome can also cause sacroiliitis

Source: Baliga RR. *Saunders/Elsevier* 2007, pages 340 and 341.

➢ Causes / associations

- Perform a focused physical examination for the causes / associations of spondyloarthritis.

- Seropositive conditions (rheumatoid factor [RF] positive)

  - o Musculoskeletal
    - – Rheumatoid arthritis
    - – Sjögren syndrome
    - – Systemic lupus erythematosus (SLE)
    - – Scleroderma

  - o Heart
    - – Subacute bacterial endocarditis (SBE)

  - o Lung
    - – Idiopathic pulmonary fibrosis

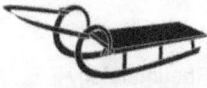

o Blood
   – Mixed cryoglobulinemia

o Infections
   – Infectious mononucleosis
   – Influenza
   – Chronic active hepatitis
   – Vaccinations
   – Tuberculosis
   – Syphilis

o Malignancy
   – Malignancies

- Give a systematic approach to the **causes of sacroiliitis**.
  o MSK
     - Ankylosing spondylitis (rheumatoid spondylitis)
     - Juvenile rheumatoid arthritis
     - Psoriasis, Psoriatic arthritis

  o GI
     - IBD (Ulcerative colitis and Crohn disease)

  o Infection
     - Reiter Syndrome
     - TB
     - Whipple disease
     - Brucellosis

Adapted from: Burton JL. *Churchill Livingstone* 1971, page114.

➢ Clinical

- Take a directed **history** for ankylosing spondylitis.

  o Back stiffness and back pain-worse in the morning, improves on exercise and worsens on rest

  o Symptoms in the peripheral joints (in 40%), particularly shoulders and knees.

  o Onset of symptoms is typically insidious, and in the third to fourth decade

  o Extra- articular manifestations:
     – Red eye (uveitis)
     – Diarrhea (GI involvement)
     – Aortic regurgitation
     – Pulmonary apical fibrosis (worse in smokers)

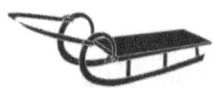

- Take a **directed history** for Spondyloarthritis.

  o Patient < 40 yr

  o The pain of ≥ 3 mon
    - Onset slow
    - ↓ with exercise
    - Getting out of bed
    - ↑ with rest, including in bed

Note:

  o If the patient has 4-5 criteria above, the sensitivity for spondyloarthritis is 77% and specificity is 92%

- Perform a focused **physical** examination for ankylosing spondylitis of the back, sacroiliac joints, and hips.

  o Loss of lumbar lordosis and thoracic kyphosis

  o Severe flexion deformity of the lumbar spine (rare)

  o Tenderness of the lumbar vertebrae

  o Reduction of movement of the lumbar spine in all directions (whole body turns)

  o Tenderness of the sacroiliac joints

  o Late involvement of cervical spine, with grating sensations on movement of neck

  o Occiput-to-wall distance (inability to make contact when heel and back are against the wall indicates upper thoracic and cervical limitation)

  o 'Question mark' posture (loss of lumbar lordosis, fixed kyphoscoliosis of the thoracic spine with compensatory extension of the cervical spine)

  o Protuberant abdomen

  o Perform Schober test- this involves marking points 10 cm above and 5 cm below a line joining the 'dimple of Venus' on the sacral promontory. An increase in the separation of less than 5cm during full forward flexion indicates limited spinal mobility

  o Finger-floor distance (a simple indicator but is less reliable because good hip movement may compensate for back limitation)

  o Chest expansion at nipple line < 5 cm (costovertebral involvement)

  o Sacroiliac tenderness

  o Postural change in advanced AS: 'question mark posture'

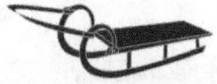

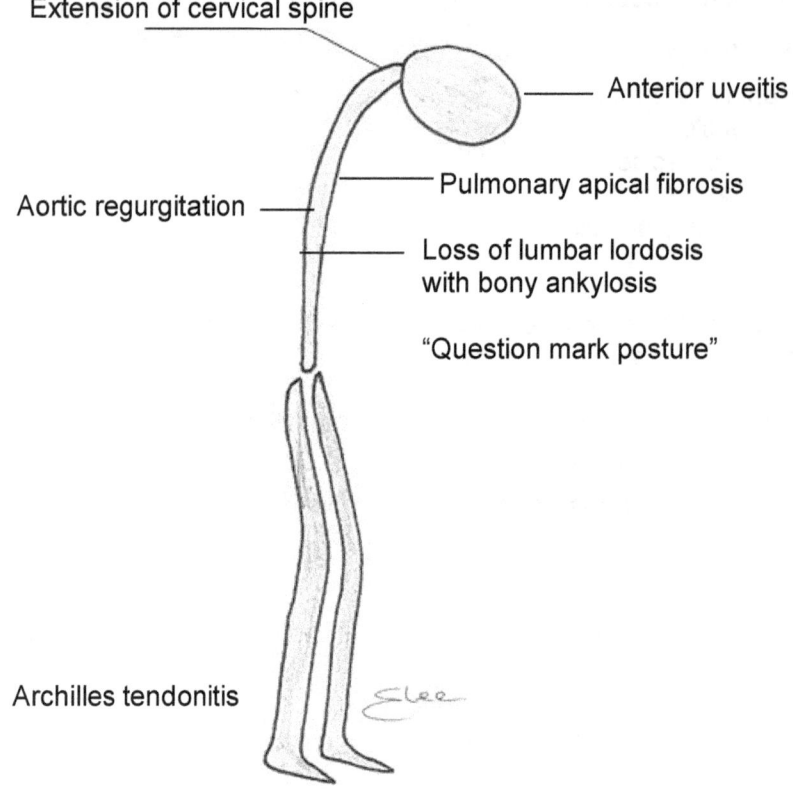

Extension of cervical spine

Anterior uveitis

Pulmonary apical fibrosis

Aortic regurgitation

Loss of lumbar lordosis
with bony ankylosis

"Question mark posture"

Archilles tendonitis

- o Distal arthritis
  - Distal arthritis occurs in up to 30% of patients and may precede
    the onset of the back symptoms. Small joints of the hand and feet
    are rarely affected.

- o Legs/ Feet
  - Achilles tendonitis
  - Plantar fasciitis
  - Cauda equine compression (rare lower limb weakness)
  - Loss of sphincter control
  - Saddle sensory loss

- o Lungs
  - Decreased chest expansion (<5 cm, suggesting costo-vertebral
    involvement)
  - Pulmonary apical fibrosis, cavities
  - Mild restrictive lung disease

- o Heart
  - Aortic regurgitation

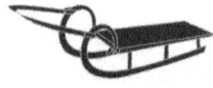

- o The eyes
  - - Acute iritis (recurrent) – painful red eye (in 10-15%)

- o CNS
  - - Tetraplegia

- o GI
  - - Ulcerative colitis or Crohn disease
  - - Hepatosplenomegaly, amyloidosis

- o GU
  - - Renal enlargement (amyloidosis)
  - - Proteinuria

Adapted from: Baliga RR. *Saunders/Elsevier* 2007, page 341; Talley NJ, et al. *Maclennan & Petty Pty Limited* 2003, page 289; Ghosh AK. *Mayo Clinic Scientific Press* 2008, Table 24-25, page 1009.

- • Give **extra-articular** associations of AS (Ankylosing Spondylitis).

  - o Eye   - Acute anterior uveitis

  - o Lung   - Fibrosis apical
    - - Cavitation

  - o Heart   - AV (aortic valve) regurgitation
    - - Conduction defects

  - o Spinal cord - Cauda equine syndrome
    - - Cervical spine fracture (following minor accident)

Clinical Alert

In patients with low back pain diagnosed as ankylosing spondylitis (AS), if surgical management is being contemplated, check for cervical disease, so as to avoid cervical subluxation.

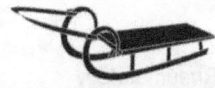

- Give the performance characteristics of the following historical components/ or AS.
    - Morning stiffness
    - Improves with exercise
    - Onset before age 40
    - Begins slowly
    - Pain persisting > 3 months

    o If ≥ 4 of the above historical points are positive, the sensitivity is 95% and specificity is 85%.

    o However, because of the low prevalence, the positive predictive value is still poor.

➤ Laboratory

    o HLA-B27 positive

    o ↑ CRP

    o HLA-B27 is neither sensitive nor specific re diagnosis of AS, or distinguishing AS from other spondylarthropathies.

Note: even if MRI is normal in the patient with back pain, HLA-B27 positive, and has two spondylitis clinical diagnostic criteria, consider the diagnosis of axial preradiographic spondyloarthritis.

➤ Diagnostic imaging

    o Radiograph or MRI positive for AS

    o Enthesis of the heel

    o Dactiylitis

- Give the diagnostic imaging changes in spondyloarthritis
➤ Early
    o Plain radiographs of spine (~40%)
        - Fuzzy iliac portion of sacroiliac joint
        - Erosions
        - Obliteration of joint space
        - Ankylosing ("bamboo spine")
        - Subchondral bony sclerosis
        - Vertebral bodies squared

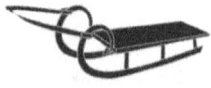

    o CT
- - Erosions
- - Sclerosis

    o MRI
- - Edema of bone marrow

    o Calcification of anterior longitudinal ligament

    o Syndesmophytes

    o Ankylosis

    o Bamboo spine (bridging of syndesmophytes along entire spine)

➢ Late disease

    o Atlantoaxial sublaxation (C1 – C2)

- Give the radiological features of Ankylosing Spondylitis.

    o Bilateral erosive SI disease (with later sclerosis)

    o Erosion in intervertebral facets and costo-vertebral joints

    o Calcified spinal ligaments

    o Erosion in limb joints (especially hips)

    o Irregularity of weight bearing surfaces

Source: Burton JL. *Churchill Livingstone* 1971, page 113.

SO YOU WANT TO BE A RHEUMATOLOGIST!

- In the context of ankylosing spondilitis, what is the normal chest expansion, what is the Schober test?

    o Normal chest expansion is 5 cm (2")
    o Schober test – 10 cm. above the dimples of venus, flex forward maximally, the extension should by 5 cm (10cm → 15cm).

Note: If DI is negative (even on MRI), then if HLA-B27+ plus two other features of spondyloarthritis, the diagnosis of AS can still be made

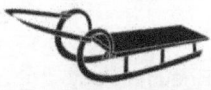

➤ Differential

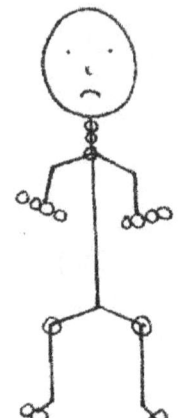

Rheumatoid arthritis

- Hands: intercarpal joints, MP joints and proximal IP joints
- Feet: tarsal and lateral MP joints
- Knees
- Small joints of cervical spine and subacromial bursae

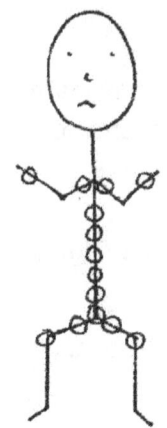

Ankylosing spondylitis

- Spine and both sacro-iliac joints
- Knees, shoulders, wrists

- Give clinical, radiological and laboratory differences which may be diagnostically useful to distinguish between **DISH** (diffuse idiopathic skeletal hyperostosis) and **AS** (ankylosing spondylitis).

		DISH	AS
o Clinical	- Men > 40 yr	+	-
o Radiology	- Flowing osteophytes across 4 contiguous vertebrae	+	-
	- Vertical bridging syndesmophytes	-	+
	- Involvement of thoracic vertebrae	+	-
o Laboratory	- HLA B27-associated (in 95%)	-	+
	- Sacroiliitis	-	+
	- ↑ IGF-1	+	-

Abbreviations: IGF-1, insulin-like growth factor 1

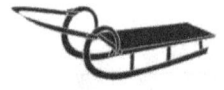

A patient with Crohn disease has received three 3-mon tapering doses of corticosteroids over the past two years. He presents with the new symptoms of hip pain. You worry about avascular necrosis of the hip, but also wish to exclude sacroiliitis / ankylosing spondylitis (AS). The radiogram is negative.

- Give the next diagnostic imaging test which should be performed.

    o MRI with gadolinium enhancement

    o Findings
        - Bone marrow edema
        - Erosions
        - Synovitis

Clinical Alert

In patients with either psoriatic arthritis or reactive arthritis who have sudden **onset of spondyloarthritis, or worsening** of previously known / diagnosed disease, think of

   o HIV infection

   o Repeated trauma

---

    o You may expect to be asked to compare and to contrast one form of spondyloarthritis (such as ankylosing spondylitis), with one of the three other spondyloarthritis conditions (such as psoriatric arthritis), reactive arthritis, or IBD-associated arthritis.

    o This is a major topic, and it is likely that you will be called upon to use MSK (musculoskeletal) factors for this comparison, or to use comparisons of changes in non-MSK systems (e.g. eye, skin, heart, lung, GI, GU, bone)

    o For a helpful reference Table, please see MKSAP 16, Rheumatology 2012, Table 15, page 29. Also a useful reference is MKSAP 16, Rheumatology 2012, Table 16, page 32, Assessment of Spondyloarthritis International Society Classification Criteria for Axial Spondyloarthritis.

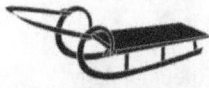

➢ Treatment

    o General – NSAIDs

    o Specific joints

      – Peripheral arthritis   – Sulfasalazine

      – Axial disease   – TNF-α inhibitor

      – Osteoporosis, osteopenia – Supplements calcium, vitamin D

    o Synovitis, enthesitis   – Bisphosphonate

    o Surgical   – Corticosteroid injections for difficult disease

      – Fusion

      – Vertebral wedge osteotomy

SO YOU WANT TO BE A RHEUMATOLOGIST!

- How does sacroilitis of psoriatic arthritis differ from ankylosing spondylitis?

    o In psoriatic arthritis, the syndesmophytes are usually from the internal and anterior surfaces of the vertebral bodies, and not from the margins of the bodies as is usually the case in ankylosing spondylitis

Source Baliga RR. *Saunders/Elsevier* 2007, page 343.

SO YOU WANT TO BE RHEUMATOLOGIST!

A young man with low back pain is suspected as having sacro-ileitis. On examination, ankylosing spondylitis (AS) is diagnosed.

- Give the GI, MSK disease and infections associated with AS.

    o GI   – Crohn disease
               – Ulcerative colitis
               – Whipple disease

    o MSK   – Juvenile rheumatoid arthritis
               – Psoriatic arthritis
               – Reiter disease

    o Infections – TB
               – Brucellosis

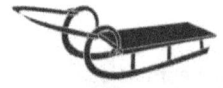

IBD-associated Arthritis

- Give the distinction between peripheral arthritis vs. sacroiliitis in Crohn disease (CD) and ulcerative colitis (UC)

	Peripheral arthritis	Sacroiliitis
o Frequency of involvement	– CD > UC (10% vs. 5%)	▪ CD > UC (30% vs. 10%)
o Relationship to B27	– 25% of type I arthritis – Type II unrelated	▪ ~ 100% of B27 positive IBD patients develop sacroiliitis
o Relationship to IBD disease extent/activity	– Yes (type I), no (type II) – Coincident bowel/joint flares in ~65% of type I, not in type II	▪ No May even precede bowel symptoms
o Responsive to DMARD (sulfasalazine first choice)	– Yes	▪ No
o Responsive to bowel resection	– UC, yes, CD no	▪ Neither CD or UC

Note: both peripheral arthritis and sacroilitis may cause an exacerbation of IBD when used to treat the associated peripheral vs axial arthropathy.

Adapted from: Davey P. *Wiley-Blackwell* 2006, page 405.

SO YOU WANT TO BE A RHEUMATOLOGIST!

- What are the radiological signs of osteomalacia (loss of mineral from bone, with normal protein matrix).

- o Milkman fracture (aka looser zone) – tongue of radiotranslucency extending from the surface into the bone
- o Usually seen upper end of femur or humerus, or lower end of tibia
- o Bending of bones
- o Later, features of osteoporosis
  - Sclerosis of cortex
  - Thinning (translucency) of bone
  - ↓ number of trabeculae
  - Sclerosis of remaining trabeculae
  - Axial bones affected more than peripheral bones

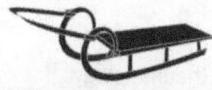

Reactive Arthritis (aka Reiter Syndrome)

➤ Definition

- o Reiter syndrome was considered to include arthritis, urethritis, and conjunctivitis. The old name for reactive arthritis is Reiter syndrome.

- o "Reactive arthritis is characterized by the presence of inflammatory arthritis that manifests within 2 months of an episode of bacterial gastroenteritis or non-gonococcal urethritis or cervicitis in a genetically predisposed person."

- o "……. an acute aseptic inflammatory arthritis that occurs 1 to 3 weeks after an infectious event originating in the GU or GI tract" …. and previously known as Reiter syndrome.

Source: Board Basics 2013, page 311; MKSAP 16, Rheumatology 2012, page 107.

➤ Causes / associations

- Give the names of **pathogens** which are commonly associated with reactive arthritis.
  - o Campylobacter
  - o Chlamydia trachomatis
  - o Chlamydophilia pneumonia
  - o Clostridium difficile
  - o HIV
  - o Neisseria
  - o Salmonella
  - o Shigella
  - o Streptococcus
  - o Yersinia

➤ Clinical
- Typical features
  - o Oligoarticular arthritis
  - o Oral ulcers
  - o Genital ulcers
  - o Skin

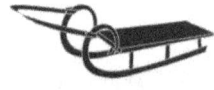

- Give the characteristic **skin lesions** associated with reactive arthritis.

  o Keratoderma blennorrhagicum
    - Palular / pustular rash on skin of palms and soles

  o Circinate balantitis
    - Shallow serpiginous ulcers, with raised edges, on the glans of the penis

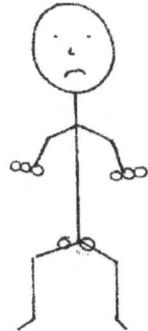

Psoriasis

- Hands, terminal IP joints
- Sacro-iliac joints
- 'Rheumatoid' pattern

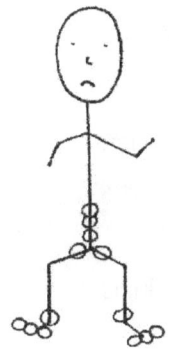

Reactive (Reiter) arthritis

- Ankles and all joints of feet
- Knees
- Hips, sacro-iliac joint and spine

- Complications

o MSK	– Calcaneal spur – calcification of plantar fascia
	– Plantar fasciitis
	– Tendonitis
	– Arthritis – usually knees & ankles
o Skin (palms, soles of feet)	– Psoriasis-like lesions (specifically, keratoderma blenorrhagia
	– Ulcer on penis (aka circinate balanitis)
o GU	– Ulcer on penis (aka circinate balanitis)
o Heart	– Aortitis
	– Myocarditis
	– Pericarditis

➤ Give the clinical features of **Stevens-Johnson syndrome.**

  o General
    - Constitutional symptoms
    - High fever

  o Eye, Ear
    - Conjunctivitis
    - Corneal ulcers
    - Uveitis
    - Otitis media

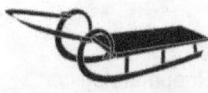

- o Mouth
  - Oral bullae
  - Hemorrhagic crusting

- o Skin
  - Maculopapular / bullous erythema multiforme

- o GI
  - Diarrhea

- o Lung
  - Bronchitis
  - Pneumonitis

- o Kidney/GU
  - Urethritis
  - Balanitis
  - Vulvovaginitis

- o MSK
  - Polyarthritis

Clinical Alert

The urate-lowering drug allopurinol may cause hepatic failure, bone marrow failure as well as Stevens-Johnson syndrome, and should be used cautiously in the presence of renal dysfunction.

Behcet disease

➤ Definition: Behcet disease is an idiopathic systemic inflammatory disorder characterized by recurrent oral ulcerations plus at least two of the following:

➤ Clinical

- o CNS
  - Meningoencephalitis
  - Basal ganglia
  - Cerebral cortex

- o Eyes
  - Uveitis anterior, posterior

- o Mouth
  - Buccal ulcers with a red areola

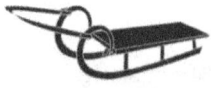

o Skin lesions
- Erythema nodosum
- Pseudofolliculitis
- Acneform nodules
- Superficial migratory
- Thrombophlebitis
- Pathergy

o MSK
- Osteoarthritis (50%)

o GI
- IBD (especially UC-like)

o GU
- Recurrent genital ulcers

o Veins
- Thrombophlebitis

o CVS/lung
- Rarely cardiac and pulmonary lesions

Adapted from: Burton JL. *Churchill Livingstone* 1971, page 114.

SO YOU WANT TO BE A RHEUMATOLOGIST OR A DERMATOLOGIST!

• In the context in Behcet disease, give an explanation of pathergy.

o Pathergy: ".......a postule-like lesion or papule appears 48 hours after skin prick by a 20- to 21-gauge needle."

Source: MKSAP 16, Rheumatology 2012, page 71.

Clinical Pearl

➢ Acute gouty arthritis

o May be proceeded by a fall in the serum concentration of uric acid

o In the presence of an inflammatory arthritis, the serum concentration of uric acid may be normal

o Therefore, a low serum urate concentration argues against but does not rule out gout.

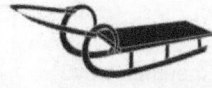

➤ Your colleague disagrees with your clinical diagnosis of Reiter syndrome, and because of the arthritis, urethritis and eye changes, suggests that the correct diagnosis is likely either Behcet syndrome (BS) or Stevens – Johnson syndrome (S-JS).

• Perform a focused physical examination which would help to distinguish **BS from S-JS**.

		BS	S-JS
o	Iritis	+	- (conjunctivitis)
o	Stomatitis	+	-
o	Genital ulcers	+	-
o	Vasculitis	+	-
o	Peripheral neuritis	+	-
o	Diarrhea	+	+
o	Fever	-	+
o	Erythema multiforme	-	+
o	Renal disease	-	+

Migratory Arthralgia

➤ Causes of a migratory arthralgia

- o Musculoskeletal
    - Rheumatic fever
    - SLE

- o Infection
    - Subacute bacterial endocarditis
    - Whipple's disease
    - Sarcoidosis
    - Brucellosis
    - Gonorrhea

- o Immune
    - Serum sickness
    - Reiters disease
    - Stevens-Johnson syndrome

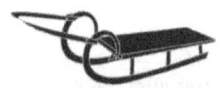

OSTEOARTHRITIS

➢ Clinical

• Give the classic **sites** of OA.

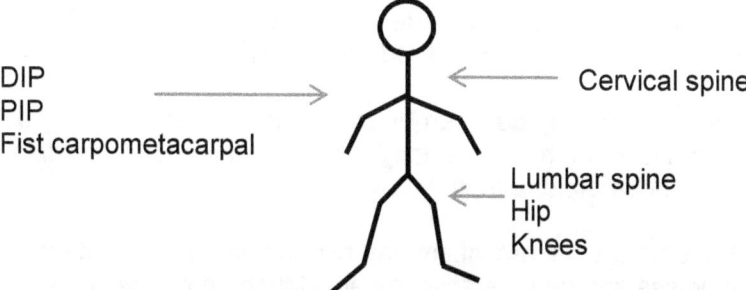

DIP
PIP
Fist carpometacarpal

Cervical spine

Lumbar spine
Hip
Knees

Abbreviation: DIP, distal interphalangeal; PIP, proximal interphalangeal

If other joints involved, consider alternate diagnosis

- o Hereditary hemochromatosis, or
- o Previous joint injury

Diagnostic Tips in OA: Other Diagnostic Considerations

- o OA of hip   – Bursitis
                                              ▪ Trochanteric
                                              ▪ Anserine

- o Carpometacarpal (CMC) OA   – de Quervain tenosynovitis
- o Metacarpophalangeal   – DIP, PID
  (MCP), OA   ▪ Think OA
                                    – MCP & PIP 2 & 3
                                      ▪ Think AH

- o Any painful & tender OA joint – Septic complication

Clinical Differential

• Give the differential diagnosis of an **acute painful calf**.

- o DVT
- o Ruptured Baker cyst (jerniation of fluid filled synovium of posterior knee)
- o Ruptured gastrocnemius muscle

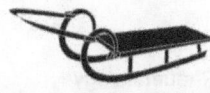

SO YOU WANT TO BE A RHEUMATOLOGIST!

- In the context of osteoarthritis (OA), how do you distinguish between Heberden and Bouchard nodes.

    o Painless nodules – Heberden nodes; DIP
                       – Bouchard nodes; PIP

- OK. Now distinguish between Bouchard nodes, which usually occur in OA, and Haygarth nodes, which usually occur in rheumatic disorders such as rheumatoid, arthritis.

    o Haygarth nodes are inflammatory and thus painful and tender, not painless and degenerative, as are Bouchard nodes in OA

    o These nodes affect

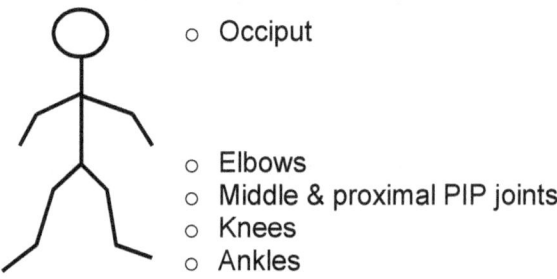

        o Occiput

        o Elbows
        o Middle & proximal PIP joints
        o Knees
        o Ankles

- In the context of reddish lesions on the palms of the hands or soles of the feet, distinguish between **Janeway lesions and Osler nodes**.

    o Janeway lesions are small and non-tendon whereas, Osler's nodes are swollen, tender. Janeway lesions arise from septic emboli or sterile vasculitis in endocarditis (with or without bacteremia, gonococcal sepsis, or lupus (SLE).

- In the context of bony swellings in a patient with osteoarthrosis, give the difference between Heberden and Bouchard nodes?

    o Heberden - TIP joints (terminal interphalangeal joints)

    o Bouchard - PIP joints (proximal interphalangeal joints)

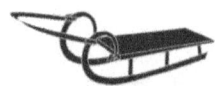

- Perform a focused **physical examination** of the hand for osteoarthritis.

  o Interphalangeal pints
    - Distal
      - Heberden nodes
    - Proximal
      - Bouchard nodes

  o Carpometacarpal pint
    - Squaring of the joint contour

  o Any hand joint which has sustained a previous injury

  o Weight loss and exercise are recommended for osteoarthritis (OA) of the knee.

  o If there are no symptoms of catching or locking to suggest a meniscal tear, knee arthroscopic lavage and/or debridement is of little benefit for the advanced knee OA.

  o Patients with symptoms, functional limitations, and radiographic findings of advanced knee OA, and who have failed to respond to conservative therapy, ".....should be referred to an orthopediatric surgeon for consideration of total bone arthroplasty".

  o OA of the MCP (metacarpophalangeal) joints or wrists in the absence of history of previous trauma → think of secondary OA from hereditary hemochromatosis.

➤ Diagnostic imaging

- Give the **"best" diagnostic imaging test** to diagnose osteoarthritis (OA).

  o Ah, the diagnosis is made clinically, but if a radiography is performed, give the expected findings in OA.

Clinical Caution: If OA does not occur in the usual **weight bearing joints**, consider the possibility of secondary disease:

  o Metacarpophalangeal joint – think of possible hereditary hemochromatosis

  o Facial and physique phenotype changes – think of possible acromegaly

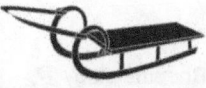

- Give the radiological features of Osteoarthrosis.
    - New bone formation
        - Osteophytes
        - Peri-articular ossicles
        - Loose bodies
    - Cartilage loss (often confined to weight bearing surface)
    - Sclerosis and subchondral cavitation
    - Subluxation of hip, shoulder, terminal IP joints
    - No ankylosis

Source: Burton JL. *Churchill Livingstone* 1971, page 113.

- Give the characteristic radiogram changes of **OA of the hand**.
    - Asymmetric narrowing of the joint space
    - Subchondral sclerosis
    - Osteophytes
    - If symptoms are in the hand, look for proximal Bouchard and distal Heberden nodes, as well as squaring of the carpometacarpal joint.

- Perform a focused physical examination for primary vs secondary osteoarthritis.

	Primary	Secondary
o Symmetrical		
o Many joints	- Many	Few
o Previously damaged joints	- No	Yes
o Fingers affected	- Yes	No
o Sites affected	- Distal (Heberden nodes) and proximal (Bouchard nodes) interphalangeal joints, and metacarpophalangeal (MCP)joints of the thumbs - Acromioclavicular joints - Small joints of the spine (lower cervical and lumbar) - Knees, - Metatarsophalangeal (MTP) joints of the great toes	Hip Knees Intervertebral disc

Adapted from: Talley NJ, et al. *Maclennan & Petty Pty Limited* 2003, page 253.

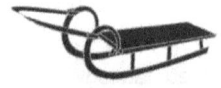

In both rheumatoid arthritis (RA) and osteoarthritis (OA), there is slow insidious onset of progressive disease, exacerbations, and the development of limitations in motion.

- Take a directed history and perform focused physical examination to distinguish RA from OA.

		Rheumatoid Arthritis *	Osteoarthritis
o	Process	– Chronic inflammation of synovial membranes – Secondary erosion of adjacent cartilage and bone – Damage to ligaments and tendons	▪ Degeneration and progressive loss of cartilage within the joints ▪ Damage to underlying bone, ▪ Formation of new bone at the margins of the cartilage
o	Common locations	– Hands (PIP, MCP), – Feet (MCP) – Wrists – Elbows – Knees – Ankles – Cervical sprue	▪ Knees, hips, hands, wrists (DIP, sometimes PIP), ▪ Cervical and lumbar spine ▪ Joints that were previously injured or diseased
o	Pattern of spread	– Progresses to other joints while persisting in the initial ones (symmetrically additive)	▪ Additive; however, only one joint may be involved
o	Swelling	– Swelling of synovial tissue in joints or tendon sheaths' – Subcutaneous nodules	▪ Effusions in the joints (especially in the knees) ▪ Bony enlargement
o	Joint inflammation	– Common	▪ Uncommon
o	Stiffness	– Prominent, often for an hour or more in the mornings, also after inactivity	▪ Frequent ▪ Usually 5-10 min) in the morning and after inactivity
o	General symptoms	– Weakness – Fatigue – Weight loss – Fever	▪ Usually absent
o	Radio-graphic changes	– Symmetric narrowing of joint space	▪ Asymmetric narrowing of joint space ▪ Osteophytes ▪ Subchondral sclerosis ▪ Cystic changes

Abbreviations: DIP, distal interphalangeal: MCP, metacarpophalangeal; OA, osteoarthritis; PIP, proximal interphlangeal; RA, rheumatoid arthritis

Adapted from: Jugovic PJ, et al. *Saunders/ Elsevier* 2004, pages 147 and 148.

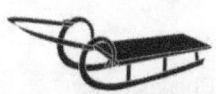

- Perform a focused physical examination for patterns of arthropathy (for the convenience of the reader, this figure has been repeated from a previous section).

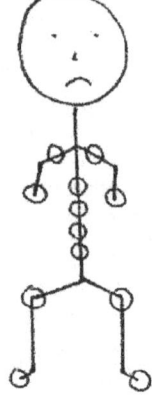

Primary osteoarthritis

Symmetrical, affecting many joints

- Great toes and thumbs: MP joints
- Fingers: terminal IP joints
- Acromio-clavicular joints

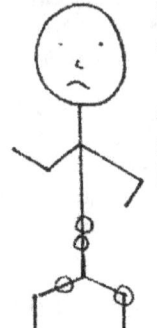

Secondary osteoarthritis

Asymmetrical, affecting weight bearing joints:

- Knees
- Hips
- Intervertebral discs

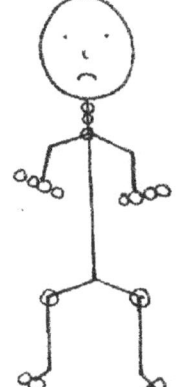

Rheumatoid arthritis

- Hands: intercarpal joints, MP joints and proximal IP joints
- Feet: tarsal and lateral MP joints
- Knees
- Small joints of cervical spine and subacromial bursae

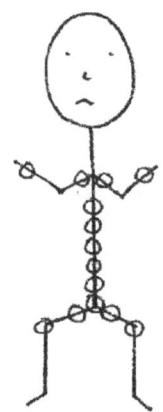

Ankylosing spondylitis

- Spine and both sacro-iliac joints
- Knees, shoulders, wrists

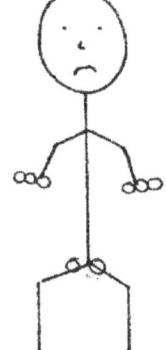

Psoriasis

- Hands, terminal IP joints
- Sacro-iliac joints
- 'Rheumatoid' pattern

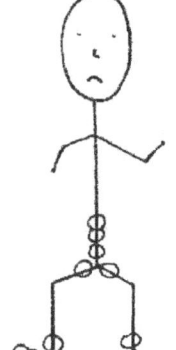

Reiter (reactive) arthritis

- Ankles and all joints of feet
- Knees
- Hips, sacro-iliac joint and spine

Source: Burton JL. *Churchill Livingstone* 1971, page 112.

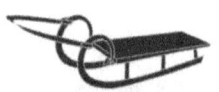

SO YOU WANT TO BE A RHEUMATOLOGIST!

- Paget disease usually causes sclerotic lesions, but the exception may be the skull. Give the bony changes in the skull in Paget disease.

  o Well circumscribed area of translucency (rarefraction) (aka osteoporosis circumscripta)
  o Platybasia-indentation of the soft skull by vertebral column (odontoid process of the axis > 5 mm above chamberlain's line [Chamberlain's line is a straight line drawn backwards from the hard palate to 5 mm above the odontoid process)

Clinical Tip

- Give the clinical and laboratory features hich help to **distinguish** between inflammatory and non-inflammatory arthritis.
  o With inflammatory arthritis, there is usually
    – Morning stiffness > 1 hr
    – Synovial fluid > 5.0×10^9 / L (> 5000 / μL)

"Adherence to guidelines reduces mortality (improves outcomes)."

James Calvin

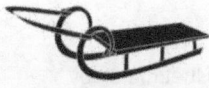

SYSTEMIC LUPUS ERYTHEMATOSIS (SLE)

➤ Definition: Systemic lupus erythromatosis (SLE) is process
".......characteized by a wide range of organ involvement, multiple
autoantibodies, and a broad spectrum of disease severity with
intermittent exacerbations and remissions"

  o For research purposes, the American College of Rheumatology has
developed criteria for the diagnosis of SLE.

  o An autoimmune disorder due to the loss of tolerance to nuclear
antigens and the development of autoantibodies.

  o This leads to a spectrum of localized or systemic disease, affecting
the skin, joints, CNS, kidneys, as well as the hematological system,
and serositis, pleuritis and pericarditis.

Source: MKSAP 16, Rheumatology 2012, page 34.

➤ Demographics

  o Prevalence ` $75/10^5$, especially in non-Caucasian females during
their reproductive years

➤ Pathogenesis

● Give the pathogenesis of SLE.

  o Female predominance
    – Possible estrogen changes from epigenetic modification of x chromosome

  o Autoantibodies
    – Against nucleic acid and/or nucleic acid binding proteins

  o ↑ type 1 interferons
    – ANA or antinuclear antigens
    – Anti-ds DNA (double stranded DNA)
    – Anti-ss DNA (single stranded DNA)

  o Deposition of immune complexes → activation of complement → tissue
damage

  o Triggering of innate immune system
    – Drugs
      ▪ Hydralazine
      ▪ Procainamide
      ▪ Methydopa
      ▪ Anti-hypertensives
      ▪ TNF-α in hibitors
      ▪ Anti-phopholipids

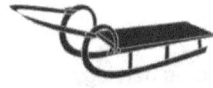

- Anti-histone
- Many others
- Infection
  - Especially viral
- Tobacco
- Sunlight

Note: Parvovirus B19 virus may cause arthralgias plus serology positive for autoantibodies

➢ Clinical

- Perform a focused physical examination for systemic lupus erythematosus (SLE) and its complications.

  o Almost all body systems are affected

  o General appearance
    - Cushingoid
    - ↑ Weight
    - Altered mental state
    - Fever

  o Head
    - CNS
      - Neuropsychiatric symptoms
      - Seizures
      - Cranial nerve lesions
    - Hair: Alopecia, lupus hairs
    - Eyes – scleritis, cystoid lesions
    - Mouth – ulcers, infection
    - Gum – bleeding
    - Butterfly rash (sun-exposed areas)
    - Cervical lymph adenopathy

  o Skin
    - Livedo reticularis
    - Purpura
    - Proximal myopathy (active disease or result steroid treatment)
    - Raynaud phenomenon
    - Follicular plugging
    - Scales
    - Telangiectasia
    - Scarring (bridge of the nose and cheeks)
    - Excessive menstrual bleeding
    - Purpura (due to thrombocytopenia)

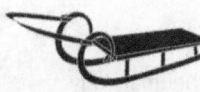

o Systemic
  - Hypertension, edema (suggesting renal involvement)
  - Fever
  - Lymph adenopathy

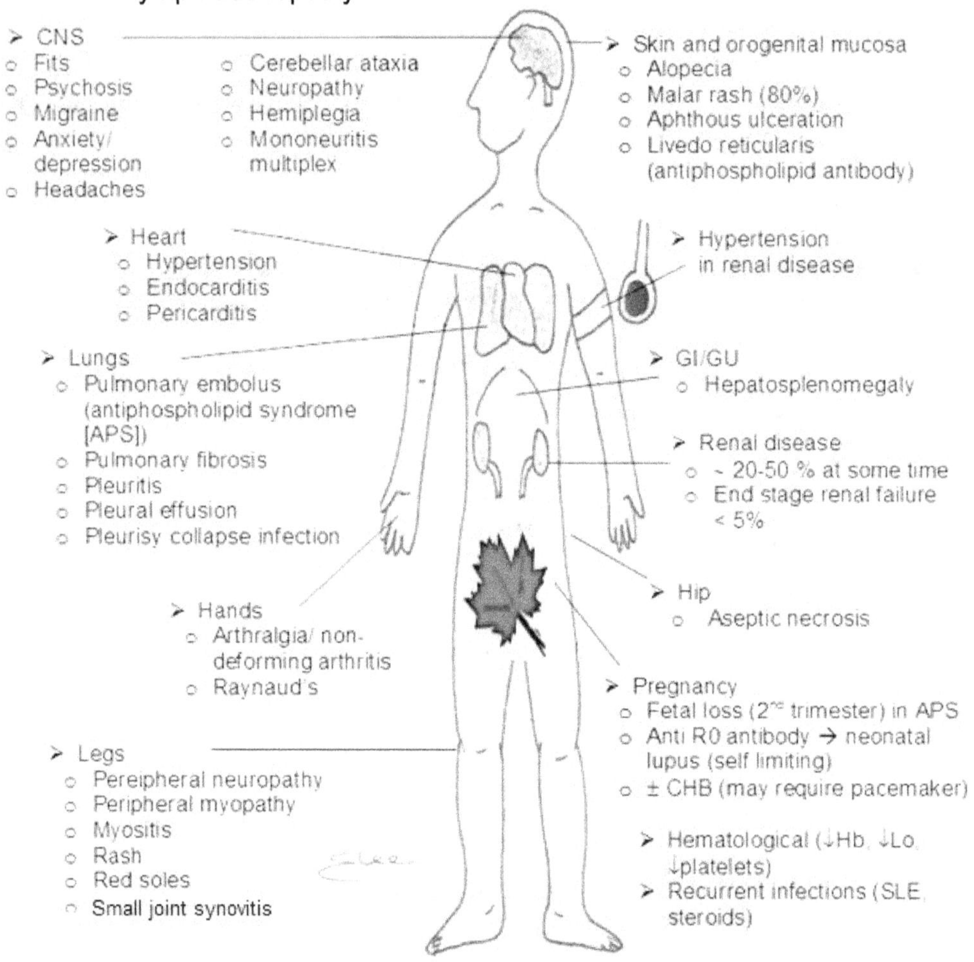

➤ CNS
o Fits
o Psychosis
o Migraine
o Anxiety/
  depression
o Headaches

o Cerebellar ataxia
o Neuropathy
o Hemiplegia
o Mononeuritis
  multiplex

➤ Skin and orogenital mucosa
o Alopecia
o Malar rash (80%)
o Aphthous ulceration
o Livedo reticularis
  (antiphospholipid antibody)

➤ Heart
o Hypertension
o Endocarditis
o Pericarditis

➤ Hypertension
  in renal disease

➤ Lungs
o Pulmonary embolus
  (antiphospholipid syndrome
  [APS])
o Pulmonary fibrosis
o Pleuritis
o Pleural effusion
o Pleurisy collapse infection

➤ GI/GU
o Hepatosplenomegaly

➤ Renal disease
o ~ 20-50 % at some time
o End stage renal failure
  < 5%

➤ Hands
o Arthralgia/ non-
  deforming arthritis
o Raynaud's

➤ Hip
o Aseptic necrosis

➤ Pregnancy
o Fetal loss (2ⁿᵈ trimester) in APS
o Anti R0 antibody → neonatal
  lupus (self limiting)
o ± CHB (may require pacemaker)

➤ Legs
o Pereipheral neuropathy
o Peripheral myopathy
o Myositis
o Rash
o Red soles
o Small joint synovitis

➤ Hematological (↓Hb, ↓Lo
  ↓platelets)
➤ Recurrent infections (SLE
  steroids)

Adapted from: Davey P. *Wiley-Blackwell* 2006, page 409 and Talley NJ, et al. *Maclennan & Petty Pty Limited* 2003, Figure 8.37, page 292.

➤ Diagnosis

  o SLE affects almost every body system.

  o The American College of Rheumatology (ACR) lists II criteria, and the presence of 4 or more of these provided good performance characteristics of the diagnosis, with sensitivity of 75% and specificity of 95%.

  o In the following, these clinical features in <u>bold form</u> components of the ACR criteria.

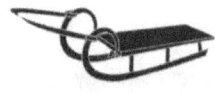

- Give the multisystem **complications** of SLE, and the ACR **criteria for diagnosis** of SLE (shown in bold).

  o Skin (90%)

  - **Malar rash** (90%, aka acute cutaneous lupus erythematosus, or butterfly rash)
  - **Discoid rash** (~20%; discoid lupus erythematosis))
  - **Photosensitivity** (> 60%)
  - **Oral ulcers**
    - Positive "lupus band test" (positive immunohistochemical staining at the dermal epidermal function of immunoglobulin and complement)
  - Subacute cutaneous lupus erythematosus
  - Lupus profundus (panniculitis)
  - Alopecia
  - Livedo reticularis (associated with anti-phospholipid antibodies and syndrome, with thrombosis and pregnancy loss)

  o CNS / PNS (15% to 95%)

  - Seizures/ psychosis
  - NPSLE (neuropsychiatric SLE, aka Lupus cerebritis [old term] please see MKSAP 16, Rheumatology 2012,Table 19, page 37

  o Heart

  - **Pericarditis** (20%)
  - Myocarditis
  - Valvular heart disease (60%)
  - Infective endocarditis
  - Non-infective (sterile) endocarditis (aka Libman Sacks Endocarditis)
  - Early atherosclerosis, including myocardial infarction

  o Lung

  - Pleuritis (~ 50%)
  - Acute pneumonitis
  - Interstitial lung disease
  - Diffuse alveolar hemorrhage
  - Pulmonary hypertension
  - Shrinking lung syndrome

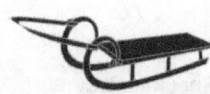

- o Musculoskeletal (90%)
  - Joints
    - Non-erosive arthritis
    - ≥ 2 joints, especially hands, wrists, knees
    - Jaccoud arthropathy
  - Tendons
    - Tendinitis
  - Muscle
    - Myositis
    - Myalgia (25%)
    - Steroid-induced myopathy
  - Bone
    - Osteoporosis (25%)
    - Osteonecrosis (10%)

- o Hematology
  - Hemolytic anemia, or
  - Leukopenia, or
  - Thrombocytopenia
  - ITP (idiopathic thrombocytopenic purpura)
  - Anti-phospholipid syndrome (in the absence of offending drugs)
  - Lymphadenopathy
    - "Although patients with SLE often have lymphadenopathy, new large and localized lymph node swelling merits further evaluation." (Source: MKSAP 16, Rheumatology 2012,Table 19, page 37)

- o GI / Liver
  - Gastroparesis
  - Vasculits
  - Protein-losing enteropathy
  - Peritonitis
  - Pancreatitis
  - Hepatitis

- o Kidney (50% to 75%)
- o Immunologic

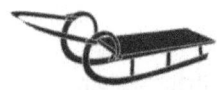

Another grouping of diagnostic criteria for SLE. Four out of eleven criteria present at any time is required for diagnosis of SLE.

Clinical	Laboratory

o Mouth
  – Oral ulcers
	o Hematological abnormalities
	  – Immunological abnormalities
	  – ANA positive (95%)

o CNS
  – Neurological involvement
  – Seizures or psychosis
	– Hemolytic anemia
	– Leukopenia
	– Thrombocytopenia
	– Positive LE cell

o Skin
  – Malar rash
  – Photosensitive rash
  – Discoid lupus rash
  – Mucosal aphthous ulceration
  – Photosensitivity
	– Anti-DNA antibody
	– False-positive

o Heart / lung	
o Kidney – Proteinuria or casts	
o Serositis: Pleuritis or pericarditis	
o MSK – Non-erosive arthritis	

Adapted from: Davey P. *Wiley-Blackwell* 2006, page 410, Table 204.1; Baliga RR. *Saunders/Elsevier* 2007, page 467.

SO YOU WANT TO BE A RHEUMATOLOGIST!

- In the context of a 30 year old woman with a butterfly molar rash and positive ANA, give the features of **Jaccoud arthropathy**.

  o Tendon inflammation → chronic non-erosive deformity of the hands seen in SLE (7%), RF (rheumatic fever), and may look like changes of RA (rheumatoid arthritis)

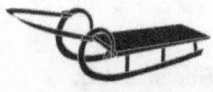

Yes, yet another (!) grouping of criteria for the Diagnosis of SLE!

For diagnosis ≥ 4 of 11 criteria are required.

Criteria	Comment
o Central nervous system	− Seizures
	− Psychosis (15%) in the absence of drugs or metabolic causes
o Serositis, pleuritis/pericarditis	− Occurs in up to 50%
o Arthritis	− Occurs in up to 80%
o Hematologic	− Antibodies to white blood cells (leukopenia), platelets (thrombocytopenia) and/or
	− Red blood cells (hemolytic anemia)
o Kidney Involvement	− Proteinuria >0.5 g/day or cellular casts, occurs in up to 40%
o Immunologic	− Antibodies to DNA, phospholipids (anticardiolipin, lupus anticoagulant) and/or Smith nuclear antigen (anti-Sm)
o Antinuclear antibodies (ANA)	− Abnormal titers of ANA in the absence of drugs known to be associated with drug-induced lupus
o Malar "butterfly" rash	− Rashes occur in 70% of individuals, often photosensitive
o Photosensitivity	− Rash on sun exposure
o Discoid rash	− Plaques
o Mucosal ulcers	

Reproduced with permission: Therapeutics Choices. Sixth Edition. Ottawa, Canada: *Canadian Pharmacist Association* 2012, Table 1, page 1057.

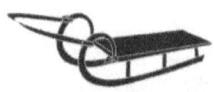

- Give the causes of **anterior uveitis** which need to be excluded in persons with SLE.

    o MSK
    - Sarcoidosis
    - Chest X ray
    - Spondyloarthritis
    - HLA-B27 positive
    - Behcet disease
    - Juvenile inflammatory arthritis
    - Granulomatosis with polyangitis
      - ANCA
    - SLE
      - Anti-ds DNA antibodies
      - Regain test
      - Tuberculin test, chest X-ray
    - SSc
      - Anti-Ro/SSA antibodies

    o Infection
    - Syphilis
    - TB
    - Histoplasmosis
    - Lyme disease

    o GI
    - IBD
      - Crohn disease
      - Ulcerative colitis

- You are observing a butterfly rash on the face of a young woman. From what you see, how do you distinguish from her having SLE versus rosacea.

    o SLE does not involve the nasolabial folds, whereas rosacea does. (Don't give me any "LIP" about "LUPUS")

- Give the reason it is critical to distinguish between the **vasculitis** and the **anti- phospholipid syndrome** in SLE.

    o Treatment
    - SLE vasculitis → anti-coagulation
    - SLE plus anti-phospholipid syndrome → anti-coagulation

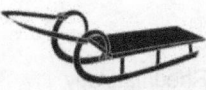

- Perform a focused physical examination for **erythema multiforme**.

➢ Definition

    o Target-shaped lesions, usually over the limbs

    o Three concentric zones of colour change – a central, dark, purple area or blister surrounded by a pale, edematous round zone which in turn is surrounded by a peripheral rim of erythema <red-white-blue

    o Pleomorphic eruption with macules, papules and bullae

➢ Causes

    o Infections (herpes simplex, mycoplasma, streptococci)

    o Drug hypersensitivity (sulphonamides, penicillin, barbiturates, salicylates, antimalarials)

    o Collagen vascular disorder (SLE, dermatomyositis, periarteritis nodosa)

    o Malignancy (carcinomas and lymphomas)

    o Multiple myeloma

    o Idiopathic – in 50% of cases no cause may be found

➢ Complications

    o Stevens-Johnson syndrome (as erythema multiforme major)
      – Fever and mucous membrane involvement (usually oral cavity, eye and genital), in addition to the eruptions of erythema multiforme

Adapted from: Baliga RR. *Saunders/Elsevier* 2007, pages 423 and 424.

- Give the **malignant complications** of SLE, and indicate which one (*) is not related to its treatment.

    o Lung   – Cancer

    o Liver   – Hepatobiliary cancer

    o Blood   – Hodgkin and non-Hodgkin lymphoma

    o Cervix   – Premalignant cervical dysplasia*

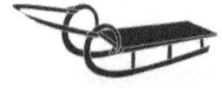

➤ Laboratory: Examples of autoantibodies in SLE

	Prevalence	Operating characteristics and clinical associations
o ANA (antinuclear antibodies)	90%	– Sensitive +++ – Not specific
o Antibodies to histones	80%	– Seen in idiopathic as well as drug-induced SLE
o Antibodies to nature DNA	60%	– Specific +++ – Linked to renal involvement

o Antibosies to SSA / R₀ and SSB / La	30%	– Linked to
		  ▪ Photosensitivity of skin
		  ▪ Drug eyes
		  ▪ Neonatal complications (e.g. congenital complete heart block)

o Antiphospholipid antibodies	30%	– Linked to
		  ▪ Thrombosis
		  ▪ Complications in pregnancy (preeclampsia, loss of fetus)

• Give the associations of the serum antibodies in SLE.

Antibody	Use / benefit
o ANA (anti-nuclear antibody)	– Sensitive
o Anti-dsDNA, anti-Sm	– Specific
o Anti-dsDNA	– Correlates with disease activity
o Anti-Ro/SSA antibodies	– Neonatal heart / block
o Anti-cardiolipin antibodies	– Livedo reticularis

o Positive: ANA and anti-histone antibody; negative: anti-dsDNA and anti-Sm antibody assays	– Drug-associated SLE, e.g.
	  ▪ TNF-α blockers
	  ▪ INH (isoniazid)
	  ▪ Hydralazine
	  ▪ Procainamide
	  ▪ Minocycline

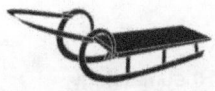

- ➢ Differential diagnosis

  - o **UCTD** (undifferentiated connective tissue disease) multisystem disease with positive ANA (autoimmune symptoms" but with < 4 criteria of the American College of Rheumatology Criteria for the diagnosis of SLE.

  - o **DILE** (drug-induced lupus erythematosis; distinguish from the phonetically similar "DILI", drug induced liver injury.
    - – DILE (Drug-Induced lupus erythematosus) may be caused by anti-TNF α drugs, and is comprised of

  - o Fever

  - o Skin rash

  - o Arthritis

  - o ANA+

  - o Antibodies for anti-ds DNA

    - – TNF-α inhibitors are curiously associated with anti-ds DNA, and rarely involve the CNS or renal system.

– Anti-hypertensives (ANA+, anti-SDNA+, anti-histone antibodies positive)	▪ Procainamide ▪ Hydralazine ▪ Methyldopa

- ➢ Treatment

- • Give the treatment of cutaneous and MSK manifestations of SLE

    - – Immunosuppressants, especially methotrexate

o Methotrexate	– Symmetric synovitis of peripheral joints and tendon sheaths – Myopathy – Do **not** use in pregnancy
o Cyclophosphamide	– Alveolitis

o Hydroxychloroquine	– Not for myositis
	– Not used in absence of lupus specific antibodies
	   ▪ Anti-ds DNA
	   ▪ Anti-Smith antibodies

o Arthritis	– NSAIDs

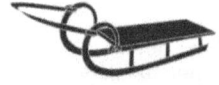

- o Arthritis plus rash
  - – Hydrochloroquine
    - ▪ ↓ flares
    - ▪ ↓ mortality
    - ▪ ↓ organ damage
    - ▪ ↓ thrombosis
    - ▪ ↓ bone loss
  - – Steroids, low dose

- o More aggressive disease (CNS, renal, blood, vasculitis) high dose steroids plus immunosuppression

- o Nephritis
  - – Cyclophosphamide
  - – Mycophenolate mofetil
  - – Belimumab

- o Raynaud phenomenon
  - – Warmth, protection from cold exposure
  - – CCB (calcium channel blockers)
  - – Anti-platelet agents
  - – Topical nitrates
  - – PD-5I (phosphodiesterase-5 inhibitor)
  - – Prostacyclin analogues (e.g. iloprost, epoprostenol)
  - – ERA (endothelin receptor antagonist), selective (ambrisentan) and non-selective (bosentan)
  - – Pain control
    - ▪ Including RSB (regional sympathetic blockage)
  - – Amputation for non-responsive and severe ulceration of digits

---

SO YOU WANT TO BE A RHEUMATOLOGIST!

- • In the context of treating severe lupus, give the mechanism of action of the biological, **belimumab**.

  - o Belimumab inhibits BAFF (B-cell activating factor)

- • Give the rationale for young women with lupus to receive **vaccination against HPV**.

  - o The risk of cervical dysplasia is markedly, increased in lupus; although the reason for this increase is not fully understood, HPV vaccination up to the age of 26 is suggested.

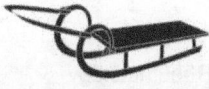

SLE and Peripartum Management

- ➢ Concerns
    - o Poor outcomes of pregnancy in a woman with lupus include
        - – Lupus nephritis (distinguish from preclampsia)
        - – Active disease within 6 mon
        - – Anti-phospholipid antibodies

- • Give the peripartum management of SLE.
    - o The prenatal care of a woman with lupus and team care with a rheumatologist and a high-risk obstetrician is recommended.
    - o While this is an advanced learner topic, the basis of care needs to be known by all internists.
- ➢ General approach
    - o Do **not** use methotrexate
    - o Maintain use of hydroxychloroquine, prednisone and azathioprine, as needed
    - o Anti-phospholipid antibody positive SLE mother
        - – ↑ risk of fetal loss
        - – History of pregnancy loss
        - – ASA (low-dose aspirin)
        - – Heparin
    - o Anti-Ro / SSA, and anti-La / SSB antibody positive SLE mother (20%)
        - – Anti-Ro / SSA, anti-La / SSB
        - – Specific ribonucleoproteins
        - – Associated with
            - ▪ Sjogren syndrome
            - ▪ NLE (neonatal lupus erythematosus)
            - ▪ SCLE (Subacute cutaneous lupus erythematosus – only with anti-Ro / SSA)
    - o ↑ risk of NLE (neonatal lupus erythematosus)
        - – Changes for 6 mon
            - ▪ Rash
            - ▪ ↓ platelets
            - ▪ ↑ liver enzymes
        - – Congenital heart block
            - ▪ Dexamethasone
            - ▪ Pacemaker

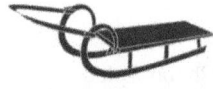

A.B.R. Thomson

- o SLE / Vasculitis
  - – Vasculitis may be associated with urticarial, rather than with pain and ulcers of the skin.
  - – This urticarial vasculitis is often associated with SLE.
  - – In the pregnant woman with urticarial plagues showing small vessel vasculitis on skin biopsy who is ANA+ plus ↓ complement, give the treatment of choice.
    - ▪ Hydroxychloroquine is the treatment of choice for the urticarial vasculitis associated with SLE.
    - ▪ Hydroxychloroquine is FDA C, and may be used during pregnancy.

- ➢ Contraception in SLE

  - o Anti-phospholipid antibody (APA) – negative
    - – OCP, combination of estrogen and progesterone

  - o Positive
    - – OCP, **progesterone only** (no estrogens)
    - – Barrier method

Buzz words

"pregnancy loss, plus arterial or venous thrombosis"

Suspect APS (**anti-phospholipid syndrome**)

Lab findings
- – Lupus anti-coagulant positive
- – ↑ anti-cardiolipin antibodies
- – ↑ anti-B2-glycoprotein I
- – R/O SLE (rule out systemic lupus erythematosus

- ➢ Hormone replacement therapy (HRT)

  - o ↑ risk of flares

  - o Anti-phospholipid antibody (APA)
    - – Positive – avoid
    - – Negative – use cautiously for severe vasomotor symptoms

- ➢ Prognosis

  - o 10-yr survival rate > 90%
    - – Active SLE
    - – Infection

  - o Later mortality
    - – Accelerated atherosclerosis
    - – Complications of immunosuppression

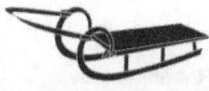

VASCULITIS

➢ Background

   o The patient with systemic vasculitits may have systemic symptoms, signs/symptoms of

   – Aassociated inflammation of the wall of the blood vessels (including narrowing / obstruction / ischemia, dilation/ aneurysm/ rupture), as well as

   – Clues pertaining to a secondary cause of the vasculitis.

   o Once these have been excluded, then there are numerous "primary vasculitis diseases" which are described on the basis of the size of the involved blood vessels.

➢ Pathogenesis
   o Vasculitis
   – Inflammation of blood vessels ⟶ Narrowing of vessels
      ▪ Ischemia
      ▪ Aneurysms
      ▪ Hemorrhage

➢ Types

• Give the name of 8 types of vasculitis, give the "**buzzwords**" associated with the condition and state the treatment.

	Name	Buzzwords	Treatment
• Large vessel			
o GCA	-Giant cell arthritis	•Headaches with scalp tenderness and jaw cladication	P
o PR	-Polymyalgia rheumatic	•AM pain / stiffness of proximal muscles, shoulders and hips	P
o TA	-Takayasu arteritis	•Arm / leg claudication, pulse deficit, asymmetric BP, bruits	P

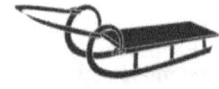

- Medium vessel

	Name	Buzzwords	Treatment
o GPA	-Granulomatosis with polymyiitis (aka Wegner granulomatosis)	•Positive for C-ANCA and anti-proteinase-3 antibody	P+C
o CSS	-Churg-Strauss syndrome	•Asthma, eosinophilic, lung infiltrate	P+C
o MPA	-Microscopic polyangiitis	•Lung infiltrate, glomerulonephritis (GN)	P+C
o HSP	-Henoch-Schonlein purpura	•Purpura, involvement of GI, joint, GN	P
o LCV	-Leukocytoclastic vasculitis	•Lower leg purpura associated with Ca, viral infection	NSAIDs*
o CV	-Cryoglobulinemia vasculitis	•HCV, purpura, GN	Rx HCV
o BS	-Behcet syndrome	•Oral / genital ulcers, uvetis, asymmetric oligoarthritis	Corticosteroids, azathioprine, biologics
o CS	-Cogan syndrome	•Acute ↓ hearing, keratitis, aortitis	C Colchicine (thalidomide)

* Leukpcytoclastic vasculitis may be treated with NSAIDs, anti-histamines, colchicine, or dapsone

Note: Treat associated conditions,

Abbreviations: C, cyclophosphamide; P, prednisone; HBV, hepatitis B virus; HCV, hepatitis C virus

➢ Chapel Hill consensus on the **nomenclature** of systemic vasculitis

- o Large-vessel vasculitis
  - - Giant cell (temporal) arteritis
  - - Takayasu arteritis
- o Medium-size vessel vasculitis
  - - Classic polyarteritis nodosa
  - - Kawasaki disease

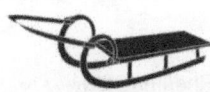

- o Small-vessel vasculitis
  - Microscopic polyangiitis*
  - Wegener granulomatosis*
  - Churg-Strauss syndrome*
  - Henoch-Schönlein purpura
  - Essential cryoglobulinemic vasculitis
  - Cutaneous leukocytoclastic vasculitis
  - Anti-glomerular basement membrane disease

➤ Other causes of small – vessel vasculitis

- o Systemic vasculitis
  - Polyarteritis (primary and secondary)
  - Takayasu arteritis
  - Serum sickness
  - Goodpasture syndrome

- o Nonsystemic
  - Hypocomplementemic urticarial vasculitis
  - Leukocytoclastic vasculitis related to:
    - Rheumatoid arthritis
    - Sjögren syndrome
    - Systemic lupus erythematosus
    - Other connective tissue diseases
  - Drug-induced and postinfectious angiitis
  - Malignancy-associated vasculitis
  - Inflammatory bowel disease
  - Organ transplant-associated vasculitis
  - Hypergammaglobulinemic purpura of Waldenström

* Strongly associated with antineutrophil cytoplasmic autoantibody (ANCA).

Chapel Hill consensus nomenclature, quoted in Ghosh AK. *Mayo Clinic Scientific Press* 2008, Table 18-1, page 695, and adapted from page 994.

"We learn something from everyone who passes through our lives. Some lessons are painful, some are painless… but, all are priceless."

Unknown

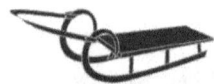

Primary Vasculitis Diseases

➤ Causes

- Give conditions **associated** with primary vasculitis

  - ○ Large
    - GCA (giant cell arteritis)
    - PMR (polymyalgia rheumatic) thought to be part of GCA, or may develop in to elderly-onset RA [rheumatoid arthritis]
    - Takayasu arteritis
  - ○ Medium
    - PAN (polyarteritis nodosa)
    - Kawasaki disease

  - ○ Small
    - Granulomatosis with polyangiitis (aka Wegener granulomatosis)
    - Microscopic polyangiitis
    - CSS (Churg-Strauss syndrome
    - HSP (Henoch Schonlein purpura)
    - Essential
      - Cryoglobulinemic vasculitis
    - Cutaneous
      - Leukocytoclastic vasculitis

  - ○ Note: this is not really a good classification system, since both PAN and Kawasaki disease may affect both medium as well as small-caliber arteries. Continuing with this theme, the small vessel vasculitis granulomatosis with polyangiitis, (aka Wegner granulomatosis), microscopic polyangiitis and CSS (Churg Strauss Syndrome) would be better discussed as ANCA (anti-neutrophil cytoplasmic antibody) associated vasculitis.

➤ Clinical

- Take a directed history and perform a focused physical examination for systemic vasculitis

  - ○ General
    - Fever
    - Fatigue
    - Weight loss

  - ○ CNS
    - Seizures
    - Cerebrovascular accident
    - Mononeuritis multiplex
    - Peripheral neuropathy (mononeuritis multiplex)

  - ○ Eye/ sinuses
    - Retinal hemorrhage
    - Necrotizing (hemorrhagic) sinusitis

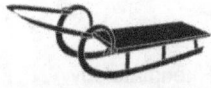

- o CVS   - Coronary artery disease

- o Lung   - Interstitial pneumonitis
  - Hemoptysis
  - Pulmonary infiltrates or nodules

- o MSK   - Myalgia
  - Arthralgia
  - Arthritis

- o GU   - Focal necrotizing glomerulonephritis
  - Abnormal renal sediment
  - Hypertension
  - Testicular pain

- o GI   - Ischemic bowel

- o Skin   - Palpable purpura
  - Livedo reticularis
  - Cutaneous infarctions
  - Nodules
  - Ulcerations

Adapted from: Ghosh AK. *Mayo Clinic Scientific Press* 2008, page 695, and 988.

- Give secondary causes of vasculitis.

  - o Infection   - Sepsis
    - Endocarditis
    - HIV
    - Hepatitis
      - HAV
      - HBV
      - HCV
    - Parvovirus B19
    - During rash of meningococcemia, scarlatina, typhus fever
      - Extension of perivascular inflammation (e.g., cellulites, abscess, meningitis)
      - Septicemia, septic emboli

  - o Infiltration   - Lymphoma
    - Hematologic / solid malignancies
    - Hairy cell leukemia (PAN); polyarteritis nodosa
    - Atrial myxoma

  - o Drugs / toxins   - CNS
    - Psychotropic drugs
    - Anti-convulsants

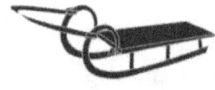

- Lung
  - Anticoagulants
- Heart
  - Antiarrhythmics
  - Diuretics
  - Sympathomimetics
- Endocrine
  - Antithyroid drugs
- MSK
  - NSAIDs
  - Leukotriene inhibitors
  - Allopurinol
  - Anti-TNF agents
- Hematology
  - Hematopoietic growth factors
  - Cryoglobulinemia
  - Paraproteinemia
  - Behcet syndrome
- Infection
  - Antimicrobials
- Cancer
  - Anti-neoplastics

o Immune
  (autoimmune)
  disorders
- MSK
  - Rheumatic and collagen vascular diseases
    - Rheumatoid arthritis
    - Sjogren syndrome
    - Ankylosing spondylitis
    - Rheumatic fever
    - Henoch- Schonlein purpura
    - SLE
    - Dermatomyositis
    - Systemic sclerosis
  - Relapsing polychondritis
  - Inflammatory myopathies
- GI / Liver
  - IBD (inflammatory bowel disease)
  - PBC (primary biliary cirrhosis)
- *Polyarteritis nodosa* and related disorders
  - Polyartheritis nodosa (20% associated with HBV)
  - Cranial arteritis
  - Aortic arch syndrome (incl. Takayashu disease)
  - Polymyalgia rheumatica (giant cell arteritis)
  - Wegener granuloma and lethal midline granuloma
  - Allergic granulomatosis (Churg)
  - Hypersensitivity angiitis (Zeek)

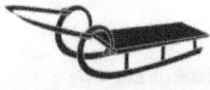

- o Blood
  (coagulopathy)
  - DIC (disseminated intravascular coagulation)
  - APS (anti-phospholipid syndrome)
  - TTP (thrombocytopenic purpura)

- o Miscellaneous
  - Multiple cholesterol emboli (severe atherosclerosis)

➢ Ulceration

- o *Endarteritis obliterans*
  - Any chronic ulcer (e.g., peptic ulcer, ulcerative colitis)
  - Syphilis
  - TB
  - Buerger syndrome
  - HBV

- o Cutaneous vasculitis
  - Henoch-schonlein purpura
  - Erythema nodosum
  - Nodular vasculitis
  - Erythema induratum
  - Malignant atrophic papulosis

➢ Drugs

Adapted from: Burton JL. *Churchill Livingstone* 1971, page 111.

➢ Differential

• Give **syndromes** which may **mimic vasculitis**.

- o CVS
  - Cardiac myxoma with embolization
  - Infective endocarditis
  - Atheroembolism: cholesterol or calcium emboli
  - Arterial coarctation or dysplasia

- o Blood
  - Thrombotic thrombocytopenic purpura
  - Antiphospholipid syndrome

- o MSK
  - Pseudoxanthoma elasticum
  - Ehlers-Danlos type 4

- o Infection
  - Lyme disease
  - Rickettsial infection
  - HIV infection

Adapted from: Ghosh AK. *Mayo Clinic Scientific Press* 2008, page 988.

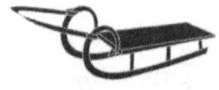

Giant Cell Arteritis (GCA) **and Polymyalgia Rheumatica** (PMR)

➢ Definition

  o "Polymyalgia rheumatic (PMR) and giant-cell arteritis (GCA) are related conditions that effect elder individuals and may reflect 2 ends of a spectrum of the same disease………

  o PMR is characterized by aching and stiffness in the muscle groups of the neck, pectoral and pelvic girdles and thighs…..characterized pathologically by low grade synovits of the proximal joints…with proximal muscle tenderness but not weakness.

  o GCA is a chronic vasculitis of large and medium-sized arteries with a predominance for the cranial branches of the arteries originating from the aortic arch" characterized pathologically by granulomatous inflammation with giant cells affecting arterial walls. (Hanley JG, et al. In: Therapeutic Choices. Grey J, Ed. 6th Edition, *Canadian Pharmacists Association*: Otttawa, ON, 2011, page 1002).

  o Common symptoms include headache, jaw claudication and vessel loss.

  o About 20% of PMR patients develops GCA concurrently or subsequent to the diagnosis of PMR; conversely,
    - About 50% of GCA → PMR

➢ Pathology (biopsy temporal arteries)

  o Lymphocytic plasma infiltration of large carliber extracranial blood vessels (e.g. temporal arteries, thoracic aorta and major branches), with

  o Destruction of the internal elastic membranes

  o As well as, multinucleated giant cells within the vessels or adventia

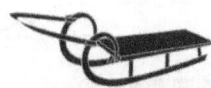

➢ Laboratory
  o Blood
    – ↑ ESR
    – ↑ CRP
    – ↓ hemoglobin
    – ↑ platelets

  o Diagnostic imaging
    – CTA / MRA (CT / MR angiography)
    – Fusiform narrowing of arteries
      ▪ Aorta
      ▪ Arotid
      ▪ Innominate
      ▪ Subclavian

- Give the role of **ultrasound-guided biopsy** in the patient with GCA (giant cell arthritis).

  o Physical examination of the temporal arteries for GCA is neither sensitive nor specific,so the site at which an arterial biopsy is taken may miss the pathology.

  o The lesions of GCA may be patchy

  o If the patient has been on corticosteroids several days before the biopsy is performed, the biopsy may be non-contributory.

  o If the clinical suspicion for GCA is high but the initial biopsy of one temporal artery is unexpectedly negative, then perform ultrasound of the non-biopsied artery and take a sample from an area which on ultrasound shows
    – Transmural thickening
    – "halo sign" in the vessel

  o If GCA is suspected but the biopsies of the but the biopsy of the temporal arteries are normal, perform CTA (CT angiogram) of the neck and chest, looking for changes compatible with GCA in the aortic arch, common carotid, innominate, and subclavian arteries

➢ Treatment
  o Tapered doses of prednisone (1 mg/kg per day po) over 4 wk

  o If recurrent attacks requiring corticosteroids immunosuppressants

  o ASA (low-dose aspirin)

  o Follow-up to detect possible aortic regurgitation / aneurysm

Abbreviations: SBP, systolic blood pressure

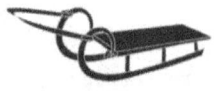

Takayasu Arteritis

➤ Definition

    o Pathological process similar to GCA affecting aorta and its major vessels, and pulmonary arteries

➤ Clinical

    o Early phase
- Active disease
  - Bruits over affected vessels
  - Fever, fatigue, malaise, myalgia, arthralgia

    o Late
- Pulseless phase
  - Differential between arms in SBP, pulse rate
- Vascular insufficiency
  - Claudication
    - Upper and lower limbs
    - Hypertension

➤ Diagnosis

    o Diagnostic imaging stenosis in affected vessels shown on angiography, CTA or MRA

➤ Treatment

    o Acute inflammatory phase
- Corticosteroids

    o Acute inflammatory phase
- Corticosteroids
- Severe / refractory disease
  - Daily
  - Cyclophosphamide
- Weekly
  - Methrotrexate
  - TNFα inhibitor
  - ASA (low-dose aspirin)
  - Statins (for associated hypercholesterolemia)

    o Revasculization surgery

"As a doc', you don't want to be an Outlier."

James Calvin

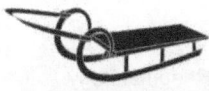

Polyarteritis Nodosa (PAN)

➤ Definition
- o Neutrophilic and mononuclear cell infiltration of wall of medium and small caliber blood vessels
- o This leads to
  - – Necrotizing arteritis, resulting in constitutional symptoms
  - – Myalgia and arthralgia
  - – Abdominal and rarely cardiac pain
  - – Neurological symptoms of
    - ▪ mononeuropathy
    - ▪ mononeuritis multiples

➤ Clinical
- o Skin
  - – Papable purpura
  - – Painful nodules
  - – Ulcers
  - – Livedo reticularis
- o Liver
  - – ~50% of PAN patients have recent HBV infection
- o Kidney
  - – Renovascular hypertension

➤ Diagnosis
- o Angiographic demonstration of stenosis or aneurysms of mesenteric or renal arteries
- o Typical biopsy findings from affected areas such as sin, muscles or nerve (sural nerve if abnormal by nerve conduction studies)

Clinical Caution

Even though renal arteries may be shown to be abnormal on angiographic studies, or the patient suspected as having PAN (polyarteritis nodosa) has hypertension, the diagnosis must **not** be obtained by attempting a kidney biopsy.

- Give the reason to **avoid performing a kidney biopsy** in the patient with suspected PAN.

  - o In PAN, the renal arterioles often show aneurysms, which would readily bleed if renal biopsy were attempted.

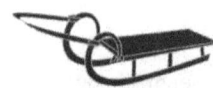

➢ Treatment

- Give the treatment of PAN (polyarteritis nodosa).

  o Mild / moderate disease

  o Non-responsive or severe disease (heart, GI, kidney, CNS)

    - Cyclophosphamide

  o If associated with recent HBV infection

  o Prednisone, for PAN, using high dose for 2 wks

  o Entecavir, for HBV

  o 50% will enjoy

    - Resolution of PAN

    - Conversion of HBeAg+ → HBeAg- (seroconversion)

  o Avoid rituximab (B cell depletion) or inhibitors of TNF-α in patients with PAN plus HBV? Why?

    - Rituximab↑ replication of HBV

Kawasaki Disease

➢ Definition

  o Systemic vasculitis of medium- to small caliber arteries

  o Usually seen in children, or adults with HIV infection

➢ Clinical

- Give the **clinical features** which raise the suspicion of Kawasaki disease.

  o Constitutional symptoms, plus

  o Eyes
    - Conjunctivitis, without exudate

  o Mouth
    - Mucositis

  o Skin rash
    - Pleomorphic
    - Erythematous
    - Periungual areas, hands, feet

  o Cervical lymphadenopathy

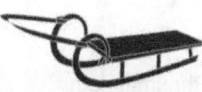

- o Joints
  - – Oligoarticular, or
  - – Polyarticular
- o Extremities
  - – Edema
  - – Erythema
- o Testicles
  - – Pain

➢ Diagnostic imaging

SO YOU WANT TO BE A RHEUMATOLOGIST MARRIED TO A CARDIOLOGIST!

- Give the reason why **coronary angiography** is performed after the patient has recovered from Kawasaki disease.

  - o Kawasaki disease may involve the coronary arteries and lead to aneurysmal dilation

---

➢ Treatment
  - o ASA – high dose
  - o IVIG (intravenous immune globulin)
  - o Severe or non-responsive corticosteroids

Small Vessel Vasculitis

  - o The small vessel vasculitis affect both small and medium- caliber arteries, and would be better described as being p-ANCA-associated vasculitis, or leukocytoclastic vasculitis. Furthermore, the medium-caliber vasculitis PAN and Kawasaki disease also affect the small-caliber vessels.

➢ Types of ANCA (based on anti-neutrophilic cycloplasmic antibodies

  - o C-ANCA, which has a cytoplasmic immunofluorescence pattern reflecting antibodies to serine protease-3 and suggesting granulomatosi ith polyangitis; and

  - o p-ANCA, where there are ANCA antibodies to myeloperoxidase and suggesting the diagnosis of microscopic polyangitis, or CSS (Churg-Strauss Syndrome)

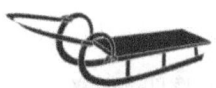

Granulomatosis with Polyangiitis (GP; aka Wegener granulomatotsis [now archaic])

➢ Definition: A systemic necrotizing vasculitis most commonly affecting the upper pulmonary and renal systems, as well as the eye, skin and nerves.

    ○ While c-ANCA is both sensitive and specific for granulomatosis with polyangiitis, it may also occur with p-ANCA and with antibodies to myeloperoxidase.

➢ Clinical

Guess what I'm thinking!

A patient with rhinitis (e.g. runny nose, itchy nose, sneezing) also has sinusitis, and a deformity of the nose with ulceration.

• Give the likely associated systemic disease

    ○ Granulomatosis with polyarteriris (GP, aka Wegener granulomatosis [WG])

    ○ Respiratory   – Upper (70%)
        ▪ Inflammation of ear, nose, throat, sinuses
        ▪ Perforation of nasal septum → saddle-shaped nose
    – Lower
        ▪ Infiltrates
        ▪ Nodules
        ▪ Bleeding

    ○ Renal (80%)   – Glomerulonephritis
    – Non-immune complexes "pauci-immune"
    – Necrotizing
    – Focal segmental or diffuse

    ○ Eye   – Kelatitis
    – Scleritis
    – Uveitis
    – Retro-orbital pseudotumor
    – Proptosis
    – Strabismus

    ○ Skin   – Ulcers
    – Purpura

    ○ Nerve   – Mononeuritis multiplex

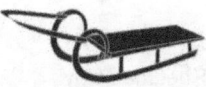

➢ Diagnosis: Biopsy of lung or kidney showing anti-proteinase-3 antibodies

• Give the preferred diagnostic test for allergic rhinitis.

  o Skin test, not in vitro IgE antibody assay

➢ Treatment
  o Initial
    – Corticosteroids, high-dose, plus
    – Cyclophosphamide po for 3-6 mon, or
    – Rituximab
  o Maintenance
    – Immunosuppression (azathioprine or methotrexate [for upper airway disease only] for a further 18 mon, plus
    – Trimethoprim-sulfamethoxazole od for prophylaxis against Pneumocystis infection
    – While 90% achieve remission, recurrent attacks will occur despite maintenance therapy

Churg Strauss Syndrome

➢ Definition: Churg-Strauss Syndrome (CSS) is "……..a systemic vasculitis in the spectrum of hypereosinophilic disorders that most often occurs in the setting of antecedent asthma, allergic rhinitis, or sinusitis."

➢ Clinical

• Give the clinical features of CSS (churg-strauss syndrome)
  o pANCA+
    – Kidney
      ▪ Glomerulonephritis
    – PNS
      ▪ Mononeuritis multiplex
  o pANCA-
    – Lung
      ▪ Infiltrates
    – Heart
      ▪ Eosinophilic cardiomyopathy
    – Skin
      ▪ Purpura

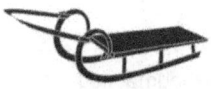

> Diagnosis

   o Serology   – pANCA, specific for myeloperoxidase (in ~40%)
                                        – pANCA + → glomerulonephritis, mononeuritis multiplex
                                        – pANCA - →pneumonitis cardiomyopathy

   o Biopsy   – Infiltration of tissue with eosinophils
                                        – Necrotizing small-vessel vasculitis (arteries or veins)

Cryoglobulinemic Vasculitis

> Clinical   o Skin – purpura
                           o Nerve – mononeuritis multiplex
                           o Kidney – immune complex glomerulonephritis

> Laboratory   o ↑ type II cryoglobulins
                           o ↓ C3, ↓ C4
                           o HCV (80%)
                           o HBV
                           o HIV

> Treatment

- Give the treatment of Cryoglobulinemic Vasculitis

   o Associated HBV, HCV

   o Acute vasculitis
      – Corticosteroids
      – Cyclophosphamide

   o Severe disease
      – Digital gangrene
      – Glomerulonephritis
      – Neurological disease
      – Plasma exchange

   o Refractory disease
      – Rituximab (depletion of T cells)

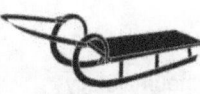

Henoch-Schonlein Purpura

➢ Demography

   o Usually in children

   o In adults
     – More severe

   o In males > 50
     – Associated with myelodysplastic syndrome, or solid neoplasms

➢ Pathogenesis

   o Idiopathic (40%)

   o Secondary (60%)   – Infection
                         – Neoplasms
                         – Autoimmune
                         – Drugs

➢ Clinical

• Give the clinical presentation of HSP (Henoch-Schonlein Purpura).

   o Recurrent episodes
     involving

   o Skin   – Leukocytoclastic vasculitis (IgA deposits)
                           ▪ Palpable purpura (lower extremities)
                           ▪ Tender nodules
                           ▪ Urticarial
                           ▪ Shallow ulcers

   o Joints   – Arthritis

   o GI   – Abdominal pain

   o Renal   – Hematuria, proteinuria
                     – Glomerulonephritis IgA deposits → diffuse
                       proliferative glomerulonephritis
                     – Progressive renal failure

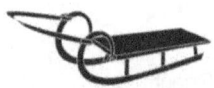

> Treatment

- Give the treatment of Henoch –Schonlein Purpura (HSP).

  - o Treat secondary causes of vasculitis, e.g.
    - – infection: HAV, HBV, HCV, HIV
    - – neoplasms: lymphoma, hairy cell leukemia
    - – autoimmune: SLE, RA, IBD, PBC
    - – drug

  - o Mucosal lesions (mouth, colon)

  - o Topical
    - – Corticosteroids
    - – Colchicine
    - – Thalidomide

  - o Eye-corticosteroids
    - – Topical
    - – Intraocular
    - – Systemic

  - o Skin, joint symptoms
    - – Prednisone 20 to 40 mg / day, short course

  - o Leukocytoclastic vasculitis
    - – Anti-histamine, plus H1/H2 blockers
    - – Hydroxychloroquine if ↑ ANA
    - – For refractory disease corticosteroids
    - – For corticosteroids resistance immunosuppressives (azathioprine, methotrexate)

  - o Proliferative glomerulonephritis
    - – High-dose corticosteroids, plus
    - – Cyclophosphamide, monthly

  - o Visceral disease
    - – Azathioprine
    - – Cyclosporine
    - – Cyclophosphamide
    - – Anti-TNFα agents

  - o Males over 50 yr
    - – Assess for occult malignancy (e.g. solid tumor, or myelodysplastic syndrome)

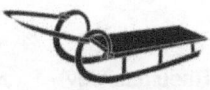

Relapsing Polychondritis

➢ Definition: Relapsing polychondritis is a clinical diagnosis characterized by chondritis of the ENT system, eye inflammation, plus non-erosive serocognitive inflammatory peripheral polyarthritis

➢ Clinical
- o Chondritis
  - Bilateral auricular chondritis
  - Nasal chondritis
  - Laryngotrachela disease
    - Stridor
    - Hoarseness

- o Eye
  - Conjunctivitis
  - Episcleritis
  - Scleritis
  - Uveitis
  - Retinal vasculitis

- o MSK
  - Peripheral joints non-erosive, serronegative inflammatory polyarthritis
  - Inflammation parasternal joints
- o Heart
  - AI (aortic insufficiency)
  - MI (mitral insufficiency)

➢ Treatment
- o Mild
  - NSAIDs
  - Dapsone
  - Corticosteroids

- o Severe
  - Azathioprine
  - Methotrexate
  - Cyclosporine
  - Cyclophosphamaide
  - Anti-TNFα drugs

• Give the investigation of choice in a patient with relapsing polychondritis who develops mild strider.

- o In relapsing polychondtis, there may be autoimmune destruction of the cartilage of the upper airway as well as the bronchi.

- o PFT (pulmonary flow testing) with flow volume loops is needed to determine is obstruction to flow is occurring.

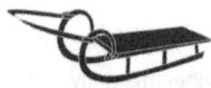

SYSTEMIC SCLEROSIS (SSC)

➢ Definition: systemic sclerosis (aka) is "....... a disease of unknown causes characterized by microvasculae injury and connective tissue deposition" (Board Basics 2013, page317).

  o "Systemic sclerosis is a disorder of unknown cause characterized by vasculopathy with [early perivascular infiltration of lymphocytes, proliferation of fibroblasts, ↑ synthesis / secretion of collagen and other matrix proteins, leading to] proliferation in small arterioles and fibrosis of the dermis and visceral organs".

Adapted from: MKSAP 16, Rheumatology 2012, page 41.

➢ Types
  o Based on diffuse or limited skin involvement
  o The types of lung disease, as well as the presence f renal disease (crisis) and CREST (calcinosis, Raynaud phenomenon) esophageal dysmotility, sclerodactyly and telangiectasia) also varies between the diffuse and limited types.

| Clinical | Cutaneous SSc | |
	Diffuse	Limited

o Skin thickening relative to
  – Elbows / knees
  – Face
	Proximal
	+++
		Distal
		+

o Lung	Interstitial lung disease	Pulmonary hypertension (PH)
o Renal crisis	+	-
o CREST syndrome	-	+

• Give the forms of **systemic sclerosis**, based on location of skin involvement.

  o LC SSc plus Crest syndrome
    – CREST (calcinosis, Raynaud phenomenon, esophageal dysmotility, sclerodactyly, and telangiectasia) syndrome
    – Note that the CREST sysndrome is a subset of LC SSc ↑ risk of pulmonary arterial hypertension (PAH)

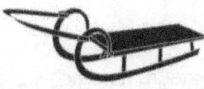

- o LC SSc (limited cutaneous systemic sclerosis)
  - – Non-progressive involvement of skin of face and distal extremities (sclerodactyly)
    - ▪ Stiff, shiny, hard, with soft-tissue defects and scarring pulp space of the distal digits, aka terminal digital pitting or ulceration)
  - – Early pruritis; late dermal calcifications at pressure points
  - – Autoantibodies
    - ▪ Anticenromere (ANA in centromere)
    - ▪ Anti-h1 (ANA in nucleoli)
  - – ↑ risk of PAH (pulmonary arterial hypertension)

- o DC SSc (diffuse cutaneous systemic sclerosis)
  - – Skin involvement moves proximal to involvement in LC SSc (i.e., proximal to distal forearms and knees)
  - – ↑ risk of
    - ▪ Lung
    - ▪ ILD (interstitial lung disease)
    - ▪ Kidney disease
    - ▪ Serositis (e.g. pericarditis, pleuritis)
    - ▪ MSK (muculoskeletal)
    - ▪ Raynaud phenomenon
    - ▪ GI / Liver
  - – Antibodies
    - ▪ Anti-Sci-70, with speckled ANA pattern
    - ▪ Anti—U3-RNA, with speckled ANA pattern

- o SSSS (Systemic sclerosis sine scleroderma)
  - – ↑ risk of involvement of
    - ▪ Lung
    - ▪ Kidney
    - ▪ Serisitis
  - – No (sine, without) skin involvement

- • Give the scleroderma **spectrum disorders**.

  - o Morphea
    - – Scleroderma-like plaques in torso of body as well as proximal extremities
    - – Pathology of morphea plaques is similar to SSc
    - – No Raynaud phenomenon
    - – No visceral associations

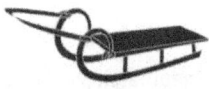

- o Scleroderma
  - – Similar to morphea ≥ 1 scleroderma-like plaque in neck, shoulder, arms
  - – Even in insulin-dependent diabetes

- o Eosinophilic fasciitis
  - – Peripheral eosinophilia
  - – Lymphoplasmotic infiltration of fascia
  - – Hardening of extremities, not including
    - ▪ Face
    - ▪ Hands

- o Scleromyxedema
  - – Papules over thickened skin of face
    - ▪ Face
    - ▪ Shoulders
    - ▪ Arms
  - – Pathology
    - ▪ Stellate-shaped fibroblasts in dermis of skin
  - – Associations
    - ▪ ↑ IgG λ (paraproteinemia)
    - ▪ Multiple myeloiditis
    - ▪ Inflammatory myopathy

- o Nephrogenic systemic fibrosis
  - – Patient with ↓ GFR (glomerular filtration rate) undergoes a MRI study with contrast)gadolinium)
  - – Hyperpigmentation of skin of
    - ▪ Torso
    - ▪ Extremities (but not the digits)
  - – Skeletal muscles contraction fibrosis
  - – Cardiac muscle

➤ Clinical

- Perform a focused physical examination for scleroderma and its complications.
  - o General appearance
    - – 'Bird-like' facies
    - – Weight-loss (malabsorption)
    - – Fever

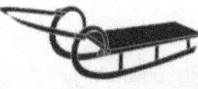

A.B.R. Thomson

- o Head
  - – Hair
    - ▪ Alopecia
    - ▪ Hair loss
  - – Eyes
    - ▪ Loss of eyebrows
    - ▪ Difficulty opening eyes
  - – Mouth
    - ▪ Difficulty smiling / raising forehead skin
  - – Skin
    - ▪ Tight
  - – Ischemia, end of nose
  - – Pigmentation
  - – Telangiectasia
  - – Neck muscles
    - ▪ Wasting and weakness
    - ▪ Pale and dry skin (anemia and Sjogren syndrome, respectively)

- o Chest

- o Heart
  - – Cor pulmonale
  - – Pericarditis
  - – Heart failure
  - – Hypertension

- o Lungs
  - – Intestinal lung disease
  - – Pulmonary hypertension
  - – Fibrosis
  - – Reflux aspiration pneumonitis
  - – Recurrent chest infections
  - – Alveolar cell carcinoma, vasculitis

- o GI
  - – GERD
  - – Dysphagia
  - – Delayed gastric emptying (succussion splash)
  - – Small bowel bacterial overgrowth [SIBO]
  - – Diarrhea,
  - – Malnutrition
  - – Malabsorption
  - – Wide-mouthed colonic diverticulae

- o Renal
  - – Proteinuria

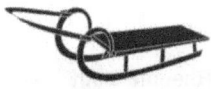

- o MSK
  - General
    - Arthritis
    - Polyarticular
    - Non-erosive
  - Finger
    - Sclerodactyly
    - Pitting of fingers
    - Raynaud phenomenon
  - Arms
    - Edema (early)
    - Skin thickening and tightening
    - Pigmentation
    - Vitiligo
    - Proximal myopathy
  - Hands
    - CRST syndrome
      - Calcinosis
      - Raynaud (atrophy distal tissue pulp)
      - Sclerodactyly
      - Telangiectasia
    - Dilated capillary loops in nailfolds
    - Small joint arthropathy and tendon crepitus
    - Fixed flexion deformity
    - ↓ hand function
  - Legs
    - Skin lesions
    - Vasculitis
    - Small joint arthropathy
    - Patellar crepitus

Adapted from: Talley NJ, et al. *Maclennan & Petty Pty Limited* 2003, page 295.

- o Making the **diagnosis** of SSc
  - Stiff, shiny, hardened skin distal to metacarpophalangeal joints
  - ≥ 2 of the following
    - Sclerodactyly
    - Terminal digitalis pitting, or ulceration
    - Basilar interstitial fibrosis on chest pallateral, representing ILD (interstitial lung disease)
    - Note that > 95% of patients with SSc (LC SSc, CREST, DC SSc) are positive for ANA (anti-nuclear antibody)

Although not a diagnostic part of SSc, **scleroderma renal crisis** is a serious component of diffuse cutaneous SSc.

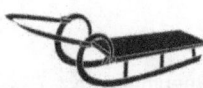

- Give the components of scleroderma renal crisis.

  - Microangiopathy
    - Hemolytic anemia
    - Thrombocytopenia

  - Kidney
    - Proteinuria
    - AKI (acute kidney injury)
    - Normal, or ↑ BP (blood pressure)

Systemic Sclerosis (SSc) is a **multi-system disease**.

- Give a differential for each of the following components of SSc.
  - Lung
    - Restrictive lung disease: no changes in
      - Skin
      - GI
      - Raynaud
  - Skin
    - Thickening of skin: eosinophilic fasciitis: Eosinophilic fasciitis
      - No involvement of hands or feet
  - SLE feature, arthritis
    - Mixed connective tissue disease
      - May have anti-RNP antibodies

- Give **cardiac associations** with Systemic Sclerosis (SSc)

  - Related to PAH (pulmonary arterial hypertension)
    - Dilated RV (right ventricle)
    - R-HF (right-sided heart failure)
    - Right-sided valves regurgitation murmurs

  - Not related to PAH
    - Pericarditis
    - Pericardial effusion
    - Pericardial tamponade
    - Myocardial fibrosis (contraction band necrosis)
    - Cardiomyopathy
      - Systolic dysfunction
      - Diastolic dysfunction
    - Arrhythmias

Pulmonary arterial hypertension (PAH: ↓ Deco, ↑ S2, split S2) is common in persons with SSc, even in the absence of other pulmonary complication.

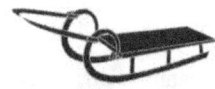

- Give **pulmonary associations** of SSc.

  - ○ Pleural   – Pleuritis

  - ○ Alveolae   – Alveolitis

  - ○ Interstitium   – Interstitial lung disease (ILD)
    -                  – Aspiration pneumonia → fibrosis

  - ○ Bronchi   – Endobronchial telangiectasias → bleeding
    -                  – Lung cancer

- Give common MSK (musculoskeletal) associations with SSc.

  - ○ Joints   – Inflammatory, non-erosive arthritis of small and large peripheral joints
    -                  – ↓ joint mobility, especially interphalangeal joints, wrists, ankles
    -                  – Tendonitis, with palpable friction rub over extensor surfaces
  - ○ Myopathy   – Inflammatory or non-inflammatory

- Give common **gastrointestinal** (dysmotility) / **hepatic associations** with SSc.

  - ○ ↓ LES (lower esophageal sphincter) → GERD (gastroesophageal reflux disease, including severe esophagitis)

  - ○ Gastroparesis

  - ○ UGIB (upper GI bleeding)

  - ○ GAVE (gastric antral vascular ectasia)

  - ○ Slow small bowel motility → SIBO (small intestinal bacterial overgrowth)

  - ○ Colon
    - – Constipation
    - – Wide-mouthed diverticulae

  - ○ Liver
    - – PBC (primary biliary cirrhosis)

- ➢ Laboratory

  - ○ ANA (anti-nuclear antibody)

  - ○ Anti-Sci-70 antibodies

  - ○ Anti-centromere antibodies

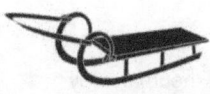

➢ Treatment

Corticosteroids are **not** part of the therapy of systemic sclerosis (SSc).

- Give a major adverse effect related to the kidney which may occur with the inappropriate administration of corticosteroids to the patient with SSc.

  ○ Corticosteroids may precipitate a scleroderma renal crisis (aka, acute kidney injury) with normal blood pressure.

The management of SLE is that of its complications.

➢ Renal

- Give the criteria for the use of ACE inhibitors in patients with scleroderma renal crisis.
  ○ For acute crisis
    – Regardless of level of serum creatinine
  ○ For chronic renal disease
    – Continue ACE inhibitor

➢ MSK

- Differentiate between the treatment of acute digital ischemia using the intravenous prostacyclin analogue epoprostenol and the maintenance use of bosentan to reduce the frequency and severity of digital ulcers in the person with Raynaund phenomenon.

- Give the MSK conditions which respond to treatment with **sulfasalazine**.
  ○ Reactive arthritis
  ○ IBD-associated arthritis
  ○ Psoriatic arthritis
  ○ Ankylosing spondylitis

➢ Lung

- Give the **treatment** of alveolitis (diagnosed on chest CT scan)
  ○ Cyclophosphamide po/IV for 1 yr, then
  ○ Azathioprine maintenance

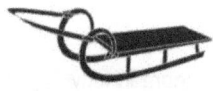

➢ GI

- Give the earliest system / sign which suggests that a patient's dysphagia for liquids is caused by Scleroderma.

  o Scleroderma (SSc) may cause dysmotility associated dysphagia early in the esophageal mucosa, such as erosions, ulcers or strictures.

  o Early in the course of SSc, even before dysphagia occurs, dysmotility may be found in the esophagus on testing of motility.

  o These changes in motility +/- dysphagia are always associated with Raynaud phenomenon.

Raynaud Phenomenon

➢ Definition: Paroxysmal digital ischemia, usually accompanied by pallor and cyanosis and followed by erythema (white-blue-red).

  o When a person fingers are exposed to the cold, they may become pale, then blue from the arterial vasospasm and ischemia, then with redness from reperfusion.

  o This latter phase from a decline in the spasm and therefore ischemia may be associated with pain and paresthesia as well as the redness. In some persons (20%) no cause/ association may be found, and this progression of white-blue-red is called Reynaud disease (i.e., Reynaud phenomenon, with no known underlying disorder).

  o However, the Raynaud phenomenon may be associated with a number of conditions.

➢ Causes / associations
  o General
    – Malnutrition and cachexia

  o Collagen vascular disease
    – Dermatomyositis
    – Polyarteritis
    – RA
    – Raynaud's disease
    – Sjogren disease
    – SLE
    – Systemic sclerosis
  o MSK
    – Cervical spondylosis
    – Paralysis or disuse of a limb
    – Cervical rib, hyperabduction syndrome

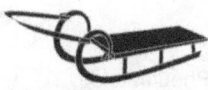

- o Blood
  - – Embolus, thrombosis or stenosis
  - – Arteriosclerosis
  - – Increased blood agglutination
    - Cold agglutinins
    - Dysproteinaemias
      - - Cryoglobulinemia
      - - Macroglobulinemia
      - - Hyperglobulinema
  - - Polycythaemia, leukemia
  - - Reflex vasoconstriction

- o Infection

- o Trauma
  - - Cold injury
  - - Frost bite
  - - Injury (Volkmann ischemia)
  - - Trench foot
  - - Vibrating machinery

- o Toxin
  - - Toxins: ergot, heavy metals, tobacco

- o Drugs – (the P's e.g. penicillin, phenothiazines, phenylbutazone, propylthiouracil, and many others

- o Allergy
  - - Allergic granulomatosis

Adapted from: Burton JL. *Churchill Livingstone* 1971, page 110; Talley N. J., et al. *Maclennan & Petty Pty Limited* 2003, Table 8.12, pages 299 and 300.

SO YOU WANT TO BE A RHEUMATOLOGIST!

- • In the context of the Raynaud phenomenon, give the meaning of the Allen test..

  - o Clench the hand and compress both the radial and the ulnar arteries
  - o Release just one, then second compression on an artery

 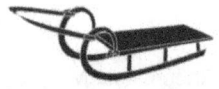

- ➢ Pathology
  - o Renal afferent arteriolar
    - – Proliferation of intima
    - – Thrombosis in lumen of afferent arterioles
    - – Ischemia of glomeruli
      - ▪ Hypertension
      - ▪ Renal failure
      - ▪ Microangiopathic hemolytic anemia

- ➢ Clinical
- • Perform a directed physical examination for the causes of Raynaud phenomenon (white->blue->red fingers/toes in response to cold temperature).

  - o Reflex
    - – Raynaud disease (idiopathic)
    - – Vibrating machinery injury (jackhammer use)
    - – Cervical sponsylosis
    - – Shoulder-hand syndrome
    - – Causalgia

  - o Connective tissue disease
    - – Scleroderma (90-100%), CRST syndrome, mixed connective tissue disease (90-100%)
    - – Systemic lupus erythematosus (SLE;15%)
    - – Polyarteritis nodosa (PAN)
    - – Rheumatoid arthritis (10%)
    - – Sjogren
    - – Mixed connective disease
    - – Polymyositis
    - – Dermatomyositis
    - – Aortic arch syndrome (Takayashu disease)
    - – Sclerodactyly
    - – Carpal tunnel syndrome
    - – Telangiectasis
    - – Lesions from digital ischemia

  - o Arterial disease
    - – Compression
      - ▪ Thoracic outlet syndrome
      - ▪ Carpal tunnel syndrome
    - – Artherosclerosis
    - – Vasculitis
    - – Prinznetal angina
    - – Embolism or thrombosis
    - – Buerger disease (thromboangiitis obliterans)
    - – Trauma (vibration-induced)

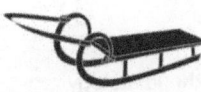

- o Neurological
  - Paralysis
  - Disuse of limb
  - Reflex sympathetic dystrophy

- o Lung
  - Pulmonary fibrosis
  - Idiopathic pulmonary hypertension

- o Endocrine
  - Hypothyroidism
  - Acromegaly
  - Addison disease

- o Hematological disease
  - Polycythemia (increased blood viscosity)
  - Leukemia
  - Dysproteinemia (cryo-, macro-, hyperglobulinemia)
  - Monoclonal gammopathy

- o Drugs/Poisons
  - Beta-blockers, ergotamine, bleomycin, vinyl chloride

- o Cold Injury

- o Malnutrition, cachexia
  - Occupational use of percussion or vibratory tools (e.g., a jack hammer)

Adapted from: Talley NJ, et al. *Maclennan & Petty Pty Limited* 2003, page 255; and Ghosh AK. *Mayo Clinic Scientific Press* 2008, page 1017.

➢ Treatment (SRC, scleroderma renal crisis)

- o ACE inhibitor (to lower the elevated renin; ACE inhibitor is superior to ARB).

- o ACE inhibitor, even the patient is an dialysis and is already on another class of anti-hypertensive

- o ACE inhibitors are FDA X category, contraindicated in pregnancy because of risk of fetal malformations, so the benefit of ACE inhibitors to the mother with SLE plus SRC must be balanced against the risk to the fetus of malformations.

- o Dialysis

BIG, BIG Reminder for the **Caution of Treating SSc**

- o Steroids – **No, No** – may precipitate SRC (scleroderma renal crisis), especially in DC SSc.
- o Say it again – Steroids are **not** used to treat systemic sclerosis

---

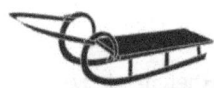

- Perform a focused physical examination for polymyositis / dermatomyositis.

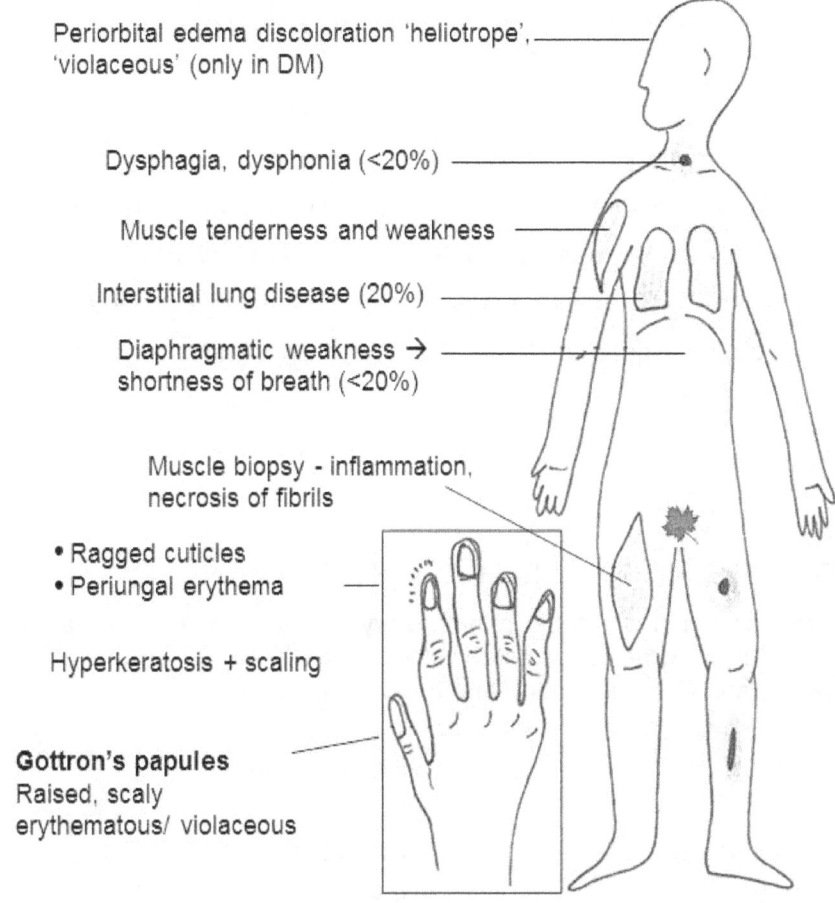

Periorbital edema discoloration 'heliotrope', 'violaceous' (only in DM)

Dysphagia, dysphonia (<20%)

Muscle tenderness and weakness

Interstitial lung disease (20%)

Diaphragmatic weakness → shortness of breath (<20%)

Muscle biopsy - inflammation, necrosis of fibrils

- Ragged cuticles
- Periungal erythema

Hyperkeratosis + scaling

Gottron's papules
Raised, scaly
erythematous/ violaceous

Adapted from: Davey P. *Wiley-Blackwell* 2006, page 412.

- In the context of dermatomyositis, give the meaning of **Gottron papules** and "**mechanic hands**".

  o Gottron papules   – Pathognomic erythematous, violaceous, clumped papules over the extensoe surface of the metacarpophalangeal joints, elbows, and knees

  o Mechanic's hands   – "roughened erythematous hyprkeratotic fissuring of the palmar and lateral aspects of fingers"

Source: MKSAP 16, Rheumatology 2012, page 59.

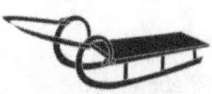

Clinical Tips

It is easy to clinically distinguish dermatomyositis (DM) from other neuromuscular diseases, since none of the following clinical features relating to muscle are seen in DM.

Clinical findings	Likely correct diagnosis
o Inflammatory myopathy	- Same
o Fasculations suggest	- Amyotrophic lateral sclerosis)
o Pericular weakness and ptosis	- Myasthenia gravis
o Muscle tenderness (proximal)	- Polymyalgia rheumatica
o Atrophy, ↓ deep tendon	- Peripheral neuropathy
o ↓ reflexes	- Hypothyroidism
	- Peripheral neuropathy

SO YOU WANT TO BE A RHEUMATOLOGIST!

- In the context of idiopathic inflammatory myopathies, give the name of the **autoantibodies** associated with ILD (interstitial lung disease), cardiac and GI involvement, and the classical rash.

  - o ILD
    - – Anti-synthetase
    - – Anti-Jo-1
  - o Cardiac, GI
    - – Antisignal recognition particle
  - o Classic rash
    - – Anti-Mi-2

➢ Diagnosis

- Give the methods to establish the diagnosis of dermatomyositis.

  - o Pathognomic Gottron papules of hand joints in dermatomyositis

  - o Blood
    - – Acute phase reactants raised (e.g. ESR and C-reactive protein)
    - – ↑ CK (creatine kinase)
    - – ↑ ALT, AST, aldolase
    - – Autoantibodies

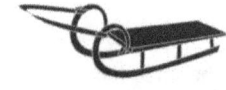

- o Diagnostic imaging (useful to identify optimal site for muscle biopsy)
    - Ultrasound with contrast
    - MRI
        - Fat-suppressed T2-weighted images
        - Short tau inversion recovering sequence
- o EMG (electromyography)

- Give the classical **triad of EMG changes** which distinguish inflammatory myositis from neuropathic disorders.

    - o "short-duration, small, low-amplitude polyphasic potentials

    - o Fibrillation patterns at rest

    - o Bizarre, high-frequency, repetitive discharges"

Source: MKSAP 16, Rheumatology 2012, page 61.

- o In the patient with inflammatory myopathies, muscle biopsy may show necrosis and regeneration.

- Give the way in which the **pattern of the lymphocytic infiltration**, the target site of the inflammation, and the cell markers help to distinguish between the main types of idiopathic inflammatory myopathies.

Type of inflammatory myopathy	Type of lymphocytic infiltration	Target site of inflammation	Additional findings
o Dermatomyositis	B cells CD-4+ T cells	– Vascular endothelium	• Perivascular • Surrounding muscle fascicles
o Polymyositis	CD-8+ T cells	– Myofibril	• More marked inflammation than in IBM
o IBM (inclusion body myositis)	CD-8+ T cells	– Myofibril	• Endomysium of muscle fascicles • Less marked inflammation than polymyositis • Filamentous tubules (very specific for IBM) • Rimmed vacuoles • Inclusion bodies

Note: the serum concentrations of the CK-MB, ALT, AST, aldolase fluctuate with the activity of the myositis.

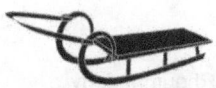

➢ Treatment

- Give the treatment of inflammatory myopathy.
    - ○ General   – Physiotherapy
        - – Exclude associated occult malignancy (especially adenocarcinoma including ovarian cancer)
        - – Skin
            - ▪ Sunscreen

    - ○ Corticosteroids, until CK (creatine kinase) is normalized

    - ○ Resistant   – Immunosuppression
        disease
        - ▪ Methotrexate
        - ▪ Azathioprine
        - – Intravenous immune globulin (IVIG)
            - ▪ Intravenous immune globulin

    - ○ Rash   – Hydroxychloroquine plus
        - – Topical corticosteroids, or
        - – Tacrolimus

A case for the Sharp Clinician !

The patient with ↑ CK, abnormal EMG, and muscle biopsy taken from an MRI-demonstrated area of maximum muscle inflammation and damage in the thigh muscle, was diagnostic with having dermatomyositis (DM), and responded well to high-dose corticosteroids. Neither an immune suppressant nor an anti-malarial were necessary. The TSH was normal. The CK levels returned to normal, and remained normal despite a recurrence of proximal muscle weakness in an area which was not previously abnormal.

- Give the likely diagnosis.
    - ○ While a recurrence of polymyosistis may be possible, the normal serum CK argues against this.

    - ○ Consider the possibility of corticosteroid-associated myopathy

    - ○ Check that the patient is not taking a statin or abusing alcohol, which may also cause a toxic myopathy.

    - ○ Review the muscle biopsy to ensure the diagnosis was inclusion body myositis, rather than DM.

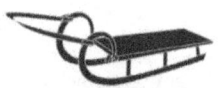

COMPLEX REGIONAL PAIN SYNDROME (CRPS)

The complex regional pain syndromes (CRPS) may occur after

- o Injury
  - – Trauma
  - – Surgery
- o CV event
  - – CVA
  - – MI

➢ Clinical

• Take a directed history and perform a focused physical examination of an extremity for CRPS (complex regional pain syndrome), and outline the therapy.

- o Pain (neuropathic)
  - – Allodynia
  - – Hyperalgesia
  - – Hyperpathia

- o ANS (autonomic nervous system) dysfunction
  - – Sweating
  - – Edema
  - – Colour change
- o Skin
  - – Swelling
  - – ↓ hair
  - – Thinning ⎤ Dystrophy
  - – Ulcers ⎦

- o Movement
  - – ↓ starting (difficulty getting started)
  - – Tremor
  - – Weakness

- o Bone
  - – Dystonia
  - – Osteoporosis

➢ Treatment

- o Physical / occupational therapy
- o Corticosteroids
- o Sympathetic blockage
- o Gabapentin
- o TCAs (tricyclic anti-depressants)
- o Bisphosphonates
  - – Useful, with or even without associated osteoporosis

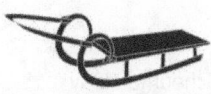

ASEPTIC NECROSIS OF THE BONE

- Take a directed history for the cause of aseptic necrosis of the bone. (acronym: **ASEPTIC**).

  o Alcohol, artherosclerotic vascular disease

  o Steroids, sickle cell anemia (Gaucher storage disease)

  o Emboli (fat, cholesterol)

  o Postradiation necrosis

  o Trauma

  o Idiopathic

  o Connective tissue disease (especially SLE), caisson disease

Abbreviations: SLE, systemic lupus erythematosus

Source: Ghosh AK. *Mayo Clinic Scientific Press* 2008, Table 24-7, page 982.

SO YOU WANT TO BE RHEUMATOLOGIST!

- Skin and muscle symptoms and signs develop in a middle aged person, who has

o Skin	– Redness	
	▪ Dorsum of fingers	
	▪ Face, chest, arms	
	– Light sensitivity	
o Muscle (myositis)	– Limb girdles	
	– Usually proximal limb muscle	
	– Rarely distal limbs	

- You make a clinical diagnosis of dermatomyositis. The person also has unintentional weight loss which tumors of the chest and abdomen may have proceeded this diagnosis?

o Chest	– Breast
	– Lung
o Abdomen	
	– Stomach
	– Ovary

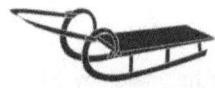

CHRONIC OSTEOMYELITIS

➢ Cause / associations
- o Monomicrobial
  - Staphylococcus aureus
  - Aerobic gram-negative bacilli
  - Pseudomonas aeroginosa – IVDU
  - Salmonella-sickle cell disease

- o Polymicrobial
  - Decubitus ulcer
  - Vascular insufficiency
  - Spread from adjacent tissue

➢ Clinical
- o Commonest site of involvement
  - Vetebrae
  - Sternoclavicular bone ⎤ Common IVDU
  - Sacroiliac bone ⎦

Abbreviation: IVDU, intravenous drug user

- Give circumstances in which you would have ↑ **suspicion of chronic osteomyelitis**.

  - o Prosthetic joint
    - Chronic pain
    - Loosening

  - o Drawing sinus tract (pathognomic)

➢ Laboratory
- o Blood
  - Positive markers for inflammation e.g. ↑ WBC, ↑ ESR, ↑ CRP
  - Cultures positive

➢ Diagnostic Imaging
- o Plain films earliest findings may take 2 wk to appear

- o Nuclear imaging
  - Sensitivity > 90%
  - Specificity low due to false positive
    - Osteoarthritis
    - Trauma
    - Surgery
    - Cancer
  - Types
    - 3-phase technetium-99m
    - Gallium-67
    - WBC-tagged

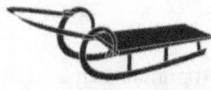

o MRI
- Imaging of choice
  ▪ Early diagnosis
  ▪ Clear demonstration of changes in
    - Bone
    - Soft tissue

o CT
- When MI is contraindicated

- Give examples in which **MRI is contraindicated**.

  o Cardiac pacemakers

  o Defibrillaters

  o Metal in body

  o Renal failure, and danger of using contrast (gadolinium)

➢ Treatment
  o Surgical debridement

  o Removal of hardware e.g. metal joints prosthesis

  o Antibiotics

  o Vacuum-assisted closure devices

  o Hyperbaric O_2

- Give the treatment in the patient who
  - Refuses surgery
  - No local / systemic signs of infection
  - Prosthesis is not loose

  o Use life-long antibiotic suppressive therapy with timethroprim-sulfamethoxazole

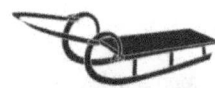

VERTEBRAL OSTEOMYELITIS

➢ Cause
- ○ Most common:
  - - S. aureus (also MRSA) and coagulate-negative Staphylococci
- ○ Less common: Streptococci, Candida, gram-negative bacilli

➢ Site
- ○ Often attacks 2 vertebral bones, plus disk space (spondylodiscitis)
- ○ Frequency: lumber > thoracic > cervical

➢ Diagnosis
- ○ Blood culture
  - - Positive in > 50%
  - - Negative → CT-directed percutaneous needle biopsy and culture
- ○ MRI
  - - Beware false-positive scan in presence of uninfected bone fracture
- ○ Nucleotide scans
  - - Even gallium scan has low specificity

➢ Treatment
- ○ Culture-directed IV antibiotics for 6 to 8 wks
  - - Vancomycin plus
  - - Ceftriaxone, or
  - - Cefepine

FAMILIAL AUTOINFLAMMATORY DISEASES

- Give the familial autoinflammatory diseases which may be distinguished by demography, genetics, clinical features and complications, as well as treatment.
  - ○ FCAS   familial cold autoinflammatory syndrome
  - ○ FMF   familial Mediterranean fever
  - ○ HIDS   hyperimmunoglobulinemia D with periodic fever syndrome
  - ○ MWS   Muckle-Wells syndrome
  - ○ NOMID   neonatal onset multisystem inflammatory disease
  - ○ TRAPS   tumor necrosis factor receptor-associated periodic syndrome

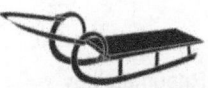

COLLAGEN DISORDERS

- o Osteogenesis imperfect
- o Ehler-Danlos syndrome
- o Marfin syndrome

Arthropathy

Useful background: Causes of **hypermobile joints**

- o Marfans
- o Ehlers-Danlos
- o Osteogenesis imperfect
- o Inflammatory polyarthritis (e.g. RA)
- o Charcot arthropathy
- o Homocystinuria
- o Hyperlysinemia
- o Idiopathic

Source: Burton JL. *Churchill Livingstone* 1971, page 113.

Marfan Syndrome (MFS)

➤ Definition: Mutations in the gene for fibrillin, leading to ↓ elastin from the dysregulation of sequestered TGF (transforming growth factor) B, resulting in overgrowth of long bones, cardiovascular and eye changes.

➤ Clinical

o Long bones	–	Arm span > height
	–	Arachnodactyly
o Brain	–	Dural ectasia
o Eyes	–	Lens dislocations (ectopia lentis)
o Face	–	High arched palate
	–	Small jaw (micrognathia)

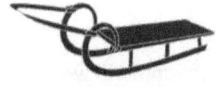

- Perform a focused physical examination for Marfan syndrome.

  o Skin
    - Small papules in the neck (Miescher elastoma)
  o Heart
    - Mitral valve prolapse
    - Aortic aneurysm
    - Aortic regurgitation

  o Chest
    - Pectus excavatum
    - Cystic lung disease

  o Hands
    - Hypermobile joints and spidery fingers (arachnodactyly)
    - Thumb sign – ask the patient to clench her/his thumb in their fist; the thumb should not exceed the ulnar side of the hand in normal subjects but because of hypermobility and laxity of the joint in Marfan disease it protrudes beyond his clenched fingers
    - Wrist sign – put the patient's fingers around his other wrist; normal subjects cannot overlap the thumb an little finger around the wrist but in Marfan's syndrome the little finger will overlap by at least 1 cm in 80%

  o Head
    – Long-headedness (dolichocephalic, with bossing of frontal eminences and prominent supraorbital ridges)
  o Eyes
    – Iridodonesis or ectopia lentis (subluxation upwards)
    – Thick spectacles
    – Blue sclera

  o Palate
    – High-arched palate

  o Spine
    – Scoliosis
    – Kyphosis

  o Limbs
    – Long arms and leg
    – Arm span (A) longer than the length (H) (A:H>1.05)

Adapted from: Baliga RR. *Saunders/Elsevier* 2007, pages 580 and 581.

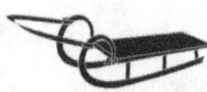

SO YOU WANT TO BE A RHEUMATOLOGIST!

- Give the way in which the diagnosis for Marfan syndrome is made.
  - o With family history: features from 2 systems
  - o Without a family history
    - Skeletal features (including pectus carinatum or excavatum, reduced lower upper-lower segment ratio, arm-span-to-height ratio > 1.05, scoliosis and reduced elbow extension
    - Involvement of at least two other systems and one of the major criteria
    - Ectopia lentis
    - Dilation of the aortic root or aortic dissection
    - Lumbosacral dural ectasia by CT or MRI

- The skeletal phenotype of homocystinuria is similar to Marfan syndrome. Give the way in which the two distinguished on physical examination.
  - o In homocystinuria the lens is dislocated downwards (and there is homocystine in the urine).

Source: Baliga RR. *Saunders/Elsevier* 2007, page 581.

- Give causes of ↑ bone density (**sclerosis**) on plain X-ray of the bones.
  - o Metastatic disease
    - Primary
    - Prostate
    - Breast
    - Reticulosis
    - Site
      - Uretelic
      - Pelvis
      - Rarely effects long bones
  - o Myelofibrosis
  - o Chronic osteomyelitis
  - o Paget disease
    - Localized or wide spread
    - Deformity (unlike metastases, in Paget disease the deformity does not grow also the surface of the bone
    - Platybasia skull is indented by vertebral column
    - Sclerosis is the usual finding except in the skull where Paget disease shows an area of decreased bone density which is well circumscribed (aka osteoporosis circumscripta)
  - o Avascular bone necrosis
  - o Osteopetrosis (aka "marble bone disease", or Albers- Schonberg disease")
  - o Fluorosis
  - o Bone cyst
    - Localized area of translucency surrounded by a rim of sclerosis

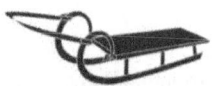

Ehlers-Danlos Syndrome (EDS)

While the classical EDS patient with mutation in gene for type V collagen is what you will likely see on a GIM (general Internal Medicine) examination, it is the type II patient with "vascular" EDS which is what you will see more often in a GI, cardiology, neurology or obstetrical practice

➢ Types

- o Classic EDS   – Skin
  - Smooth, stretchy
  - Easy bruising
  - Slow healing of wounds
  - – Joints
    - Hypermobility

- o Vascular EDS   – Blood vessels
  - Aneurysm
  - AV fistulae
  - Dissections
  - Rupture of vessels
  - – Rupture of bowel
  - – Rupture of uterus in pregnancy

Oseogenesis Imperfecta

A question for Trivial Pursuit: what genetic conditions is caused by the gene for type I collagen, resulting in brittle bones, abnormal tooth development, and blue sclera?

- o Osteogenesis impefecta, treated with bisphosphonates for increasing bone mineral mass and decreasing bone pain.

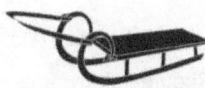

Neuroarthropathy (Charcot Joint)

➢ Definition: "a chronic, progressive arthropathy resulting from a disturbance in the sensory innervation of the joint"

➢ Causes / associations

  o Conditions associated with the development of Charcot joint
    - Diabetes mellitus
    - Tabes dorsalis
    - Syringomyalgia
    - Myelomeningocele
    - Leprosy

➢ Clinical

• Perform a directed physical examination for Charcot joint (neuroarthropathy).

  o Joint
    - Warm, swollen, tender
    - Enlarged
    - Crepitus
    - ↑ mobility

  o Cause of sensory loss to the affected joint
    - Metabolic
      ▪ Diabetes
    - Degenerative
      ▪ Syringomyelia (dissociated sensory loss)
      ▪ Myelomeningocele
    - Infections
      ▪ Syphilis
      ▪ Leprosy

  o Chronic, progressive, degenerative arthropathy arising from loss of sensory innervations of joint
    - Early redness, heat, swelling, tenderness;
    - Late enlargement of affected joint with crepitus, deformity, swelling and instability (usually hypermobile joint)
    - Associated muscle atrophy (compare joint with the normal contralateral joint)
    - Feet and ankles affected commonly, from peripheral neuropathy and local injury
    - May be complicated by osteomyelitis from skin ulcers

  o Decreased sensation (position and vibration, pain and temperature)

Adapted from: Baliga RR. *Saunders/Elsevier* 2007, pages 349 and 350.

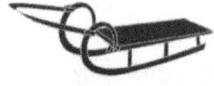

SO YOU WANT TO BE RHEUMATOLOGIST!

- In the context of severe osteoarthropathy associated with impaired sensation to pain (**Charcot arthropathy**), what are the radiological changes?
    - ○ Osteoarthropathy
    - ○ Calcification
        - Synovium
        - Intra articular base bodies
    - ○ Differentiate clinically from similar picture causes by repeated injection of steroids into the joint

SO YOU WANT TO BE A RHEUMATOLOGIST!

- In the context of the diabetic patient, give the significance of the **prayer sign**.
    - ○ Prayer sign- unability to oppose the flexor surfaces of the PIPs
    - ○ Diabetic stiff hand syndrome
    - ○ Flexion contracture and limited flexion of PIP joints
    - ○ Positive prayer sign
    - ○ Waxy, thick skin over the fingers

- In the context of diffuse swelling of a finger, what are the non-traumatic causes of a sausage-shaped digit.
    - ○ Psoriatic arthritis
    - ○ Sarcoidosis

Source: Mangione S. Hanley & Belfus 2000, page 462

SO YOU WANT TO BE A RHEUMATOLOGIST!

- What is **Behcet syndrome**?

    - ○ Aphthous ulcers in mouth and genitals, associated with arthritis, uvertis and various neurological disorders

Source: Mangione S. *Hanley & Belfus* 2000, page 67.

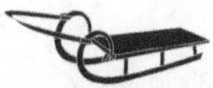

PRESSURE ULCER

➢ **Staging** of pressure ulcers

  o Stage I
  - Nonblanchable erythema of intact skin, usually over a bony prominence.
  - In darker skin types, discolouration, warmth, edema or induration may be indicator. The area may be painful, firm, soft, warmer or cooler than adjacent skin.

  o Stage II
  - Partial-thickness skin loss involving the epidermis, dermis or both
  - Clinically, this presents as
    ▪ An abrasion
    ▪ Intact or ruptured blister
    ▪ Shallow erosion with a red-pink wound bed

  o Stage III
  - Full-thickness ulceration
  - Subcutaneous fat may be visible, but none, tendon or muscle are not exposed.
  - Presents as a deep crater that may have undermining of adjacent tissue.

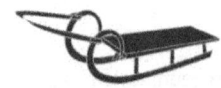

- o Stage IV — Full-thickness ulceration with exposed
  - Bone
  - Tendon
  - Fascia
  - Muscle
  - Joint capsule

  - Often includes undermining and tunneling.
  - Slough (yellow, tan, gray, green or brown) or eschar (tan, brown or black) may be present, and may cover the base of the ulcer.
  - A pressure ulcer cannot be accurately staged until enough slough and/or eschar has been removed to expose the base of the wound.
  - Pressure ulcers do not necessarily progress in order, nor do they heal by reverse staging.

Reproduced with permission: Therapeutics Choices. Sixth Edition. Ottawa, Canada: *Canadian Pharmacist Association* 2012, Table 1, page 1162.

➢ Select risk/causative factors for pressure ulcers

Local	Systemic
o Pressure, especially overlying bony prominences	– Circulatory disturbance
	– Malnutrition
o Dry skin	– Prolonged immobilization, e.g.,
o Excessive moisture	• Fractures
o Friction	• Spinal cord injury
o Shearing forces	• Stroke
	• Major surgery
	– Sensory deficit
	– Smoking

Reproduced with permission: Therapeutics Choices. Sixth Edition. Ottawa, Canada: *Canadian Pharmacist Association* 2012, Table 2, page 1163.

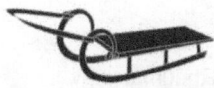

- Perform a focused physical examination for common **types of leg ulcers**.

Type of Ulcer

Feature	Venous	Arterial	Neurotrophic
➤ Onset, trauma	+/-	+	+
➤ Course	Chronic	Progressive	Progressive
➤ Location	Medial aspect of leg	Toe, heel, lateral , posterior aspect of leg, foot	Plantar
➤ Pain	- (unless infected)	+	-
○ Ulcer edges	Shaggy	Discrete	Discrete
○ Ulcer base	Healthy	Eschar, pale	Healthy or pale
○ Surrounding skin	Stasis changes	Atrophic	Callous

Adapted from: Ghosh AK. *Mayo Clinic Scientific Press* 2008, Table 25-9, page 1053.

➤ Clinical Gems:

  ○ Reiter Disease
    - "Calcaneal spur" (calcification of plantar fascia-highly suggestive of diagnosis)
    - Plantar fasciitis
    - Tendonitis
    - Periostial calcification

Source: Burton JL. *Churchill Livingstone* 1971, page 114.

SO YOU WANT TO BE A WANT A BE!

- In the context of pain along the radial side of the wrist, what is the Finkelstein sign?

    ○ Tenosynovitis of tendons of the thumb passing over the radius bone causes pain
    ○ The pain is reproduced by placing the thumb in the palm of the hand, and wrapping the fingers around the thumb.
    ○ The wrist is deviated to the ulnar side.

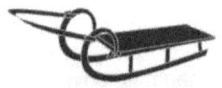

FIBROMYALGIA

➤ Definition

○ "Fibromyalgia is a central pain sensitivity syndrome characterized by widespread pain and tenderness in which the sensory processing systems are altered, producing allodynia and hyperalgesia…. neurobiologic" and psychosocial factors play a role" (MSKAP 16, Rheumatology 2012, page 26).

○ "Fibromyalgia is characterized by chronic widespread pain, increased tenderness at specific points known as "tender points", fatigue, headache and unrefreshing sleep. Mood disorder such as depression or anxiety are commonly associated with fibromyalgia" (Finestone AM, et al. In: Therapeutic Choices. Grey J, Ed. 6th Edition, *Canadian Pharmacists Association*: Otttawa, ON, 2011, page 983).

➤ Diagnosis

Please refer to either
○ American College of Rheumatology 1990 Criteria
○ Wolfe E, et al. Arthritis Rheum 1990; 33: 160-172, or
○ 2010 Preliminary Diagnostic Criteria
  – Wolfe F, et al. Arthritis Care Res 2010; 62: 600-610.

➤ Clinical

• Take a directed history and perform a focused physical examination for causes of polymyalgia rheumatica-like syndromes.

○ MSK	– Fibromyalgia (FMN)
	– Polymyalgia rheumatica (PMR)
	– Seronegative rheumatoid arthritis (SRA)
	– Polymyositis
	– Systemic vasculitis
	– Systemic lupus erytematosus (SLE)
	– Polyarticular osteoarthritis
	– Osteomalacia (OA)
	– Remitting seronegative, symmetric synovitis and peripheral edema
○ Metabolic	– Hypo-/Hyperthyroidism
	– Hyperparathyroidism
○ Infection	– Infectious endocarditis
○ Mental health	– Depression
○ Infiltration	– Paraneoplastic syndromes
	– Systemic amyloidosis

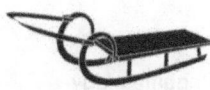

Adapted from: Ghosh AK. *Mayo Clinic Scientific Press* 2008, page 987.

PMR, FMN, SRA and polymyositis may cause pain, tenderness, and morning stiffness. In FMN the ESR is normal, and there is response to steroids in SRA and there usually is a response to steroids.

- Perform a focused physical examination to distinguish PMR from the other causes of polymyalgia-rheumatica (PMR) – like syndromes.

Characteristic	PMR	FMN	SRA	Polymyositis
o Age	> 50 yrs	Usually >50 yrs	Any age	Any age
o Physical examination	Hip, shoulder girdle tenderness and limited ROM	Tender points	Synovitis	Muscle weakness

Abbreviations: CPK, creatine phosphokinase; ESR, erythrocyte sedimentation rate; FMN, fibromyalgia; N, normal; PMR, polymyalgia rheumatica; RA, rheumatoid arthritis; ROM, range of motion; SRA, seronegative rheumatoid arthritis.

Adapted from: Ghosh AK. *Mayo Clinic Scientific Press* 2008, page 987.

➤ Differential

- Give the differential diagnosis of polymyalgia rheumatica (PMR).

Diagnosis	Distinguishing Features From PMR
o Myositis	– Muscle weakness on physical examination – ↑ CPK – Abnormalities on EMG and muscle biopsy
o Fibromyalgia	– Usually seen in younger patients – Widespread pain and tenderness at a significant number of soft tissue sites – Not limited to the shoulders and hips – Normal ESR and CRP

Diagnosis	Distinguishing Features From PMR
o Rheumatoid Arthritis	– Synovitis distal to the wrist and ankle – Seropositivity for rheumatoid factor (RF) – Consider an-CCP antibodies if RF negative – Inadequate response to low-dose prednisone therapy – Radiographic erosions
o Malignancy	– As directed by clinical examination, laboratory evaluation (e.g., iron deficiency anemia) and lack of response to conventional therapy – The incidence of malignancy is not increased in PMR or GCA

Abbreviations: anti-CCP = anti-cyclic citrullinated peptide; CPK = creatine phosphokinase; CRP = C-reactive protein; EMG = electromyography; ESR = erythrocyte sedimentation rate

Reproduced with permission: Therapeutics Choices. Sixth Edition. Ottawa, Canada: *Canadian Pharmacist Association* 2012, Table 1, page 1004.

➤ Treatment

• Give the treatment of fibromyalgia

  o Non pharmacological
    – Education
    – Reassurance
    – Exercise
    – Cognitive behavioural therapy

  o Pharmacological
    – SNRIs (serotonin-norepinephrine reuptake inhibitors)
    – TCAs (tricyclic anti-depressants)
    – Anti-epileptic medications (e.g. pregabalin)
    – Note: do **not** use narcotics

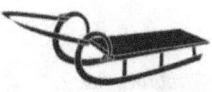

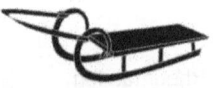

ONLINE RESOURCES:

- ○ *MELD, Model for End-Stage Liver Disease, available online calculator: www.mayoclinic.org/meld/mayomodel7.html

- ○ AGA educator resources: http://www.gastro.org/gi-fellowship/educator-resources

- ○ CAPstone: http://www.giandhepatology.com

- ○ CCFA: http://www.ccfa.org

- ○ CCFC (Crohn's and Colitis Foundation of Canada): www.ccfc.ca

- ○ Home parenteral Nutrition: www.oley.org

- ○ http://mayoclini.org/meld/mayomodel6.html

- ○ http://www.accessdata.fda.gov/drugsatfda_docs/label/2011/201917lbl.pdf

- ○ http://www.accessdata.fda.gov/drugsatfda_docs/label/2011/201917lbl.pdf

- ○ http://www.accessdata.fda.gov/drugsatfda_does/label/2011/201917lbl.pdf

- ○ http://www.aidsinfo.nih.gov/guidelines/

- ○ http://www.fda.gov/Drugs/DrugSafety/PostmarketDrugSafetyInformationforPatientsandProviders/ucm213038.htm.

- ○ http://www.fda.gov/Drugs/DrugSafety/ucm291119.htm

- ○ http://www.fda.gov/Drugs/DrugSafety/ucm291119.htm

- ○ http://www.fda.gov/NewsEvents/Newsroom/PressAnnouncements/ucm256299.htm

- ○ http://www.fda.gov/Safety/MedWatch/SafetyInformation/SafetyAlertsforHumanMedicalProducts/ucm291144.htm

- ○ http://www.fda.gov/Safety/MedWatch/SafetyInformation/SafetyAlertsforHumanMedicalProducts/ucm211796.htm

- ○ http://www.gastro.org/practive/medical-osition-statements

- ○ http://www.mayoclinic.org/gi-risk/mayomodel2.html

- ○ http://www.pathology.pitt.edu/lectures/gi

- ○ http://www.pathologyatlas.com

- ○ IBS Support group: www.ibsgroup.org

- ○ International Association for the Study of Obesity: http://www.iaso.org

- ○ Intestinal transplantation: http://www.intestinaltransplant.org

- ○ Liver and intrahepatic bile ducts. www.PathologyOutlines.com

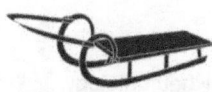

- Me'decins San Frontieres: http://www.msf.org
- MedEdPORTAL: https://www.mededportal.org/
- Medical council of Canada. Weight Gain/Obesity. http://mcc.ca/Objectives_Online/
- Medical Council of Canada. Weight Loss/ Eating Disorders/ Anorexia http://mcc.ca/Objectives_Online/
- Medical council of Canada. Weight loss/Eating Disorders/Anorexia. http://mcc.ca/Objectives_Online/
- MedicineNet: www.medicinenet.com/irritable_bowel_syndrome/article.htm
- National Endoscopy Program : www.grs.nhs.uk
- National Endoscopy Program : www.grs.nhs.uk
- Natural Comprehensive Cancer Network (NCCN) guidelines: www.nccn.org
- Portal of online geriatric education: http://www.pogoe.org/
- Recommendations about chemoprophylaxis for malaria. Also see http://www.nc.cdc.gov/travel/yellowbook/2012/chapter-3-infectious-disease-related-to-travel/malaria.htm
- UpdateToDate: www.uptodate.com/patients/index
- www.aasid.org/practiceguidelines/Page/default.aspx
- www.aasld.org/practiceguidelines/Page/default.aspx
- www.gastro.org/practice/meicacl-osition-statements
- www.motherisk.org/women/index.jsp
- www.orl.cz/ehorroby/ustni/vestibulum/veozena

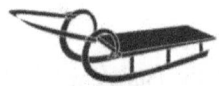

INDEX

Note: Page number followed by f and t indicates figure and table respectively.

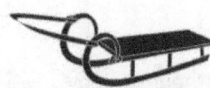

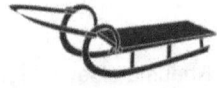

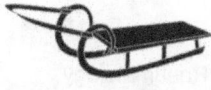

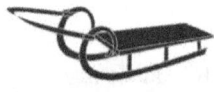

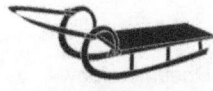

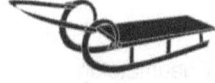

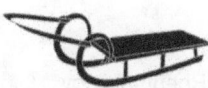

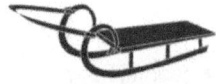

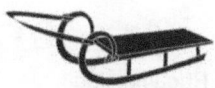

M

Mallet finger/thumb, 16t, 17f
Marfan syndrome (MFS), 29–30
    clinical, 196–198, 197f
    definition, 196
Methotrexate, 105
MFS. *See* Marfan syndrome
Microorganisms, causes
    bacterial arthritis, 71–72
    fungal arthritis, 73
    Lyme disease, 73
    tuberculosis, 72
Midfoot fracture, 67t
Migratory arthralgia, causes, 132
Morton neuroma, feet, 68t
Motor examination, MSK, 2t
Motor neuropathy, 4
MSK. *See* Musculoskeletal
Musculoskeletal (MSK) system
    abnormal articular findings and diagnosis, 10t–13t
    abnormal physical findings and definition of, 2t–3t
    disorder, history for, 2
    motor examination, 2t
    motor/sensory neuropathy, physical examination for, 4
    non-steroidal anti-inflammatory drugs, side effects of, 8–9, 10t
    physical examination for, 5t–8t
    sensory examination, 2t–3t
Myxoma, arterial, 161

N

Neck
    movements and myotomes, 14t
    swan neck deformity, 16t, 17f
Neer impingement sign, 37f
Neuroarthropathy
    causes/associations, 200
    clinical, 200–202
    definition, 200
Non-steroidal anti-inflammatory drugs
    MSK, side effects of, 8–9, 10t

O

OA. *See* Osteoarthritis
Oligoarthritis
    arthropathy patterns, 88f
    causes of, 87

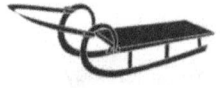

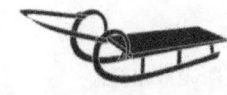

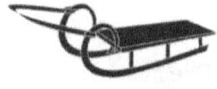

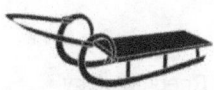

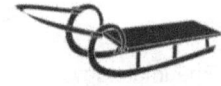

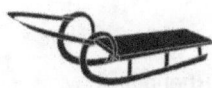

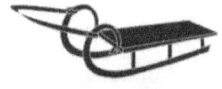

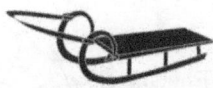

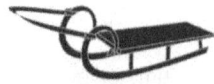

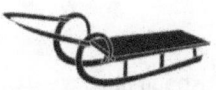

Wrists, 14–27
 abnormal articular findings and diagnosis, 5t, 11t
 arthritis in OA, 25t
 arthritis in RA, 25t
 deformities, 19t–20t, 21, 21f–22f
 motion, range of, 14t, 23t
 movements, 26f
 physical examination
  for rheumatoid arthritis, 29

Y
Yergason sign, 37f, 42

 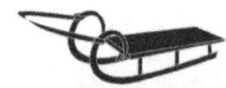

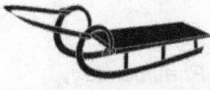

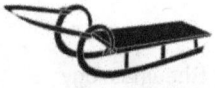

INTERNAL MEDICINE
Mastering The Boards and Clinical Examinations

ENDOCRINOLOGY

A.B.R. Thomson

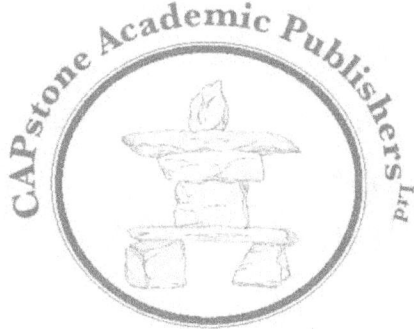

CAPstone (Canadian Academic Publishers Ltd) is a not-for-profit company dedicated to the use of the power of education for the betterment of all persons everywhere.

"The Democratization of Knowledge"

2016

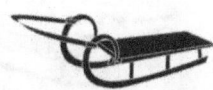

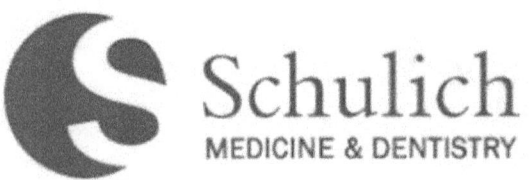 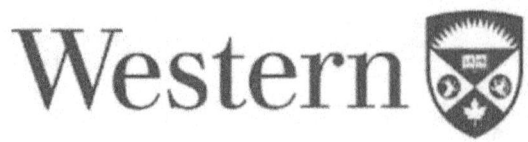

THE WESTERN WAY

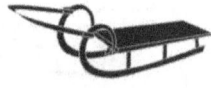

TABLE OF CONTENTS

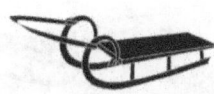

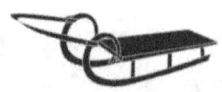

MASTERING THE BOARDS AND THE CANMED OBJECTIVES

Medical expert
The discussion of complex cases provides the participants with an opportunity to comment on additional focused history and physical examination. They would provide a complete and organized assessment. Participants are encouraged to identify key features, and they develop an approach to problem-solving.

The case discussions, as well as the discussion of cases around a diagnostic imaging, pathological or endoscopic base provides the means for the candidate to establish an appropriate management plan based on the best available evidence to clinical practice. Throughout, an attempt is made to develop strategies for diagnosis and development of clinical reasoning skills.

Communicator
The participants demonstrate their ability to communicate their knowledge, clinical findings, and management plan in a respectful, concise and interactive manner. When the participants play the role of examiners, they demonstrate their ability to listen actively and effectively, to ask questions in an open-ended manner, and to provide constructive, helpful feedback in a professional and non-intimidating manner.

Collaborator
The participants use the "you have a green consult card" technique of answering questions as fast as they are able, and then to interact with another health professional participant to move forward the discussion and problem solving. This helps the participants to build upon what they have already learned about the importance of collegial interaction.

Manager
The participants are provided with assignments in advance of the three day GI Practice Review. There is much work for them to complete before as well as afterwards, so they learn to manage their time effectively, and to complete the assigned tasks proficiently and on time. They learn to work in teams to achieve answers from small group participation, and then to share this with other small group participants through effective delegation of work. Some of the material they must access demands that they use information technology effectively to access information that will help to facilitate the delineation of adequately broad differential diagnoses, as well as rational and cost effective management plans.

Health advocate
In the answering of the questions and case discussions, the participants are required to consider the risks, benefits, and costs and impacts of investigations and therapeutic alliances upon the patient and their loved ones.

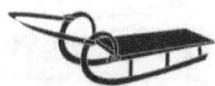

Scholar
By committing to the pre- and post-study requirements, plus the intense three day active learning Practice Review with colleagues is a demonstration of commitment to personal education. Through the interactive nature of the discussions and the use of the "green consult card", they reinforce their previous learning of the importance of collaborating and helping one another to learn.

Professional
The participants are coached how to interact verbally in a professional setting, being straightforward, clear and helpful. They learn to be honest when they cannot answer questions, make a diagnosis, or advance a management plan. They learn how to deal with aggressive or demotivated colleagues, how to deal with knowledge deficits, how to speculate on a missing knowledge byte by using first principals and deductive reasoning. In a safe and supportive setting they learn to seek and accept advice, to acknowledge awareness of personal limitations, and to give and take 360^0 feedback.

Knowledge
The basic science aspects of gastroenterology are considered in adequate detail to understand the mechanisms of disease, and the basis of investigations and treatment. In this way, the participants respect the importance of an adequate foundation in basic sciences, the basics of the design of clinical research studies to provide an evidence-based approach, the designing of clinical research studies to provide an evidence-based approach, the relevance of their management plans being patient-focused, and the need to add "compassionate" to the Three C's of Medical Practice: competent, caring and compassionate.

"They may forget what you said, but they will never forget how you made them feel."

Carl W. Buechner, on teaching.

"With competence, care for the patient. With compassion, care about the person."

Alan B. R. Thomson, on being a physician.

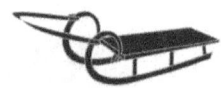

PROLOGUE

HREs, better known as, High Risk Examinations. After what is often two decades of study, sacrifice, long hours, dedication, ambition and drive, we who have chosen Internal Medicine, and possibly through this a subspecialty, have a HRE, the [Boards] Royal College Examinations. We have been evaluated almost daily by the sadly subjective preceptor based assessments, and now we face the fierce, competitive, winner-take-all objective testing through multiple choice questions (MCQs), and for some the equally challenging OSCE, the objective standardized clinical examination. Well we know that in the real life of providing competent, caring and compassionate care as physicians, as internists, that a patient is neither a MCQ or an OSCE. These examinations are to be passed, a process with which we may not necessarily agree. Yet this is the game in which we have thus far invested over half of our youthful lives. So let us know the rules, follow the rules, work with the rules, and succeed. So that we may move on to do what we have been trained to do, do what we may long to do, care for our patients.

The process by which we study for clinical examinations is so is different than for the MCQs: not trivia, but an approach to the big picture, with thoughtful and reasoned deduction towards a diagnosis. Not looking for the answer before us, but understanding the subtle aspects of the directed history and focused physical examination, yielding an informed series of hypotheses, a differential diagnosis to direct investigations of the highly sophisticated laboratory and imaging procedures now available to those who can wait, or pay.

This book provides clinically relevant questions of the process of taking a history and performing a physical examination, with sections on Useful background, and where available, evidence-based performance characteristics of the rendering of our clinical skills. Just for fun are included "So you want to be a such-and-such specialist!" to remind us that one if the greatest strengths we can possess to survive in these times, is to smile and even to laugh at ourselves.

Sincerely,

Alan Thomson

Emeritus Distinguished University Professor, U of A
Adjunct Professor, Western University

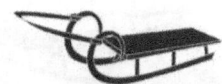

DEDICATION

In the memory of Jim and Dorothy

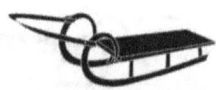

ACKNOWLEDGEMENTS

Patience and patients go hand in hand. So also does the interlocking of young and old, love and justice, equality and fairness. No author can have thoughts transformed into words, no teacher can make ideas become behaviour and wisdom and art, without those special people who turn our minds to the practical - of getting the job done!

Thank you, Naiyana and Duen for translating those terrible scribbles, called my handwriting, into the still magical legibility of the electronic age. Thank you, Sarah, for your creativity and hard work.

My most sincere and heartfelt thanks go to the excellent persons at JP Consulting, and CapStone Academic Publishers. Jessica, you are brilliant, dedicated and caring. Thank you.

When Rebecca, Maxwell, Megan Grace, Henry and Felix ask about their Grandad, I will depend on James and Anne, Matthew and Allison, Jessica and Matt, and Benjamin to be understanding and kind. For what I was trying to say and to do was to make my professional life focused on the three C's - competence, caring, and compassion - and to make my very private personal life dedicated to family - to you all.

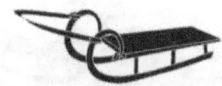

DISCLAIMER

The primary purpose of this publication is education. The author, editor and publisher acknowledge that the development of new material opens to way for possible errors – what is correct today might not be the standard of care tomorrow. Readers are advised to ensure that the doses of drugs which they use are in compliance with their country's product information, and that the use of any therapeutic agent, be it a pharmaceutical or a technology, should be guided by local guidelines. There is often a wide diversity of professional opinion, and guidelines from one country are not always congruent with another.

The author, editor and publisher do not guarantee the safety, reliability, accuracy, completeness or usefulness of this material.

They disclaimer any and all liability for damage and claims that may result from the use of information, publications, technologies, products, and for series provided in this publication.

We have made every attempt to trace the holders of copyright for material reproduced in this book. If by some oversight we have omitted a copyright holder, please contact us.

Thank you

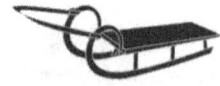

ARE YOU PREPARING FOR EXAMS IN GASTROENTEROLOGY AND HEPATOLOGY?

See the full range of examination preparation and review publications from CAPstone on Amazon.com

Gastroenterology and Hepatology

First Principles of Gastroenterology and Hepatology in Adults and Children - Volume I – Gastroenterology (ISBN: 978-1494345624)

First Principles of Gastroenterology and Hepatology in Adults and Children - Volume II - Hepatology and Paediatrics (ISBN: 978-1494345501)

Medical Mini Review Series in Gastroenterology and Hepatology: Efficient Refresher for the Busy Clinical Gastroenterologist (ISBN: 978-1502472199)

Medical Mini Review Series in Gastroenterology and Hepatology: Efficient Refresher for the Busy Clinical Gastroenterologist (ISBN: 978-1502472199)

Practice Review in Gastroenterology (ISBN: 978-1500855321)

Practice Review in Hepatopancreatobiliary Diseases and Nutrition (ISBN: 978-1500855734)

Endoscopy and Diagnostic Imaging - Part I: Skin, Nail and Mouth Changes in GI Disease; Esophagus; Stomach; Small intestine; Pancreas (ISBN: 978-1477400579)

Endoscopy and Diagnostic Imaging - Part II: Colon and Hepatobiliary (ISBN: 978-1477400654)

Scientific Basis for Clinical Practice in Gastroenterology and Hepatology (ISBN: 978-1475226645)

The Physiology and Pathophysiology of Gastrointestinal and Hepatopancreaticobiliary Disorders: Preparing for Professional Competence. (ISBN: 978-1500298265)

General Internal Medicine

Achieving Excellence in the OSCE - Part One: Cardiology to Nephrology (ISBN: 978-1475283037)

Achieving Excellence in the OSCE - Part Two: Neurology to Rheumatolgy (ISBN: 978-1475276978)

Mastering the Boards and Clinical Examinations in Internal Medicine, Part I: Cardiology, Endocrinology, Gastroenterology, Hepatology and Nephrology (ISBN: 978-1461024842)

Mastering The Boards and Clinical Examinations In Internal Medicine, part II: Neurology, Respirology and Rheumatology (ISBN: 978-1478392736)

Bits and Bytes: Surviving Morning Rounds (ISBN: 978-1478295365)

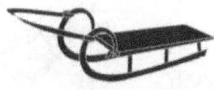

Mastering the Boards: Endocrinology   A.B.R. Thomson

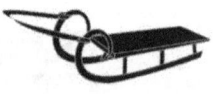

ENDOCRINOLOGY

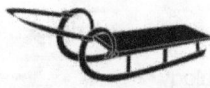

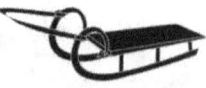

METABOLIC SYNDROME / OBESITY

- Give the diagnostic criteria for metabolic syndrome, and the metabolic targets for these criteria in non-pregnant diabetes.

Diagnostic criteria metabolic syndrome		Metabolic targets in DM (non-pregnant)
o Waist circumference		
M	> 102 cm (> 40 in)	
F	> 88 cm (> 35 in)	
o HDL-cholesterol		
M	< 1.04 mmol/L (40 mg/dL)	> 1.04 mmol/L (> 40 mg/dL)
F	< 1.30 mmol/L (50 mg/dL)	> 1.30 mmol/L (50 mg/dL)
o LDL-cholesterol	-	< 2.59 mmol/dL (< 100 mg/dL)
o Triglycerides	≥ 1.70 mmol/L (≥ 150 mg/dL)	< 1.70 mmol/L (< 150 mg/dL)
o Blood pressure	≥ 130 / ≥ 85 mm Hg	< 130 / 80 mm Hg
o Blood sugar		
- Fasting	≥ 5.6 mmol/L (≥ 100 mg/dL)	3.9 – 7.2 mmol/L (70-130 mg/dL)
- PC	-	< 10.0 mmol/L (< 180 mg/dL)
o Hemoglobin AIC	-	< 7.0%

Abbreviations: M, male; F, female; PC, after meals

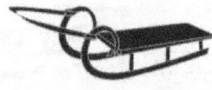

OBESITY

- Give the WHO Classification of overweight and obesity in adults according to body mass index.

Classification	BMI[a]	Risk of Comorbidities[b]
o Underweight	< 18.5	Mildly increased
o Normal	18.5-24.9	Average
o Overweight	25-29.9	Mildly increased
o Obese	≥ 30	
− Class I	30-34.9	Moderate
− Class II	35-39.9	Severe
− Class III	≥ 40	Very severe

[a] Values are aged and gender independent]

[b] Both BMI and a measure of fat distribution (e.g., waist circumference) are important in estimating the risk of comorbidities (type 2 diabetes, hypertension, dyslipidemia)

Reproduced with permission: Therapeutics Choices. Sixth Edition. Ottawa, Canada: *Canadian Pharmacist Association* 2012, Table 1, page 412.

DIABETES MELLITUS

➢ Definition

- o A chronic metabolic disturbance.....a heterogeneous syndrome

- o Characterized by fasting and/or postprandial hyperglycemia

- o Caused by an absolute or relative lack of insulin, resistance to the action of insulin, or both

- o Complications involving small blood vessels (microangiography), larger blood vessels (macroangiopathy) and nerve damage (neuropathy), affecting multiple organs and systems.

- o Classification
  - − T1DM (Type 1 diabetes mellitus)
    - ▪ Autoimmune destruction of pancreatic beta cells, resulting in an absolute deficiency of insulin
    - ▪ Often presents with acute metabolic symptoms

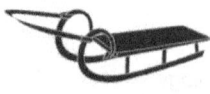

- T2DM
  - Insulin resistance, with some insulin deficiency
  - (GDM) gestational diabetes mellitus – "….onset ot recognition of glucose intolerance in pregnancy…."
  - MODY (maturity-onset diabetes of the young
  - Damage / loss of pancreas from disease, drugs, infection, metabolic disorders, trauma, surgery

➢ Pathogenesis

• Give the pathogenesis of the types of Diabetes.

   o Type I : destruction of pancreatic B cell, leading to absolute insulin deficiency
   - Autoimmune
   - In > 90% of type 1A
     - There are autoantibodies against B-cells or their metabolic products
     - These include
       - Anti-glutamic acid decarboxylase
       - Anti-islet cell autoantigen
       - Anti-insulin antibodies
   - In type 1B
     - No autoimmune markers (idiopathic)
     - Asia / African heritage
   - Idiopathic
     - Linkage to HLA DQ-A and DQ-B genes
     - More common in persons of Asian or African descent
   - Late onset autoimmune DM of adulthood – DM in older lean persons with anti-islet cell antibodies
   - Note
     - Age and obesity do not exclude DMT1 (type 1 diabetes)
     - DMT1 is characterized by deficiency of insulin due to an autoimmune or idiopathic destructive process of the pancreatic B-cells
   o Type II
   - Insulin resistance, plus
   - Relative insulin deficiency
   - Remember spectrum: insulin resistance → ↑ insulin secretion (hyperinsulinemia) and normal glucose concentration → ↓ B cell insulin secretion → ↑ glucose

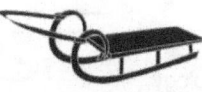

- When insulin deficiency eventually develops, type II DM is called "insulin requiring type 2 diabetes".
- 50% of women with gestational DM develop type II DM within 10 year

o Gestational
  - 7% of pregnancies
  - Diagnosis
    - 50 g glucose po → if BS > 140 mg/dL (7.8 mmol/L) at 1 hr :
    - 100 g glucose po → after 12 hr fast and carbohydrate > 150 g/day
  - Requires insulin, metformin, sulfonylurea with exacting attention to BS target ("tight" glycemic control = prevent microvascular disease, i.e. kidney eyes, peripheral nerves)
  - BS targets
    - AC 3.3-5.0 mmol/L (60-90 mg/dL)
    - PC < 6.7 mmol/L (< 120 mg/dL)
    - For values at 2 and 3 hr, see MKSAP 15, Endocrinology and Metabolism, 2009, Table 5, page 3.

o MODY (maturity-onset diabetes of the young)
  - Young persons at presentation
  - Mutation of
    - Gene for glucokinase Crate-limiting enzyme in glycolytic pathway
    - Gene for transcription factors which in turn regulate the gene for insulin
  - Autosomal dominant
  - Genetic defects in B-cell function (enzymes, transcription factors)
    - Secondary causes (e.g. pancreatic endocrine, liver disease, drugs, infection should be suspected of patient presents with
    - Atypical features
    - Rapid onset on DM without risk factors

From the OGTT (oral glucose tolerance test) result, distinguish between impaired glucose tolerance vs. type 2 DM.

- Impaired glucose tolerance	- 2 hr mark of OGTT
- Type 2 diabetes	- Blood glucose concentration ≥ 11.1 mmol/L (7.8 -11.0 mmol/L (140-199 mg/dL)

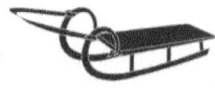

> A Gem and a Pearl: If hyperglycemia is found in a hospitalized patient, repeat the testing once the patient has recovered from their illness and are at home

➢ Clinical

• Take a directed history for diabetes mellitus.

  o Glucose control

    – Method and frequency of glucose monitoring, and by whom (patient, caregiver, health care worker)

    – Typical levels of HbA1c, blood glucose at different times

    – Dietary pattern, spacing of meals and snacks, quality and quantity of intake (CDA diet/calories/day); alcohol.

    – Hypoglycemic reactions (frequency, symptoms); anxiety, tremor, seizures, palpitations, sweating, hunger

    – Hyperosomolar non-ketotic coma (HONC)

    – Diabetic ketoacidosis (DKA)
      ▪ Symptoms of hyperglycemia (polyuria, polyphagia, polydypsia)
      ▪ Anorexia, nausea, vomiting, abdominal pain
      ▪ Fatigue
      ▪ Kussmaul breathing
      ▪ Precipitation: D/C insulin, infection, altered exercise/diet

    – Medications (type, dose, frequency and adverse effects) Insulin, oral hypoglycemics, antagonistic medications (thiazides, corticosteroids)

  o Causes/associated conditions

    – Hormone-induced states (rare)
      ▪ Acromegaly
      ▪ Cushing syndrome
      ▪ Glucagonoma
      ▪ Pheochromocytoma

    – Drugs
      ▪ Oral contraceptive agents
      ▪ Steroids
      ▪ Streptozotocin, diazoxide, phenytoin, thiazide diuretics

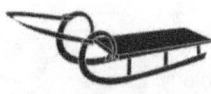

- Pancreatic disease
  - Chronic pancreatitis, carcinoma
  - Hemochromatosis

- Syndromes
  - Lipoatrophic diabetes (characterized by generalized lipoatrophy, hyperglycemia, hepatomegaly, hirsutism, acanthosis nigricans, hyperpigmentation and hyperlipidemia)

- Family history
  - Having one sibling or parent with T2 diabetes increases the lifetime risk for developing T2 diabetes to 10-15 %
- Complications
  - Hyperglycemia
    - Blurred vision
    - Polyphagia
    - Weight changes
    - Polydipsia (+/- nocturia)
    - Polyuria
    - Yeast infections
  - Hypoglycemia (adrenergic symptoms and signs)
    - Hunger
    - Palpitations
    - Sweating
    - Anxiety
    - Tremors
    - Seizures
  - Neuropathy
  - ANS neuropathy
  - Impotence
  - Neurogenic bladder: retention overflow incontinence
  - Orthostasis hypotension (gastroparesis),
  - Bowel dysmobility (diarrhea/constipation)
  - PC bloating, fullness
  - Autonomic neuropathy
    - Orthostatic hypotension
    - Gastroparesis (nausea, vomiting, postprandial bloating and early satiety)
    - Diarrhea / constipation, neurogenic bladder (retention and overflow incontinence)
    - Impotence

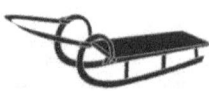

- Sensory neuropathy
  - Vibration sense (first lost), proprioception and light touch in glove-and-stocking distribution, Charcot's joints, foot ulcerations
- Radiculopathy
  - Shooting or burning pain, often radiating down lower extremities
- Mononeuropathy
  - Cranial nerve (CN) palsies; often CN III (but pupils spared), CN IV, CN VI
- Amyotrophy
  - Atrophy of the pelvic girdle and large leg muscles that can spontaneously remit
  - Often affects older males
- Mononeuritis multiplex
  - Peripheral nerve palsies that can cause sensory or motor neuropathies such as foot drop
- Peripheral neuropathy
  - Anesthetic/paresthetic/hyperesthetic feet
  - Sensory: vibration, proprioception, light touch (glove-in stocking)
  - Charcot joints
- Retinopathy
  - Fundoscopic examinations; visual acuity – blurred vision; cataracts
- Nephropathy
  - Known renal disease or proteinuria, date of last urinalysis
- Cardiovascular
  - Cardiac: angina, MI, Hx or symptoms of CHF or pulmonary edema
  - Peripheral vascular disease: claudication, rest pain, foot ulcers or infections, amputations, foot care

Abbreviation: CN, cranial nerve

Adapted from: Davey P. *Wiley-Blackwell* 2006, page 280; and Talley NJ, et al. *Maclennan & Petty Pty Limited* 2003, Table 9.17, page 336.

What's "the best"? The "best" clinical findings for diabetic foot in a diabetic patient are a foot ulcer >2cm, a foot ulcer with bone exposed, or a positive probe test.

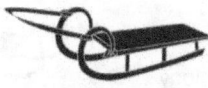

➢ Risk factors

• Give the risk factors of diabetes mellitus.

  o Presence of complications associated with diabetes
  o Vascular disease (coronary cerebrovascular or peripheral)
  o Abdominal obesity
    – Overweight
  o Acanthosis nigricans
  o Age ≥ 40 years
  o Dyslipidemia[a]
  o First degree relative with T2DM
  o History of
    – Delivery of a macrosomic infant
    – IFG or IGT
    – Gestational diabetes mellitus
  o Hypertension
  o Member of high-risk population
    – Aboriginal
    – Hispanic
    – South Asian
    – Asian
    – African descent
  o Polycystic ovary syndrome
  o Schizophrenia

[a] Associated with insulin resistance

Abbreviations: IFG, impaired fasting glucose; IG, impaired glucose tolerance; T2DM, type 2 diabetes mellitus

Reproduced with permission: Therapeutics Choices. Sixth Edition. Ottawa, Canada: *Canadian Pharmacist Association* 2012, Table 2, page 383.

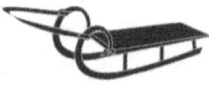

- GIve the management of the risks of diabetes.

  o Modifiable risk factors
    - Hypertension
    - Smoking
    - Hyperlipidemia
    - Obesity
    - Diet
    - Lifestyle
    - Exercise
    - Substance abuse
    - Personal history of gestational diabetes
  o Management
    - Diet
      - Caloric intake
      - Amount and types of fats, protein, fibre, and sugar
    - Lifestyle
      - Weight
      - Smoking
      - Alcohol or substance use
      - Exercise (type and amount)
    - Drug treatments
      - All medications
      - Insulin (type, amount, dosing schedule, side effects)
      - Hypoglycemic agents (type, frequency, side effects)
      - Monitoring (type [blood/urine], frequency, HbA_{1c})
      - Adherence to recommendations
      - Family history of diabetes

Adapted from: Jugovic PJ, et al. *Saunders/ Elsevier* 2004, pages 20 and 21.

What's "the best"? The "best" clinical tests for hypothyroidism are: slow speech, cool, dry and course skin, and brachycardia or a Billewicz diagnostic scale ≥ 30 points.

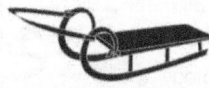

Diabetic Foot

➢ Definition

  o The diabetic foot refers to the development of diabetic peripheral neuropathy leading to reduced sensation, leading to trauma, ulceration, infection, gangrene, and deformities (Charcot arthropathy) may develop.

➢ Clinical

• Perform a focused physical examination of the diabetic foot.

  o Skin (look between toes)
    - Dry cracked skin
    - Necrobiosis diabeticorum
    - Blisters, corns, bunions
    - Ingrown or dystrophic nails
    - Cellulitis
    - Ulcers
    - Infection between toes
  o Vascular insufficiency
    - Pallor, red cool skin
    - Loss of hair
    - Ulcers, with or without infection
    - Gangrene or amputations
    - Reduced posterior tibial and dorsalis pedis pulses
  o Neuropathy
    - Sensory
      ▪ Reduced vibration sense (use 128 Hz fork)
      ▪ Reduced pin prick/fine touch (5.07 monofilament)
      ▪ Glove/stocking distribution in legs
    - Motor
      ▪ Claw-hammer toes, foot drop, pes cavus, ankle deformity
    - Reflex
      ▪ ↓ ankle jerk

Adapted from: Baliga RR. *Saunders/Elsevier* 2007, page 554; McGee SR. *Saunders/Elsevier* 2007, pages 605 to 609.

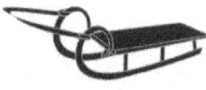

- Give the performance characteristics of clinical tests for the diabetic foot.

Finding	PLR
o Predictors of subsequent foot ulceration	
– Unable to sense the 5.07 monofilament	2.4
o Predictors of osteomyelitis, in patients with foot ulcers	
– Ulcer area >2 cm	7.2
– Positive probe test	4.3
– Ulcer depth >3 mm or bone exposed	3.6

Abbreviations: PLR, positive likelihood ratio

Adapted from: McGee SR. *Saunders/Elsevier* 2007, Box 51-1, page 608.

- Give the management of the diabetic foot.

  - o Prophylaxis
    - – Standard thorough diabetic foot care, including regular inspection of feet
    - – Extra precaution in diabetic with
      - Vascular disease
      - Neuropathy
      - Immunodeficiency

  - o Clinical
    - – Beware of possibility of osteomyelitis

  - o Treatment
    - – Mild-empiric antibiotics
    - – Usual organisms
      - Staphylococci
      - Streptococci
      - Enteric gram-negative bacilli
      - Anaerobes
      - Pseudomonas aeruginosa
    - – Severe infections may lead to imputation
    - – Continued careful glycemic control

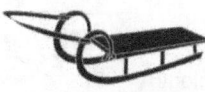

Clinical Caution

Your diabetic patient has peripheral sensory neuropathy, and a bony abnormality in the foot which you cleverly think might represent Charcot changes arising from repeated trauma from the sensory neuropathy.

Be careful, be on your guard!
   Osteomyelitis arise from foot infection in the diabetic may mimic Charcot changes

---

- In the setting of a diabetic with a foot infection, give the criteria for a limb-threatening infection, and appropriate empirical antibiotics to be given in conjunction with debridement.

    o Suggestion of a limb-threatening infection
        - Deep ulcers
        - Cellulitis extending far beyond ulcerative area
        - Evidence of tissue ischemia
        - Sepsis

    o Likely organisms
        - Polymicrobial
        - Staphyococci
        - Streptococci
        - Pseudomonas aeruginosa
        - Gram-negative enteric rods
        - Anaerobes

    o Empiric antibiotics
        - Vancomycin plus meropenem

Osteomyelitis in the Diabetic

- In the patient with osteomyelitis and a draining wound or sinus-tract, give the reason why the antibiotic chosen should not be based upon those organisms cultured from these sites, but rather from a cultured bone biopsy.

    o The organisms in the bone causing the osteomyelitis are not necessarily reflected by the microbiological isolates from the cultures of the superficial lesions, i.e. wound or sinus tract.

    o High index of suspicion for underlying osteomyelitis
        - Foot ulcers
            - 2 cm ulcer present for > 2 wk with visible bone or positive probe-to-bone test

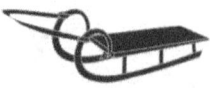

- - Other lesions
    - Tender
    - Red
    - Warm
    - Purulent
    - Discharge
    - Sinus tract
    - Crepitus
    - Bullous formation   gas → necrotizing fasciitis
    - Change in skin colour
    - Gangrene

- ➤ Treatment

  - o Surgical debridement

  - o Culture to direct antibiotics
    - Vancomycin plus cephalosporin, e.g. ceftriaxone, or cefipime, or
    - Fluoroquinolone, e.g. ciprofloxacin, or levofloxacin plus metronidazole, or clindamycin

  - o Possible amputation

- Give the **skin lesions** seen in diabetes.

  - o Acanthosis nigricans

  - o Chronic pyogenic infections and carbuncles

  - o Eruptive xanthomata

  - o Granuloma annulare

  - o Leg ulcers and gangrene

  - o Lipoatrophy and lipohypertrophy

  - o Necrobiosis lipoidica diabeticorum*

  - o 'Pebbles' on the dorsal aspect of the fingers

  - o Peripheral anhidrosis (due to autonomic neuropathy)

  - o Vulval candidiasis

* Sharply demarcated plaques with shiny surface, yellow waxy centres, and red margins with surrounding to angiectasia, sometimes complicated by ulceration of plaque, usually seen on the shin

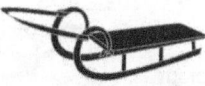

- Give the skin lesions seen on **shins** in diabetes.
  - o Diabetic dermopathy
  - o Erythema ab igne
  - o Erythema nodosum
  - o Livedo reticularis
  - o Necrobiosis lipodica diabeticorum
  - o Pretibial myxedema

Printed with permission: Baliga RR. *Saunders/Elsevier* 2007, pages 442 and 443.

- Give 8 classes of drugs that may cause dysglycemia*.
  - o Atypical antipsychotic agents, e.g.
    - – Clozapine
    - – Olanzapine
    - – Paliperidone
    - – Quetiapine
    - – Risperidone
  - o Beta-adrenergic antagonists, e.g.
    - – Atenolol
    - – Metoprolol
    - – Propranol[a]
  - o Diazoxide
  - o Glucocorticoids, e.g. prednisone
  - o Interferon-alfa
  - o Isoniazid
  - o Niacin
  - o Pentamidine
  - o Protease inhibitors (eg., amprenavir, atazanavir, darunavir, fosamprenavir, indinavir, lopinavir, nelfinavir, ritonavir, saquinavir, tiprenavir)
  - o Tacrolimus
  - o Thiazide or loop diuretics, e.g.,
    - – Furosemide
    - – Hydrochlorothiazide

[a] Medication-induced dysglycemia should not preclude the use of these medications if clinically indicated

Reproduced with permission: Therapeutics Choices. Sixth Edition. Ottawa, Canada: *Canadian Pharmacist Association* 2012, Table 1, page 381.

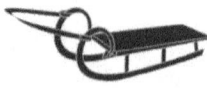

- Give a **classification** of oral hypoglycemic agents.

  o 2-glucosidase inhibitor

  o Amylinomimetics

  o Biguanides

  o DDP-4 inhibitor

  o GLP-1 mimetics

  o Meglitinides

  o Sulfonylureas

  o Thiazolidinediones

- Give the **mechanism(s) of action** of types of oral hypoglycemic drugs used to treat type II DM.

  o Gut
  - A-glucosidase inhibitor
    - ↓ / slow CHO absorption
  - Incretin modulators
    - GLP-1 mimetics
      - Activate GLP-1 receptors
      - ↓ glucagon
      - ↑ insulin secretion (glucose dependent)
        - ↓ gastric emptying
        - ↑ satiety
      - ↓ Hg A1C
      - May be given by injection to supplement a combination of oral agents to result in
        - ↓ body weight
        - ↓ blood sugar, with hypoglycemia
    - DPP-IV inhibitors
  - Bile acid sequestration
    - Mechanism of hypoglycemia unknown
  o Liver
  - Biguanides
    - ↓ hepatic production of glucose
  - Thiazolidinediones
    - ↓ hepatic production of glucose
    - ↑ PPAR γ → ↑ peripheral sensitivity to insulin

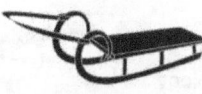

- Note
    - NYHA class II HF (heart failure) – not recommended
    - Class III or IV HF – contraindicated

- Pancreas
    - Sulfonylureas (long-acting)
        - Bind to sulfonylurea receptor on B-celss
        - ↑ insulin release
    - Glinides (short acting)

Abbreviations: DPP-IV, dipeptidyl peptidase IV; GIP, gastric inhibitory peptide; GLP-1, glucagon-like peptidase I, PPAR γ, peroxisome proliferator-activated receptor-γ

Tips to using insulin, based on the source of the sugar

- Fasting BS (intrinsic)
    - Hepatic production of glucose
        - Use long-acting insulin (glargine, detemir)

- PC BS
    - Absorbed glucose (extrinsic)
        - Use rapid-acting insulin (lispro, aspart, glulisine) ~ 1 insulin unit per 15 g CHO intake 1-2 units for every 2.2-2.8 mmol/L (40-50 mg/dL) above target premeal BS
        - ↓ risk of hypoglycemia (when correct dose is given, of course)

- If there are troublesome postprandial fluctuations of blood sugar concentration, consider adding a rapid-acting insulin and analogue (such as lispro, aspart, glulisine)

- May need to be used in T2DM with fasting hyperglycemia despite combined oral agents

Abbreviations: BS, (plasma) blood sugar concentration; PC, after meal

---

A Gem and a Pearl: The sulfonylurea (glyburide) and the biguanide (metformin) should **not** be used in the diabetic with kidney disease.

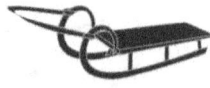

A.B.R. Thomson

- Give the definition of the "**dawn phenomenon**" in type I diabetes mellitus; provide the pathogenesis and the recommended treatment.

  - Definition "An increase in the blood glucose levels during the early moving hours (4am-8 am)"

  - Pathogenesis
    - Early am ↑ GH and other insulin "counterregulatory hormones"

  - Management
    - Use NHP insulin at bedtime rather than at supper
    - Continuous SC insulin infusion

Diabetic Ketoacidosis (DKA)

➢ Definition
   - Arterial blood pH ≤ 7.30
   - HCO_3^- ≤ 15 mEq/L
   - Glucose ≥ 250 mg/dL
   - Anion gap
   - Serum ketones

A Gem and a Pearl

In DKA, the hyperglycemia may be only modest; it is the anion gap (AG) acidosis which is so important. So, "follow the AG" (Anion Gap) closely to "close the gap".

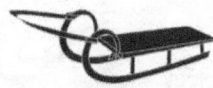

➢ Pathogenesis

- Give the pathogenesis of diabetic ketoacidosis (DKA).

    o May occur in both type I and II DM.

    o Simplified pathogenesis

    o $\downarrow\downarrow$ insulin → ↑ glucagon → ↑ BS

    o Muscle
      – ↓ Uptake of glucose

    o Liver
      – ↑ production of glucose
      – ↑ FFA → ↑ B-hydroxybutyrate⌐ → metabolic acidosis (anion group)
      ⌊ ↑ acetoacetate → diuresis

Plus K^+ (K^+ Use potassium ↑ hosphate), 20 mmol/L (20 mEq/L) unless K^+ > 5.0 mmol/L (5.0 mEq/L)

➢ Treatment
    o IV fluids to correct dehydration and ↓ risk of hypokalemia as K^+ moves into cells as acidosis is corrected.

    o IV insulin to correct
      – ↑ BS, ↑ FFA, ↑ ketones, ↑ H^+ (metabolic acidosis)
      – No more ketones
      – No more anion gap

A type 1 diabetic with DKA is treated with insulin and glucose infusions which is effective reducing the acidosis and ketones. The infusion are stopped when the anion gap is 16 mEq/L and the ketones are falling, but the DKA relapses.

- Give the explanation for the relapse of the DKA.

    o In DKA, ↓insulin → ↑ ketones → ↑ AG (anion gap)

    o When Na^+ is ↑/N, switch to 5% D / 0.45% saline

    o Insulin infusion plus glucose infusion until the AG < 12 mEq/L

    o In this patient the insulin / glucose infusion was stopped before the ketones were completely cleared; reducing the insulin before the ketones are cleared will cause a relapse of DKA.

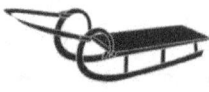

- Perform a focused physical examination to differentiate DKA from HONC.

	DKA	HONC
o CNS	– Normal, to coma	Drowsy CVA
o CVS	– Hypotension (including postural changes) – Tachycardia	Myocardial infarction Peripheral vascular disease DVT
o Respiratory	– Rate ↑ – Depth ↑ (Kussmaul breathing) – Ketotic breath	Pulmonary embolus
o GI	– Succussion splash (gastroparesis)	

Abbreviations: CVA, cerebrovascular accident; DKA, diabetic ketoacidosis; DVT, deep vein thrombosis; HONC, hyperosmolar non-ketotic coma

Adapted from: Davey P. *Wiley-Blackwell* 2006, page 282

Patients with diabetes acidosis have a metabolic acidosis with respiratory compensation (**Kussmaul breathing**)

- Give the reasons why it is **not recommended** to administer HCO3⁻ when the arterial pH < 7.0 (risk of cardiac dysfunction).

    o Possible development of ↓↓ K+, leading to arrhythmias

    o Risk of developing respiratory alkalosis if too much HCO3- is given, thereby removing the drive for the respiratory compensation of the metabolic acidosis.

    o Correction alkalosis may occur once production of ketone bodies stops

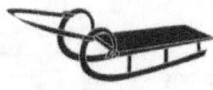

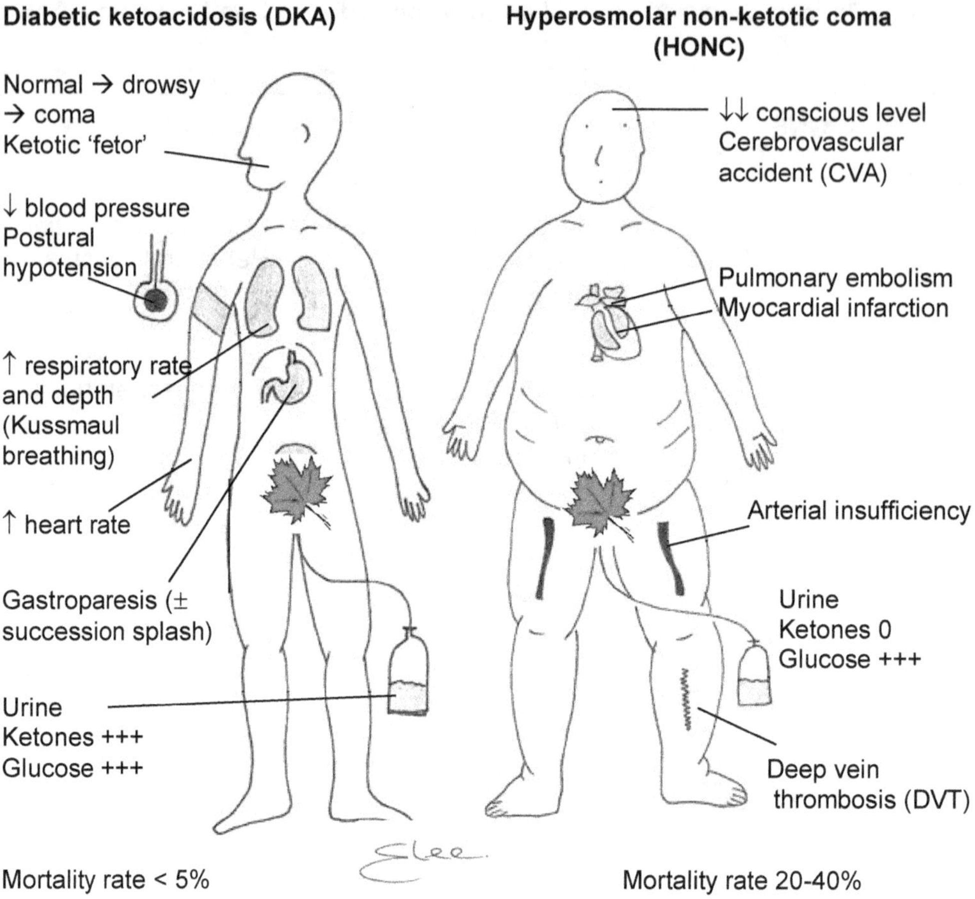

Diabetic ketoacidosis (DKA)

Hyperosmolar non-ketotic coma (HONC)

Normal → drowsy
→ coma
Ketotic 'fetor'

↓↓ conscious level
Cerebrovascular
accident (CVA)

↓ blood pressure
Postural
hypotension

Pulmonary embolism
Myocardial infarction

↑ respiratory rate
and depth
(Kussmaul
breathing)

↑ heart rate

Arterial insufficiency

Gastroparesis (±
succession splash)

Urine
Ketones 0
Glucose +++

Urine
Ketones +++
Glucose +++

Deep vein
thrombosis (DVT)

Mortality rate < 5%

Mortality rate 20-40%

Management of DKA
IV fluids
IV insulin
IV KCl (after insulin
and fluids)
Treatment of
underlying cause

Investigations	DKA	HONC
Glucose	↑	↑↑
Na	→	↑↑
Urea	↑	↑↑
pH	↓	→
Serum osmolality	↑	↑↑

Abbreviations: CVA, cerebrovascular accident; DVT, deep vein thrombosis

Adapted from: Davey P. *Wiley-Blackwell* 2006, page 282.

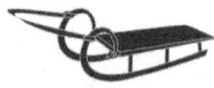

Hyperglycemic Hyperosmolar Syndrome (HHS)

- o Elderly type II diabetes with altered nutrition plus dehydration

- o Precipitory factor → counter regulatory factors → hyperglycemia → ↑ fluid loss by kidneys → ability of kidneys too excrete glucose is exceeded → ↑↑ BS, ↑↑ osmolality

- ➢ Definition
  - o Plasma
    - – > 320 mOsm/ Kg H_2O
    - – > 600 mg/dL glucose
    - – No / few ketones
  - o Arterial pH / HCO_3 near normal

- • Give the treatment of HHS (hyperglycemic hyperosmolar syndrome).

  - o Identify and correct precipitating cause

  - o Correct extracellular space 0.9% saline

  - o Correct intracellular space when normal
    - – BP (blood pressure)
    - – UO (urine output)
    - – Hypotonic solution

  - o Insulin
    - – IV once BP/UO corrected and treatment has begun to correct intravascular space
    - – SC once
      - ▪ Plasma glucose < 200 mg/dL
      - ▪ Patient conscious and eating

Diabetic Nephropathy

- ➢ Terms
  - o Microalbuminuria
    - – 30-300 mg/d
  - o Macoalbunuria
    - – > 300 mg/d
  - o Nephrotic syndrome
    - – > 3,500 mg/d

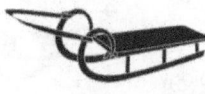

➢ Treatment
- o Angiotension-converting enzyme inhibitor (ACE) or angiotensin-II receptor blockers (ARBs) are for
  - – Normal BP plus microalbuminuria, or
  - – Hypertension, and
  - – ARB for macroalbuminemia

- o Note: avoid ACEI / ARB if renal dysfunction is already present

- o Close control of blood sugar

Diabetic Neuropathy

➢ Types
- o Mononeuropathies
  - – Cranial nerve
  - – Peripheral nerve
- o Polyneuopathies
- o Radiculopathies (spinal nerve roots)
- o Autonomic neuropathic

• Perform a focused physical examination for diabetic neuropathy.

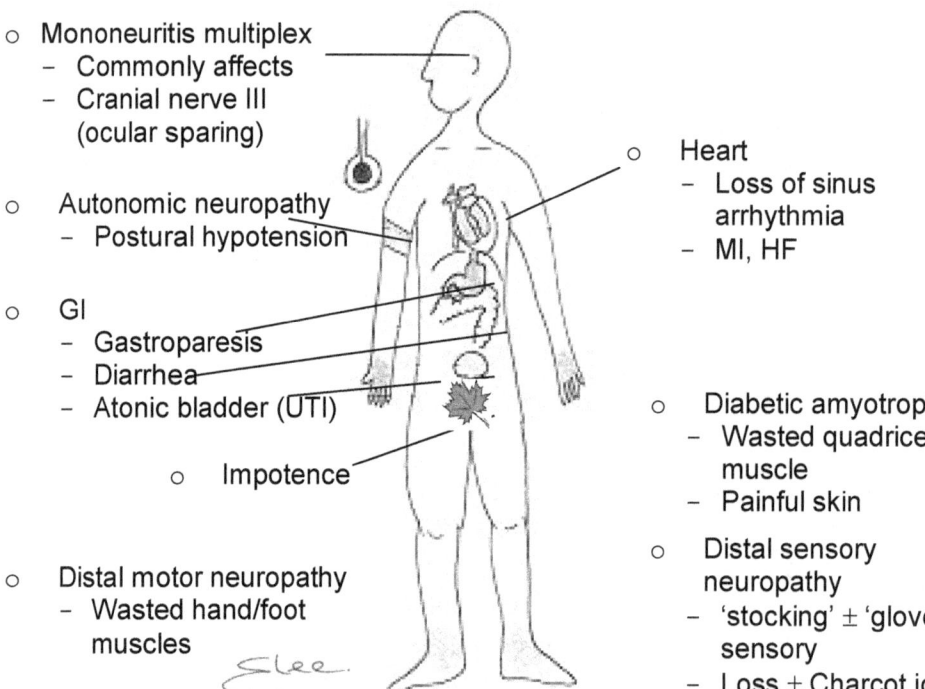

- o Mononeuritis multiplex
  - – Commonly affects
  - – Cranial nerve III (ocular sparing)

- o Autonomic neuropathy
  - – Postural hypotension

- o GI
  - – Gastroparesis
  - – Diarrhea
  - – Atonic bladder (UTI)

  - o Impotence

- o Distal motor neuropathy
  - – Wasted hand/foot muscles

- o Heart
  - – Loss of sinus arrhythmia
  - – MI, HF

- o Diabetic amyotrophy
  - – Wasted quadriceps muscle
  - – Painful skin

- o Distal sensory neuropathy
  - – 'stocking' ± 'glove' sensory
  - – Loss ± Charcot joint

Abbreviations: HF, heart failure; MI, myocardial infarction; UTI, urinary tract infection

Adapted from: Davey P. *Wiley-Blackwell* 2006, page 280.

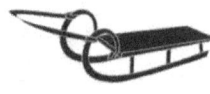

- Give the **symptom complexes** suggesting autonomic neuropathy.

  - o CVS
    - – Resting tachycardia
    - – Failure of ↑ HR in response to Valsalva maneuver, standing, deep breathing
    - – Orthostatic hypotension
    - – SCD (sudden cardiac death)

  - o GI
    - – Gastroparesis
    - – Diarrhea

  - o GU
    - – Atonic bladder
    - – Erectile dysfunction

A Gem and a Pearl: In the diabetic with autonomic (cardiovascular) neuropathy, investigate for unrecognised coronary artery disease

---

➤ Treatment

- Give **classes of medication** to treat the pain of neuopathy.

  - o SSRI / SSHRI (selective serotonin reuptake inhibitors / partial serotonin and norepinephrine reuptake inhibitors)
  - o TCA (tricyclic antidepressants)
  - o Antiseizure drugs
    - – Gabapentrin
    - – Phenytoin
    - – Carbamazepine

Quick reminder: **All** DM > 40 yr should be on daily ASA.

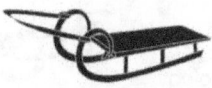

Hypoglycemia in Non-diabetics

➢ Pathogenesis

- Give the pathogenesis of hypoglycemia in non-diabetics.
  - o Postprandial (reactive) hypoglycemia
    - – Definition: Hypoglycemia within 30-60 min of a meal of particularly low-complex (simple) carbohydrates (CHO)
    - – Likely due to slow gastric emptying followed by sudden "dumping" of dietary CHO, which leads to rapid release of insulin, without normal continued emptying of CHO from stomach (mismatching of luminal CHO and insulin release)
  - o Fasting hypoglycemia
    - – Exogenous
      - ▪ Inadvertent or surreptitious use of oral hypoglycemias or insulin

➢ Causes

- Take a directed history and perform a focused physical examination in the adult to determine the causes of hypoglycemia.

  - o Hereditary
    - – Inborn errors of metabolism
  - o Starvation and exercise
  - o Reaction to glucose ingestion
    - – Early diabetes mellitus
    - – Functional
    - – Post gastrectomy
    - – Rapid gastric emptying
  - o B cell overactivity
    - – Insulinoma
    - – Islet cell hyperplasia
  - o Endocrine disease
    - – B-cell hyperplasia
    - – Early diabetes mellitus
    - – Hypoadrenalism
    - – Hypopituitarism
    - – Hypothyroidism
    - – Insulinoma

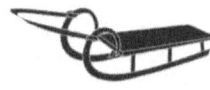

- o Drugs / toxins
  - Alcohol
  - Antihistamines
  - Insulin
  - Salicylates (ASA)
  - Sulphonylureas and diguanides
  - Tobacco
- o Sensitivity to:
  - Alcohol
  - Galactose, fructose
  - Leucine
  - Tobacco
- o Liver disease
  - Cirrhosis
  - Glycogen storage disease
  - HCC
  - Hepatoma
- o Tumors
  - Adrenal tumor
  - Hepatocellular (HCC)
  - Insulinoma
  - Sarcoma / fibrosarcoma (mediastinal, retroperitoneal)

Adapted from: Burton JL. *Churchill Livingstone* 1971, page 93.

➢ Laboratory

- Give the way in which measurement of blood C-peptide concentration helps to distinguish the fasting hypoglycemia and hyperinsulinemia of inadvertent / surreptitious use of oral hypoglycemic or insulin, versus diabetes.

	Blood concentration		
Drug use	Sugar	Insulin	C-peptide
o Insulin (exogenous) injection	↓	↑	↓
o Insulin secretagogues (endogenous insulin)	↓	↑	↑

- o Endogenous fasting hypoglycemia (↑ utilization of glucose)
  - Causes
    - Insulinoma
    - Islet cell hyperplasia (e.g. after bariatric surgery)
    - Nesidioblastosis (rapidly growing tumors)
    - Tumors producing insulin-like growth factors

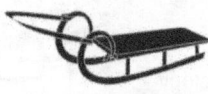

- Diagnosis (suspicion)
- Symptoms of hypoglycemia, with supervised 72-hr fast, with BS < 2.5 mmol/L (< 45 mg/dL)
- Inappropriate hyperinsulinemia > 36-43 pmol/L (> 5-6 micro U/L)
  o Find tumor
    - CT, MRI, EUS, octreotide scan
  o ↓ supply of glucose (deficiency of gluconeogenic substrate)
    - GI
      • Starvation, malnutrition
      • Alcohol
    - Liver (↓ production of glucose)
      • Sepsis
    - Endocrine
      • Addison disease
      • ↓ cortisol
      • Hypopituitarism
        – ↓ ACTH (adrenocorticotropic gland)
        – DH (growth hormone)

A Gem and a Pearl:
  o Define: "**hypoglycemia unawareness**"; give its pathophysiology and management
  o Hypoglycemia occurs without warning, with the diabetic suddenly losing consciousness
  o Definition: especially in type I DM, the usual symptoms of hypoglycemia (tachycardia, anxiety, sweating, tremor) are replaced by CNS symptoms (confusion, attend personality, loss of consciousness
  o Pathogenesis: Repeated episodes of several hypoglycemia, leading to loss of usual adrenergic symptoms of hypoglycemia.
  o Management: ↓ doses of insulin → ↓ episodes of severe hypoglycemia, allowing "...the brain to adapt to the new ambient glycemia so that the normal adrenergic responses to hypoglycemia can be re-established."
  o Treatment
    - Short term
      • Glucagon
      • Rapid acting carbohydrate
    - Long term
      • For several weeks reduce the patient's dose of insulin to "reset" sensitivity to hypoglycemia

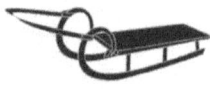

- Give the complications of hypoglycemia (Usually related to diabetic treatment).

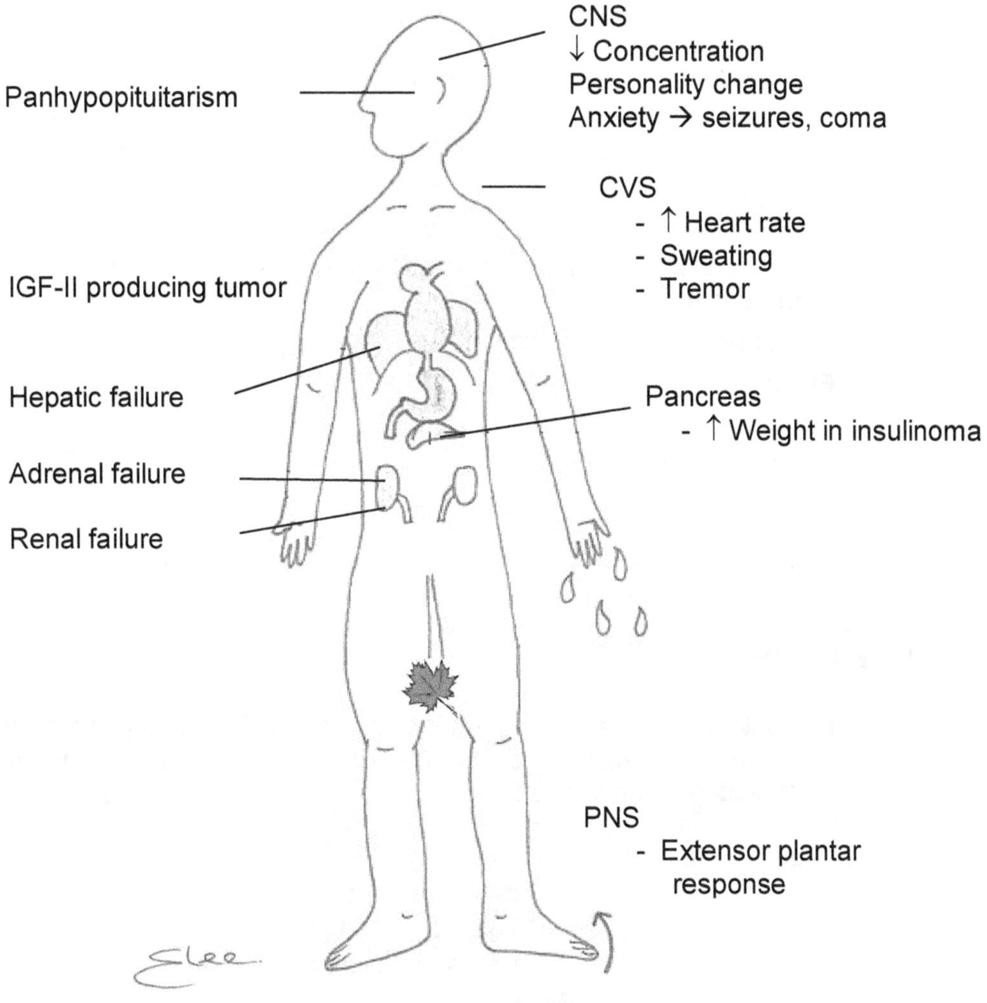

Panhypopituitarism

CNS
↓ Concentration
Personality change
Anxiety → seizures, coma

CVS
- ↑ Heart rate
- Sweating
- Tremor

IGF-II producing tumor

Hepatic failure

Pancreas
- ↑ Weight in insulinoma

Adrenal failure

Renal failure

PNS
- Extensor plantar response

ELee.

Abbreviations: CNS, central nervous system; CVS, cardiovascular system; PNS, peripheral nervous system

Adapted from: Davey P. *Wiley-Blackwell* 2006, page 280.

Yes or No, True or False

"Close control of blood glucose with insulin reduces in hospital mortality from diabetes"
YES – A reasonable ICU target of random blood sugar is 140 to 200 mg/dL.

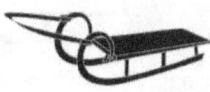

GESTATIONAL DIABETES

- Give risks of untreated gestational diabetes.

    o Mother, ↑ risk of
    - Accelerated renal dysfunction (leading to chronic renal failure (if serum Cr [creatinine] > 3 mg/dL, or CrCl [creatinine clearance] < 50 ml/min per 1.73 m^2)
    - Accelerate diabetic retinopathy
    - Future DMt2 (requires eye screening every trimester) then annually thereafter)
    - Postpartum hypothyroidism
    o Fetus
    - ↑ risk
      - Congenital malformations
      - Fetal loss

Note: Before pregnancy, **stop** ACE inhibitors, ARBs and statins.

HYPERLIPIDEMIA

- In the context of cardiac risk reduction, take a directed history and perform a focused physical examination for risk factors for which screening of the lipid-profile is recommended.

    o Age   – Children
            - Family history of
              – Hypercholesterolemia
              – Chylomicronemia
            – Men
              - ≥ 40 years
            – Women
              - > 50 years, or postmenopausal

    o Life style   – Sedentary lifestyle
                 – Alcohol
                 – Cigarette smoking (current)

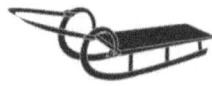

- o Skin
  - – Premature arcus conealis
  - – Psoriasis
  - – Xanthomes
  - – Xanthelasmas

- o CVS
  - – Artherosclerosis
  - – CAD in first-degree relative < 60 years
  - – Hypertension

- o Liver
  - – Cholestasis
  - – Acute intermittent porphyria

- o Kidney
  - – eGFR < 60 mL/min/1.73 m^2 (chronic renal disease)
  - – Nephrotic syndrome
  - – Renal insufficiency

- o Infection
  - – HIV treated with HAART

- o Inflammation, chronic e.g.
  - – Rheumatoid arthritis
  - – Dysglobulinemias
  - – Systemic lupus erythematosus

- o Endocrine
  - – Diabetes mellitus
  - – Hypothyroidism
  - – Metabolic syndrome
  - – Obesity

- o Medications
  - – BB (beta blockers "without intrinsic sympathomimetric or alpha-blocking activity")
  - – Corticosteroids
  - – Diuretics (thiazides)
  - – HAART (highly active antiretroviral therapy)
  - – Estrogens
  - – Progestins
  - – Anabolic steroids
  - – HRT (hormone replacement therapy)
  - – OCA (oral contraceptive agents)

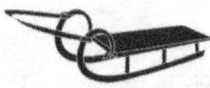

o Nutrition   – Anorexia nervosa
                           – Hypertriglyceridemia
                           – Obesity
                           – Hypothyroidism

   o Post-transplantation (possibly due to anti-rejection medication)

Abbreviations: HDL-C, high density lipoprotein cholesterol; LDL-C, low density lipoprotein cholesterol

Adapted from: Roederer GO, et al. Chapter 34. In: Therapeutic Choices. Grey J, Ed. 6th Edition, *Canadian Pharmacists Association* 2012, page 432 and 433; Ghosh AK. *Mayo Clinic Scientific Press* 2008, Table 6-4, page 233.

➢ Useful background: **International Diabetes Federation Classification** of the Metabolic Syndrome

Risk factor	Defining level
o Central obesity*	Waist circumference
– Europids	Men ≥ 94 cm; Women ≥ 80 cm
– South Asians	Men ≥ 94 cm; Women ≥ 80 cm
– Chinese	Men ≥ 94 cm; Women ≥ 80 cm
– Japanese	Men ≥ 94 cm; Women ≥ 80 cm
– Ethnic South and Central Americans, First Nations	Use South Asian recommendations until more specific data are available
– Eastern Mediterranean and Middle East (Arabic) populations, Sub-Saharan Africans	Use European data until more specific data are available
o Triglyceride level	≥ 1.7 mmol/L
o HDL-C level	
– Men	< 1.0 mmol/L
– Women	< 1.3 mmol/L
– Blood pressure	≥ 130/85 mm Hg
– Fasting glucose level	5.7-7.0 mmol/L

*Criteria: central obesity required, plus 2 or more other risk factors.

Abbreviations: HDL-C, high density lipoprotein cholesterol

Reproduced with permission: Therapeutics Choices. Sixth Edition. Ottawa, Canada: Canadian Pharmacist Association 2012, Table 2, page 436.

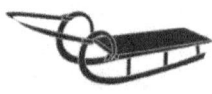

Hypertriglyceridemia and Cardiovascular Risk

- o Persons at ↑ cardiovascular risk include these with
  - – Metabolic syndrome
  - – Diabetes
  - – End-stage renal disease
  - – Renal transplantation patients
  - – Those with family history
  - – Various laboratory measures may be used to calculate a risk score, such as hsCRP, apolipoprotein B, cholesterol (LDL, HDL, non-HDL-C).

Hypertriglyceridemia is a risk factor for the development of CHD (coronary heart disease).

- Give the conditions under which the serum triglyceride concentration may be associated with increased cardiovascular risk.
  - o Atherogenic dyslipidemias (e.g. familial combined hyperlipidemia)
  - o Chronic renal failure
  - o Diabetes
  - o Insulin resistance

- Give the circumstances when moderate hypertriglyceride (2.26-5.64 mmol/L, 200-499 mg/dL) is not treated.
  - o ↑ serum triglyceride concentrations are not treated if the non-HDL cholesterol is normal

Said differently, moderate hypertriglyceride is treated if non-HDL cholesterol is elevated

- Give the difference in the LDL cholesterol (LDL-C), and the non-HDL cholesterol (non-HDL-C).
  - o Non-HDL-C = LDL-C plus 0.78 mmol/L (30 mg/dL)

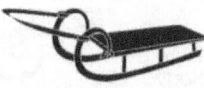

Tricks and Red Herrings
- ○ ↑ LDL-C (cholesterol) is treated with statin or statin plus bile acid sequestration (BAS)
- ○ If ↓ HDL-C
  - – Treat with nicotinic and fibrate
- ○ If ↑ TG (triglyceride)
  - – Treatment depends on LDL and level of ↑ TG

    - ↑TG   - Fibrate or nicotinic acid

    - ↑↑TG (> 400 mg/dL)   - Statin

    - ↑TG + ↑LDL-C   - Do not use BAS

DIABETES INSIPIDUS

- • Give the type and causes of diabetes insipidus.

- ➢ Types
  - ○ Central posterior pituitary defect)
    - – ↓ synthesis of AVP (arginine vasopressin)
  - ○ Nephrogenic
    - – ↓ action of AVP on kidney

- ➢ Causes
  - ○ Hypothalamic mass
  - ○ Traumatic brain injury
  - ○ Infiltration of posterior pituitary
    - – Sarcoidosis
    - – Langerhans cell histocytosis
  - ○ Drugs
  - ○ Unconsciousness (water deprivation)
  - ○ Pregnancy (↑ placental vassopressinase → ↑ breakdown of AVP)

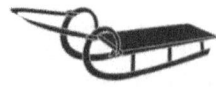

A Gem and a Pearl:

- o DI plus thickened stalk of pituitary on diagnostic imaging suspect infiltration of the hypothalamus
  - – Sarcoidosis
  - – Langerhans cell histiocytosis

➢ Diagnosis

• Give the diagnosis of DI.

- o Failure to normally increase in urinary hyperosmolality following water deprivation and desprivation and desmopressin
- o Water deprivation
  - – Normal
    > 800 mOsm/kg
  - – DI
    < 300 mOSm/kg
- o Desmopressin 5 µm intranasal
  - – Central DI
    50% ↑
  - – Nephrogenic DI
    Almost no response

A Gem and a Pearl

If a patient with DI is on a fixed dose of despressin, and by habit they continue to ingest large amounts of water, hyponatremia may occur.

"Quality is about mastery."

Research and education will never succeed without quality of patient care.

James Calvin

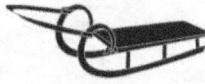

THYROID DISEASE

➢ Laboratory

- Give **tests of Thyroid Function.**
  - o Routine measurements
    - – TRH and TSH stimulate secretion of active T4 (thyroxine) from the thyroid gland, small amounts of which are acted upon by 5'-deiodinase in the periphery to T3 (triiodothyronine).
    - – Level of TSH does not necessarily correlate with symptoms
    - – When T3 and T4 are bound to proteins (albumin, prealbumin, TBG [thyroxine-binding globulin]), they are inactive.
    - – Only free T4 is available to act as a prohormone to form T3.
    - – The "gold standard" for measuring T4 is equilibrium dialysis, with confirmation if necessary using the T4 antibody assay (if the results of testing give T4 and TSH levels which do not correlate with the clinical picture, suspect that there may be antibodies to T4).
  - o Antibodies
    - – The presence in serum of anti-thyroid peroxidase antibody, and anti-thyroglobulin antibody may not sufficiently high in Hashimoto thyroiditis to cause clinical hypothyroidism (with ↑ TSH concentrations)
    - – Antibodies to the TSH receptor (anti-TSI [thyroid stimulating immunoglobulins) and anti-TBII [thyrotropin-binding inhibitory immunoglobulins]) are pathognomic for Graves disease diagnostic use
  - o Measuring TSI or TBII may be useful
    - – To predict the course of the thyroid disease
      - ▪ ↑ TSI   – Graves disease in pregnancy
                       – Euthyroid ophthalmopathy
      - ▪ ↑ TBII   – As above, plus
                       – Graves disease, in which there is hypothyroidism which fluctuates with hyperthyroid with hyperthyroidism.
  - o Serum thyroglobulin (TG)
    - – A glycoprotein used to store T4
    - – Subacute / destructive thyroidism

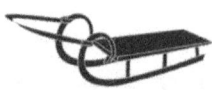

- ↓ TG
  - Surreptitious intake of T4
  - Marker for effective therapy (surgery, radioactive iodine ablation therapy) of papillary or follicular thyroid cancer.
- o Calcitonin
  - ↑ in medullary thyroid cancer

➢ Diagnostic imaging
- o RAIU (radioactive iodine uptake)

– ↑ RAIU	Thyrotoxicosis	Uptake of I* is not appropriate for the function of the thyroid – this a frequent "trick" in MCQs
– ↓ RAIU	Thyroiditis	

Surreptitious intake of T4

- o Thyroid scan
  - Pattern of uptake
    - Diffuse
  - Graves disease
    - Focal
      - Nodules
        - Solitary, often autonomous
        - Multiple-toxic multinodular gioter (TMG)

- o Thyroid ultrasound, with colour-flow Doppler
  - Useful when RAIU or scan cannot be performed, such as
    - During pregnancy
    - While breast feeding
    - Flow
      - ↑ flow
        - Hyperthyroidism
      - ↓ flow
        - Thyroiditis

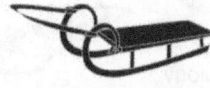

> A Gem and a Pearl: Thyroglobulin in antibodies will cause ↓ TG and give a false impression of satisfactory therapy for thyroid tumors.
>
> Learning Point: Measure serum thyroglobulin plus thyroglobulin antibodies

➤ Clinical

• Take a directed history for thyroid disease.

- o Condition
  - − Medications, allergies, smoking
  - − History of major illnesses (especially autoimmune)
  - − Hospitalizations/surgeries
  - − Radiation exposure (especially neck)
  - − Family history of multiple endocrine neoplasia, medullary cancer or other cancers/lumps
  - − Person history of goiter or nodules
  - − Family history of goitre or nodules
- o History of HIV status/risk factors, smoking, alcohol, drug usage

- o Causes /associations
  - − Diabetes mellitus
    - ▪ Polyuria, polydipsia, thirst, blurred vision, weakness, infections, groin itch, rash (pruritus vulvae, balanitis), weight loss, tiredness, lethargy, and disturbance of conscious state
  - − Hypoglycemia
    - ▪ Morning headaches, weight gain, seizures, sweating
  - − Primary adrenal insufficiency
    - ▪ Pigmentation, tiredness, loss of weight, anorexia, nausea, diarrhea, nocturia, mental changes, seizures (hypotension, hypoglycemia)
    - ▪ Acromegaly
    - ▪ Fatigue, weakness, increased sweating, heat intolerance, weight gain, enlarging hands and feet, enlarged and coarsened facial features, headaches, decreased vision, voice change, decreased libido, impotence.

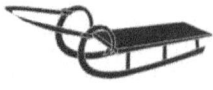

- o Complications
  - – Goiter
    - Dysphagia
    - Neck swelling
    - Stridor
  - – CNS
    - Fatigue, weakness, tremor
    - Dysphagia
  - – GI
    - Diarrhea/constipation
    - Weight change
  - – GU
    - Decreased menses or fertility
    - Polyuria
  - – Thyrotoxicosis
    - Preference for cooler weather
    - Weight loss
    - Increased appetite (polyphagia)
    - Palpitations
    - Increased sweating
    - Nervousness
    - Irritability
    - Diarrhea
    - Amenorrhea
    - Muscle weakness
    - Exertional dyspnea
  - – Hypothyroidism
    - Fatigue
    - Cold intolerance
    - Slowing of mental and physical performance
    - Hoarseness
    - Enlarged tongue
    - Slow pulse
    - Pericardial effusion
    - Anorexia
    - Weight gain
    - Constipation

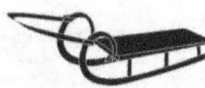

- Paresthesia
- Slow speech
- Muscle cramps
- Slow relaxation of reflexes
- Menorrhagia
- Amenorrhea
- Anovulatory cycles
- Periorbital edema
- Rough skin
- Dry coarse hair
- Anemia

➢ Differential diagnosis
- o Thyroid tumor (benign vs. malignant)
- o Goitre
- o Thyroid cyst
- o Thyroglossal duct cyst

Adapted from: Talley NJ, et al. *Maclennan & Petty Pty Limited*, 2003, Table 9.5, page 318; and Jugovic PJ, et al. *Saunders/ Elsevier* 2004, pages 152 and 153.

- Perform a focused physical examination for thyroid disease.

  - o Neck mass (goiter)
    - – Inspection
      - Nutritional status
      - General appearance
      - Anatomical landmarks of thyroid
      - Mass, tenderness
      - Effect of swallowing
    - – Palpation
      - Positioning, with and without swallowing
      - Gland size, consistency, tenderness and nodularity
      - Module location, size and number, character, tenderness
    - – Auscultation
      - Bruit

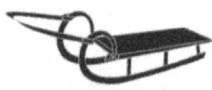

- o CNS
  - – Tremor
  - – Weakness
  - – Hypo-/ hyperreflexia

- o Eyes
  - – Chemosis (conjuntival edema) and hyperemia, periorbital edema
  - – Corneal exposure with ulceration
  - – Widening of the palpebral fissure (thyroid stare)
  - – Lid retraction (widening of palpebral fissure) or lid lag on downgaze (von Graefe sign)
  - – Exophthalmos
  - – Proptosis
  - – Double vision
  - – Visual loss from optic nerve compression and edema)

- o Voice
  - – Hoarse
  - – Stridor

- o CVS
  - – Palpitations, hypertension, tachycardia
  - – Deep tendon reflexes

- o GI
  - – Dysphagia
  - – Diarrhea/constipation
  - – Weight change

- o Skin
  - – Sweating
  - – Pretibial, myxedema
  - – Thinning of hair
  - – Pigmentation

Adapted from: Talley NJ, et al. *Maclennan & Petty Pty Limited* 2003, Table 9.1, page 308; Table 9.2, page 311, Table 9.5, page 318; Baliga RR. *Saunders/Elsevier* 2007, page 353- 356; Jugovic PJ, et al. *Saunders/ Elsevier* 2004, page 152; Mangione S. *Hanley & Belfus* 2000, pages 81 and 82.

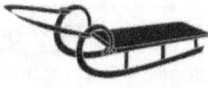

Useful background: Likelihood ratios for palpable thyroid gland indicating a goiter

Palpable thyroid	PLR	NLR
o Adults*	3.8	0.37
o Children	3.0	0.30
o Pregnancy	4.7	0.08

* Sensitivity 70% (95% CI 68%-73%), Specificity   82%   (95% CI 79%-85%)

Source: Simel DL, et al. *JAMA* 2009 Chapter 21, Table 21-10, page 287.

Some useful stats

	↑ size of thyroid nodules
o Benign	≤ 1/3 ↑ in size
o Malignant	Suspect when size ↑ > 50%

CLINICAL CHALLENGE

A patient presents with a firm but painful thyroid gland after a recent viral infection. There are no autoimmune markers. There were both symptoms and signs of hyperthyroidism.

- Give the likely cause of and mechanism for the clinical presentation.

  o Destruction of thyroid from de Quervain non-autoimmune thyroiditis
  o The destruction from thyroiditis releases preformed thyroid hormone into circulation
  o ↑ Circulating thyroid hormone →hyperthyroidism

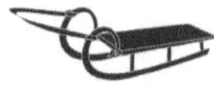

Thyroid Nodule and Goiter

➢ Definition of Goiter
  o A chronically enlarged thyroid gland due to hypertrophy or degeneration
  o Not due to neoplasia or inflammation
  o The term goiter does not reflect the functional status of the gland.
    – The performance characteristics of physical examination for detecting goiter are good
    – Sensitivity 70% (95% CI = 68 to 73%)
    – Specificity 82% (95% CI = 79 to 85%)
    – PLR = 3.8
    – NLR = 0.37

	For assessing thyroid size PLR
▪ Normal (0-20 gm)	0.15
▪ Small (1-2x normal: 20 to 40 gm)	1.9 (size tends to be overestimated)
▪ Large > 2x normal (> 40 gm)	25 (size tends to be underestimated)

  o Note
    – These characteristics are not influenced by the presence of thyroid nodules.

• Give the meaning of sensitivity, specificity, PLR, NLR.

  o PLR (positive likelihood ratio) = sensitivity/ (1-specificity) [PID/ (1-NIH)] the finding is more likely with than without the target disorder (probability of disease increases)
  o NLR (negative likelihood ratio) = 1- sensitivity/ specificity [(1-PID)/ NIH] the finding is less likely without than with the target disorder (probability of disease decreases
  o Sensitivity – PID (positive in disease)
  o Specificity – NIH (negative in health)

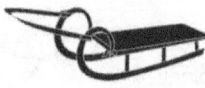

- Take a directed history and perform a focused physical examination to determine if a thyroid nodule is likely to be malignant.

➢ History
  o Age < 30 years old or > 60 years old
  o Single nodules
  o History of head or neck irradiation
  o Compressive symptoms (pain, dysphagia, stridor, hoarseness)

➢ Physical exam
  o Fixed and firm solitary nodule with enlarged regional lymph nodes

- Give the types of thyroid nodules / goiter and their causes.

➢ Type of thyroid disease
  o Benign nodules
    - Follicular adenoma
    - Hashimoto thyroiditis
    - Hürthle adenoma
    - Multinodular goitre
  o Malignant nodules
    - Papillary
    - Follicular
    - Medullary, anaplastic
    - 1° lymphoma
    - Metastatic (breast or kidney tumors)

➢ Causes of a diffuse goitre (patient often euthyroid)
  o Idiopathic (majority)
  o Puberty or pregnancy
  o Thyroiditis
    - Hashimoto
    - Subacute (gland usually tender)
  o Simple goitre (iodine deficiency)
  o Goitregens, e.g. iodine excess, drugs (lithium, phenylbutazone)
  o Inborn errors of thyroid hormone synthesis, e.g. Pendred syndrome (an autosomal recessive condition associated with nerve deafness)

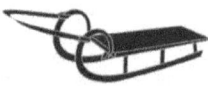

- Give the causes of solidary and diffuse types of thyroid nodules / goiter.

  o Benign
    - Dominant nodule in a multinodular goiter
    - Degeneration or hemorrhage into a colloid cyst or nodule
    - Follicular adenoma
    - Simple cyst (rare)
  o Malignant
    - Carcinoma – primary or secondary)e.g. renal wall carcinoma)
    - Lymphoma (rare)

- Give the changes on ultrasound of the neck / thyroid of the neck / thyroid which suggest thyroid nodule.
  o Solitary nodule
  o Irregular halo
  o Hypoechoic
  o Punctuate calcification
  o Increased blood flow

Adapted from: Scenarios for directed histories and physical examinations, Fundamental clinical situations, page 152 and 153; Talley N. J., et al. Clinical Examination: a Systematic Guide to Physical Diagnosis. *Maclennan & Petty Pty Limited*, East gardens, Australia, 2003, Table 9.3, page 314.

SO YOU WANT TO BE AN ENDOCRINOLOGIST!

- Give the meaning of the Pemberton sign, in the context of a thyroid mass.
  o " a reversible superior vena cava obstruction produced by a retroclavicular goitrous thyroid rising into the thoracic inlet"
  o If after raising the hands above the head for 3 minutes the person does not develop signs or symptoms of SVC obstruction, the sign is negative.
  o Other causes of SVC obstruction, such as lymphoma, or other tumors causing reversible may cause a positive Pemberten's sign, with blue/ pink face, dizziness, nasal congestion, obstruction of the thoracic outlet, dyspnea.

Source: Mangione S. *Hanley & Belfus* 2000, page 157

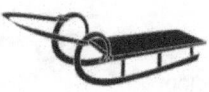

SO YOU WANT TO BE AN ENDOCRINOLOGIST!

- Give the circumstances may a bruit be head over a carcinoma of the thyroid.
  - When the uptake of radioactive iodine into the papillary or follicular carcinoma has been enhanced by increasing the blood supply to the thyroid with a drub such as carbimazole.

- Give the way on physical examination, when you find a midline mass, in the neck, to distinguish between a thyroid lesion and a thyroglossal cyst.
  - Both move on swallowing, but only the thyroglossal cyst moves when the tongue is protruded.

- Give the way to demonstrate a laryngocele.
  - A laryngocele may be demonstrated by performing the valsalva maneuver ("forced expiration against a closed glottis [bearing down], which increases intrathoracic and central nervous pressure, pushing on the diverticulum and making it more prominent in the area of the hyoid and thyroid cartilages.

- Give the ways to distinguish clubbing and bony enlargement from thyroid acropachy from pulmonary hypertrophic osteoarthropathy (periostits)
  - Thyroid periostitis – hands and feet, asymptomatic
  - Pulmonary hypertrophic osteoarthropathy – long bones

Source: Mangione S. *Hanley & Belfus* 2000, page 163.

In the context of thyroid disease, give the meaning of Berry sign.

Berry sign is the loss of the carotid pulse due to a thyroid malignancy causing enlargement of the thyroid to the point of blocking the carotid artery.

- Give the usual cause of unilateral proptosis.

  - Malignancy, not Graves disease (bilateral in 95%, thus unilateral in only 5%)

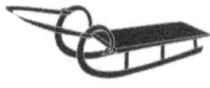

STRUCTURAL DISORDERS OF THE THYROID

- Give a classification of structural disorders of the thyroid.

  - Aberrant disorder
  - Cancer
  - Goiter
  - Nodules

Thyroid nodules

The patient with a thyroid nodule may have a normal, increased or decreased TSH level. A thyroid scan and a FNAB (fine needle aspiration biopsy) may be necessary to help determine if the nodule is malignant, and if surgical resection is indicated. It is suggested to "....consider surgery if 2 or more risk factors for malignancy are present" (Lochnan H, et al. Chapter 30. In: Therapeutic Choices. Grey J, Ed. 6th Edition, *Canadian Pharmacists Association* 2012, page 372).

- Give the risk factors for thyroid cancer.

  - The patient   –   < 20 or > 60 years of age
    -        – Male
    -        – Previous
      - Malignancy
      - Radiation exposure
    -        – Family history of thyroid cancer

  - The nodule   –   Nodule
    - \> 4 cm
    - Becoming rapidly larger
    - Fixed to soft tissue
    -        – Spread
      - Vocal cord paralysis
      - Lymphadenopathy

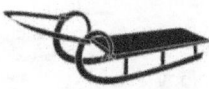

- Give a classification of **Thyroid Nodules**.

  o Benign
    - Adenoma
      - Nodule (cancer risk, 10%)
      - Hyperplasia
      - Follicular
      - Hurthle cell
      - Hyalinizing trabecular
    - Thyroglossal duct cyst
    - Pyramidal lobe
    - Lipoma
    - Dermoid cyst
    - Teratoma
    - Branchial cyst
    - Cervical nodes

  o Malignant
    - Papillary
    - Follicular
    - Medullary
    - Anaplastic
    - Lymphoma
    - Sarcoma
    - Metastatic
      - Melanoma
      - Breast
      - Kidney

Adapted from: MKSAP 15, Endocrinology and Metabolism, 2009, page32.

A thyroid hormone nodule is usually benign, but the risk of cancer is still 5-10%.

- Give factors associated with ↑ **risk of cancer** in a thyroid nodule.

  o Patient
    - Age < 20 - < 60
    - Males
    - Compression; hoarseness (vocal cord involved), dysphagia, dyspnea
    - Head and neck cancer (especially with radiation exposure)

  o Nodule
    - Rapid growth
    - Hard
    - Fixation
    - Cervical adenopathy

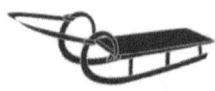

Even in the absence of clinical factors which suggest a malignant nodule, thyroid ultrasonography should be performed, with possible FNA biopsy of the nodule.

- Give the changes in a thyroid nodule seen on **thyroid ultrasound,** which suggests that the lesion may be malignant.

Feature	Malignant	Benign
o > 3 cm	+	-
o Echogenicity	Hypo ($\downarrow$)	Hyper ($\uparrow$)
o Border	Irregular	Hypolucent halo
o Shape	H > W*	Cyst
o Calcification	Micro'	"comet tail"
o $\uparrow$ vascularity	Centre	Periphery

*height > width on sagittal view

Note: use the size of the nodule and the characteristics to determine which nodule to be biopsied, including in a multi-nodular goiter

Abbreviation: FNA, fine needle aspiration

- Give the **rationale** for giving L-thyroxine to the patient with thyroid malignancy.

- Giving L-thyroxine causes $\downarrow$ TSH, and a $\downarrow$ TSH is associated with $\downarrow$ recurrence of the cancer

Toxic Goiter with Single or Multiple Adenomas

➤ Pathogenesis: ".... a somatic mutation in the Gs α-subunit or TSH receptor causing constitutive activation in one or more nodule(s), which leads to autonomy of function and secondary thyrotoxicosis"

Source: MKSAP 15, Endocrinology and Metabolism, 2009, page 28.

➤ Clinical
   o CancerGoiter plus one toxic adenoma, or multiple nodules (toxic multinodular goiter), with / without clinical hyperthyroidism, and with / without obstructive symptoms
   o Often precipitated by recent exposure to iodine

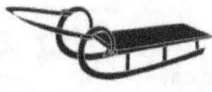

- ➢ Diagnostic imaging
  - o Scan single "hot" nodule, or patchy beware the "cold" nodule
  - o Ultrasound, to correlate clinical findings with scan

- ➢ Treatment
  - o Antithyroid drugs, maintenance
  - o I^{131}
  - o Surgery
    - – Toxic adenoma partial thyroidectomy (remove involved lobe)
    - – Toxic multinodular goiter total thyroidectomy

SO YOU WANT TO BE AN ENDOCRINOLOGIST!

In the patient with thyroid autonomy associated with either a toxic multinodular goiter or a toxic adenoma, give the meaning of the **Jod-Basedow phenomenon.**

- o The patient with thyroid autonomy from a toxic adenoma or a toxic multinodular goiter may be asymptomatic, but develop adrenergic symptoms upon intake of iodine.

Goiter

- ➢ Useful background:
  - o A normal thyroid gland weighs <20 gm (in iodine non-deficient regions), and is usually not palpable
  - o Goiter does not reflect function or neoplasia
    - – Goiter is hypertrophy or degeneration of the thyroid gland
    - – With normal or abnormal thyroid function.
  - o Pemberton sign
    - – Hands above the head for 30 min causing
      - ▪ Blue/ pink face/ neck from venous stasis and ↑JVP
      - ▪ Head congestion, dizziness, stiffness

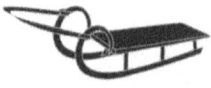

- From a retrosternal goiter, or any cause of reversible SVC syndrome (tumor)
- Compression complications of a thyroid goitre
  - Trachea (stridor)
  - Esophagus (dysphagia)
  - Recurrent laryngeal nerve (dysphonia)

➢ Clinical

• Take a directed history for the factors which increase the pretest probability of a goiter being present.

  o Children, especially those in endemic iodine deficiency locales
  o Pregnant and lactating women
  o Elderly patients
  o Symptoms of hyperthyroidism or hypothyroidism
  o Patients with excessive radiation exposure
  o Patients with Down Syndrome

Source: Simel DL, et al. *JAMA* 2009 Chapter 21, page 287.

• Take a directed history for **multinodular goiter**.
  o Face – redness upper raising arms above head (Permberten's sign, suggesting a retrosternal goiter)
  o Ears VIII involvement → deafness
  o Larynx   – Hoarseness → pressure on/ damage to recurrent laryngeal nerve

  o Trachea   – Stridor

  o Esophagus   – Dysphagia

  o Thyroid   – Multinodular goiter
                              – May have painful enlargement
                              – Symptoms of thyrotoxicosis (mention atrial fibillation)

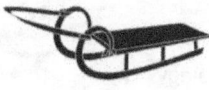

HYPOTHYROIDISM

➢ Definition: "Hypothyroidism is a clinical syndrome that usually results from a deficiency of thyroid hormone, [OR] rarely it can be due to resistance to thyroid hormone". (Lochnan H, et al. Chapter 30. In: Therapeutic Choices. Grey J, Ed. 6th Edition, *Canadian Pharmacists Association* 2012, page 365).

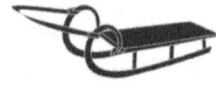

➢ Laboratory

xxxxxxxxxxxxxxxxxxxxxxxxxxxxxxxxxxxxxxxxxxxxxxxxxxxxxxxxx

SO YOU WANT TO BE A ENDOCRINOLOGIST!

An increased serum TSH (thyroid-stimulating hormone) is usually a sensitive indicator of hypothyroidism.

- Give two clinical situations in which the patient may be clinically hypothyroid, but the TSH concentration is normal or low, rather than increased.
  - o In the patient with clinical hypothyroidism, the TSH may be normal or low in disease of the pituitary (secondary hypothyroidism) or hypothalamus (tertiary hypothyroidism).

- Give the definition of "subclinical hypothyroidism", give 4 indications for it to be treated.

➢ Definition: "Subclinical hypothyroidism is defined by an elevated TSH with normal thyroid hormone levels" (Lochnan H, et al. Chapter 30. In: Therapeutic Choices. Grey J, Ed. 6th Edition, *Canadian Pharmacists Association* 2012, page 365).

➢ Indications for treatment of subclinical hypothyroidism:
  - o ↑↑ TSH (> 10 mU/L)
  - o Symptoms of hypothyroidism
  - o Anti-TPO (anti-thyroid peroxidase) positive
  - o Abnormal lipid profile
  - o Planned pregnancy

On the basis of TSH (thyroid-stimulating hormone), anti-TPO (thyroid peroxidase antibodies), fT_3 (free triiodothyronine) and fT_4 (free thyroxin), distinguish primary (1°), hypothyroidism from secondary (2°) and tertiary (3°) hypothyroidism, and from resistance to thyroid hormone.

	Causes of Hypothyroidism		
	1°	2° / 3°	Resistance
TSH	↑	↓ / N	↑
Anti-TPO	+	-	
fT_4	↓	↓	↑

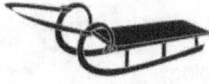

- ➢ Causes

- Give a systematic approach to the causes of hypothyroidism.

    - o Thyroid
        - – Primary failure
        - – Hashimoto disease (autoimmune thyroiditis)
    - o Pituitary
        - – Primary failure, causing hypothyroidism
    - o Treatment/ surgery
        - – Thyroidectomy
        - – Treatment of hyperthyroidism
    - o Diet
        - – Long-term iodine deficiency
    - o Hereditary
        - – Autosomal recessive
        - – Homozygote has thyromegaly and hypothyroidism
    - o Iatrogenic
        - – Surgical removal
        - – I^{131} treatment
        - – External radiation of bed of thyroid
    - o Drugs similar to those which may cause hyperthyroidism
    - o Postpartum thyroiditis
        - – Hypothyroid phase
    - o Subacute thyroiditis
        - – Recovering phase

SO YOU WANT TO BE AN ENDOCRINOLOGIST!

We all know that amiodarone may cause thyrotoxicosis. Give 3 drugs / chemicals which may cause hypothyroidism.

- o Amiodarone (↑ and ↓ TSH)
- o IFN (interferon)
- o Lithium
- o IL-2

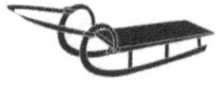

- Give the types of hypothyroidism.

  - Primary
    - Without a goitre (decreased or absent thyroid tissue)
      - Idiopathic atrophy
      - Treatment of thyrotoxicosis, e.g. iodine, surgery
      - Agenesis or a lingual thyroid
      - Unresponsiveness to TSH
      - Elderly persons; inhibitory autoantibody to TSH
    - With a goiter (decreased thyroid hormone synthesis)
      - Chronic autoimmune diseases, e.g. Hashimoto's thyroiditis
      - Drugs, e.g. lithium, amiodarone
      - Inborn errors (enzyme deficiency)
      - Endemic iodine deficiency or iodine-induced hypothyroidism
      - Riedel thyroiditis
  - Secondary
    - Pituitary lesions
  - Tertiary
    - Hypothalamic lesions
  - Transient
    - Thyroid hormone treatment withdrawn
    - Subacute thyroiditis
    - Postpartum thyroiditis

Adapted from: Talley NJ, et al. *Maclennan & Petty Pty Limited* 2003, Table 9.5, page 318; Davey P. *Wiley-Blackwell* 2006, page 284.

- Give the causes of hypothyroidism.

Cause	Comments
o Hashimoto thyroiditis	– Most common cause
	– Anti-PO leels very high
o Hypothyroid phase of subacute thyroiditis	– Usually transient

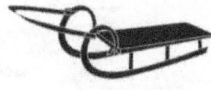

Cause	Comments
o Congenital	– Aplasia of thyroid – Dyshormogenesis
o Iodine deficiency	– Rare in North America
o Recovering phase of non-thyroidal illness	– Transiently elevated TSH
o Pituitary disorder	– Secondary hypothyroidism – TSH low or normal – fT_4 usually low
o Hypothalamic disorder	– Tertiary hypothyroidism – TSH low or normal – fT_4 usually low
o Resistance to thyroid hormone	– High TSH, fT_3 and fT_4

Abbreviations: anti-TPO, thyroid peroxidase antibodies; fT_3, free triiodothyronine; fT_4, free thyroxine

Reproduced with permission: Therapeutics Choices. Sixth Edition. Ottawa, Canada: *Canadian Pharmacist Association* 2012, Table 1, page 366.

CLINICAL PEARL

- Give the likely explanation why a patient with hypothyroidism treated with L-thyroxine may become hypotensive.
  - o The hypothyroidism was associated with adrenal insufficiency,, which became clinically apparent (hypotension) as the hypothyroidism was corrected.

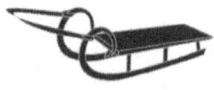

➢ Clinical

• Perform a focused physical examination for HYPOTHYROIDISM.

- o Face
  - – Weight gain
- o Eyes
  - – Periorbital and facial puffiness, lose of outer portion of eyebrows
- o Skin/hair
  - – Coarse, sandpaper like , dry, hair breaks easily
- o Nails
  - – Thick
- o Hands
  - – Doughy skin (glucosaminoglycan deposit)
- o Mood
  - – Lethargic, disinterested
- o CNS
  - – Slow reflex relaxation
  - – Cerebellar syndrome
  - – Psychosis
  - – Coma
  - – Unmasking of myasthenia gravis
  - – Cerebrovascular disease
  - – High cerebrovascular fluid protein
  - – Nerve deafness
  - – Peripheral neuropathy
- o MSK
  - – Entrapment, carpal tunnel, tarsal tunnel
  - – Muscle cramps
  - – Proximal myopathy
  - – Hypokalemic periodic paralysis
- o CVS
  - – Bradycardia
  - – Heart failure (HF)

Adapted from: Talley NJ, et al. *Maclennan & Petty Pty Limited* 2003, Table 9.5, page 318; Table 9.6, page 319; and Mangione S. *Hanley & Belfus* 2000, page 164.

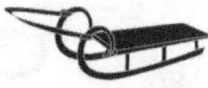

Tricky Tricks

- Give conditions associated with hypothyroidism in which there is normal or ↓ TSH concentrations.
  - Central hypothyroidism
  - Intake of exogenous thyroid hormone e.g. L-thyroxine

- Perform a focused physical examination for hypothyroidism.

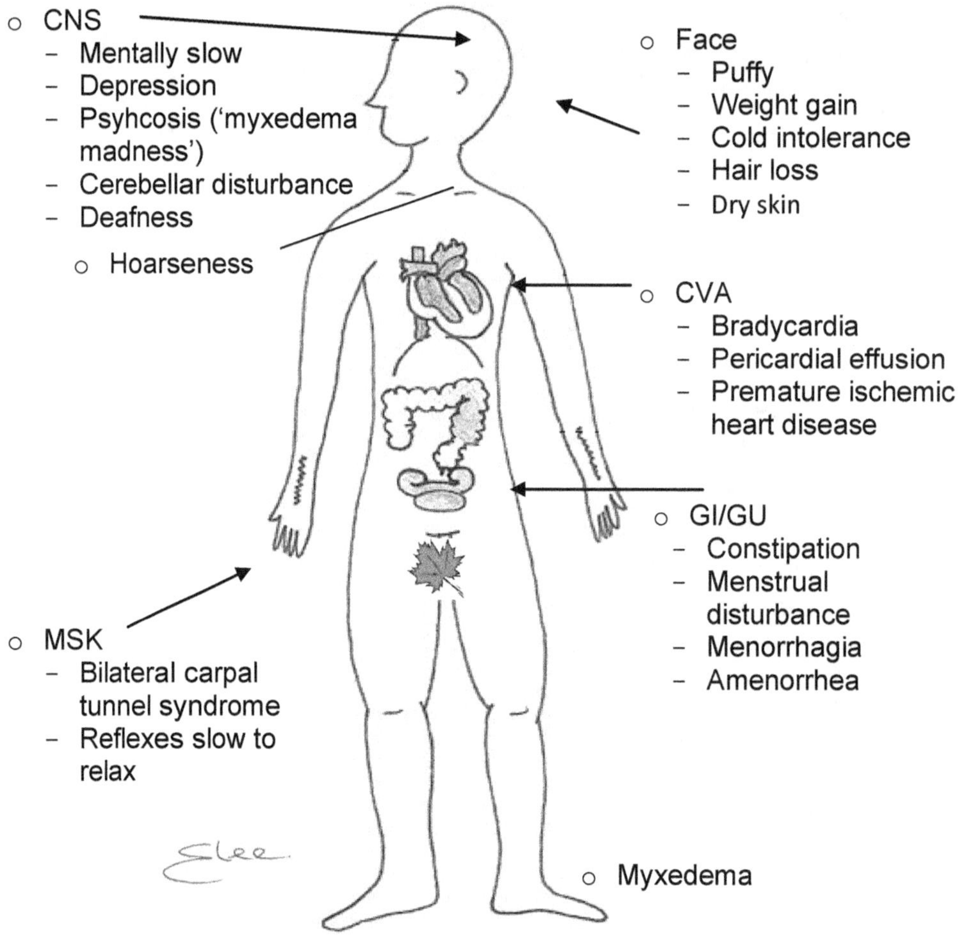

- CNS
  - Mentally slow
  - Depression
  - Psyhcosis ('myxedema madness')
  - Cerebellar disturbance
  - Deafness

    - Hoarseness

- Face
  - Puffy
  - Weight gain
  - Cold intolerance
  - Hair loss
  - Dry skin

- CVA
  - Bradycardia
  - Pericardial effusion
  - Premature ischemic heart disease

- GI/GU
  - Constipation
  - Menstrual disturbance
  - Menorrhagia
  - Amenorrhea

- MSK
  - Bilateral carpal tunnel syndrome
  - Reflexes slow to relax

- Myxedema

Abbreviations: CNS, central nervous system; CVS, cardiovascular system; GI/GU, gastrointestinal/ genitourinary; MSK, musculoskeletal

Adapted from: Davey P. *Wiley-Blackwell* 2006, page 234.

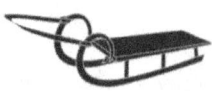

SO YOU WANT TO BE A GOOD GENERAL PHYSICIAN!

- In the context of the eyebrows, give the meaning of the Queen Anne sign.
  - o Thinning of the hair of the eyebrows

- Give conditions other than cosmetic practice and hypothyroidism, which are associated with thinning of the eyebrows.
  - o Systemic Lupus Erythematosis (SLE)
  - o Miscellaneous drugs and skin diseases

- Give how to distinguish between thinning of the brows from SLE versus hypothyroidism.
  - o In hypothyroidism, it is the later portion of the eyebrow, which is thinned.

Adapted from: Mangione S. *Hanley & Belfus* 2000, page 11.

- Give how to distinguish thyroid acropacly, and from a pulmonary etiology.

	Thyroid	Pulmonary
o Painful periostitis	No	✓
o Long bones	No	✓
o Hands, feet	✓	No

- Give the performance characteristics of physical findings for hypothyroidism.
  - o Periorbital puffiness and slow movements (> 1 minute to fold a bed sheet) are not clinically significant physical findings for hypothyroidism.

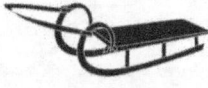

Finding	PLR
o Skin	
– Cool and dry skin	4.7
– Coarse skin	3.4
(Cold palms)	
(Dry palms)	
– Puffiness of wrists	2.9
– Hair loss of eyebrows	1.9
(Pretibial edema)	
o Speech - slow "Hypothyroid" speech	5.4
o Pulse <60 bpm	4.1
o Thyroid enlarged	2.8
o Neurologic	
– Delayed ankle reflexes	3.4

Abbreviation: likelihood ratio (LR) if finding present= positive PLR

Adapted from: McGee SR. *Saunders/Elsevier* 2007, Box 22.3, page 263.

- Give the **Billewicz diagnostic index** for hypothyroidism.

| Finding | Points scored if finding is | |
	Present	Absent
o Symptoms		
– Diminished sweating	+6	-2
– Dry skin	+3	-6
– Cold intolerance	+4	-5
– Weight increase	+1	-1
– Constipation	+2	-1
– Hoarseness	+5	-6
– Paresthesia	+5	-4
– Deafness	+2	0

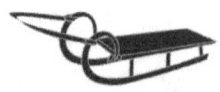

Finding	Points scored if finding is	
	Present	Absent
o Physical Signs		
– Slow movements	+11	-3
– Coarse skin	+7	-7
– Cold skin	+3	-2
– Periorbital puffiness	+4	-6
– Pulse rate <75/ min	+4	-4
– Slow ankle jerk	+15	-6

Source: McGee SR. *Saunders/Elsevier* 2007, Table 22-1, page 264.

Billewicz score	Sensitivity (%)	Specificity (%)	PLR	NLR
o Less than –15 points	3-4	28-68	0.1	-
o -15 to +29 points	35-39	…	NS	-
o +30 points or more	57-61	90-99	18.8	-

Source: McGee SR. *Saunders/Elsevier* 2007, Box 22-3, page 263.

➢ Pathology

- A patient with a ↓ TSH has a stable-sized thyroid nodule on periodic follow-up on thyroid ultrasound. Give the timing of fine needle aspiration biopsy (FNAB), and appropriate treatment choices.

  o Nodule > 1 cm with TSH normal

  o Nodule < 1 cm with

     – Risk factors for cancer
        ▪ Family history positive for thyroid cancer
        ▪ Radiation
     – In children
     – To head & neck
     – Suspicious ultrasound

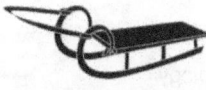

> Testing

o Hoshimoto hyroiditis, subclinical hypothyroidism-recovering phase of subacute thyroidistis, and postpartum thyroiditis – hypothyroidism ill manifest ↑ TSH, ↓ free T4 and ↓ free T3. Give the way to distinguish.

o Central (pituitary) hypothyroidism
   – ↓ TSH
   – Absent
      ▪ TPO Ab (antithyroid peroxidase antibody)
      ▪ TG Ab (thyroglobulin antibody)

> Treatment target for TSH (with L-thyroxine)

o Usual
   – 1.0 to 2.5 mU/L (1.0 – 2.5 µU/mL)

o For > 80 yr
   – 2.5 to 5.0 mU/L (2.5 – 5.0 µU/mL)

o For ↑ risk for development of clinically overt hypothyroidism
   – Pregnancy
   – Strong family history
   – Goiter
   – TPO (anti-thyroid peroxidase) Ab (antibody)

o A higher than usual range for TSH may be appropriate to treat with L-thyroxine
   – Hyperfunction
      ▪ Do not give T4-suppressing drugs for benign nodule
   – Surgery
      ▪ If suspicious for malignancy
      ▪ Growth
      ▪ Perigoiter compression by multinodular thyroid

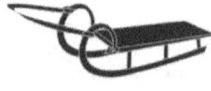

- Based on the measurements, give the **type of hypothyroirism**.

TSH	T3	T4	Type of hypothyroidism
↓	↓	↓	Hypothyroidism (secondary) due to a central cause such as hypopituitary
↑	↓	↓	Primary hypothyroidism
↑	N	N	
No symptoms			Subclinical hypothyroidism (treat when TSH > 10 micro U/mL)
↓	↓	N/↓	ESS (euthyroid sick syndrome), early (in late ESS, ↑ TSH)

Measurement of T3 is generally not necessary to make the diagnosis of clinically suspected hypothyroidism. However, T3 levels are included below for MCQ purposes (so you are not misled).

Sick Thyroid Syndrome

➤ Definition
  o The patient with severe systemic illness may have
    - Cytokine release (as well as other mediators of inflammation)
    - No symptoms of hypo - hyperthyroidism (i.e. patient is clinically euthyroid)
    - But lab' tests are abnormal (T4, unchanged; ↓↓ T3, ↑ reverse T3)

- Give the **treatment** of the Sick Thyroid Syndrome.
  o Other than treating the underlying condition, no treatment is needed for the ↓ T3 and ↑↑ RT3.

Myxedema Coma
➤ Clinical
  o Suspect myxedema coma when a clinical picture of hypothyroidism occurs with
    - Mental changes
    - Hypothermia
    - Hypoventilation
    - Hypoxemia
    - Hypercapinia

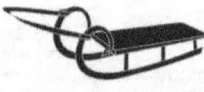

➢ Treatment
  o Thyroxine
    – IV L-thyroxine 4 μg/kg lean body mass (100-600 μg IV bolus), followed by
    – Sodium potassium iodide (SSKI, Lugol solution)
  o Hydrocortisone 50-100 mg IV q 6-8 h until stable
    – Volume monitoring and replacement
    – Assess dose of all other medications used

HYPERTHYROIDISM

➢ Causes
  o Primary
    – Graves disease
    – Toxic multinodular goiter
    – Toxic uninodular goitre: (usually a toxic adenoma)
    – Hashimoto thyroiditis (thyrotoxicosis early in its course; later H thyroiditis causes hypothyroidism)
    – Subacute thyroiditis (transient)
    – Postpartum thyroiditis (non-tender)
    – Iodine-induced ('Jod-Basedow' phenomenon – iodine given after a previously deficient diet)
  o Secondary
    – Pituitary (very rare): TSH hypersecretion
    – Hydatidiform moles or choriocarcinomas: by HCG secretion (rare)
    – Struma ovarii (rare)
    – Drugs, e.g. excess thyroid hormone ingestion, amiodarone

Adapted from: Talley NJ, et al. *Maclennan & Petty Pty Limited* 2003, Table 9-5, page 318; Table 9.6, page 319; and Mangione S. *Hanley & Belfus* 2000, page 163 and 164.

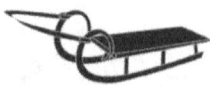

- Give the causes of hyperthyroidism.

  o Graves Disease
  o Goiter
    - Multinodular
    - Uninodular (usually an adenoma)
    - Toxic uninodular goiter (usually a toxic adenoma)
  o Thyroiditis
    - Hashimoto (transient)
    - Subacute
    - Postpartum
  o Drugs
    - Iodine (after previous dietary deficiency)
    - Thyroxine excess
    - Amiodosone
  o Tumor
    - Pituitary (TSH production)
    - Ovarian (struma ovarii; extrathyroidal T4)
    - Hydatid moles; choriocarcinoma (HCE secretion)

Adapted from: Talley NJ, et al. *Maclennan & Petty Pty Limited* 2003, page 318.

"What lies behind us and what lies before us are tiny matters compared to what lies within us."

Henry Stanley Haskins

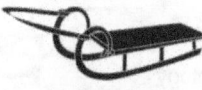

➢ Clinical

- Perform a focused physical examination for hyperthyroidism.
  - o Face
    - Anxious
    - Nervous
    - Restless
    - Frightened faces
    - Energetic
  - o Eyes
    - Stare
    - Wide palpebral fissures
    - Lid lag
    - Inability to wrinkle brow on upward gaze
    - Opthalmopathy
    - Exophthalmos (forward protrusion of eyeball >18 mm from the orbit)
    - Conjunctivitis
    - Conjunctival edema (chemosis)
    - Periorbial edema
    - Papilledema optic atrophy
    - Extraocular defects
      - Muscle weakness
      - Amblyopia
      - Impaired upward gaze
      - Impaired convergence
      - Strabismus
      - Restricted gaze and visual acuity
      - Visual field competence defects
  - o Mood
    - Apathy
    - Depressed mood (especially in elderly)

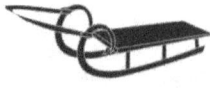

- o Skin/Hair
  - – Fine skin and hair
  - – Hyperpigmentation at pressure points
  - – Pretibial myxedema (non-pitting edema, pigmented, pruritic); note: myxedema of hypothyroidism is more general

  Warm, moist, velvety skin

- o Nails
  - – Broken
  - – Onycholysis (Plummer nails, IVth digit, separation of nail from nail bed)

- o Hands
  - – Palmar erythema
  - – Fine tremor
  - – Thyroid periostitis

- o CNS
  - – Hyperreflexia
  - – Fine tremor

- o GI/ GU
  - – Diarrhea
  - – Amenorrhea

- o Muscle
  - – Myopathy
  - – Proximal muscle weakness

- o Heart
  - – Cardiomyopathy
  - – HF (heart failure)
  - – CCF (high output)
  - – Atrial fibrillation
  - – Flow murmur
  - – Tachycardia
  - – ↑ pulse pressure

- o Lung
  - – Means-Lerman scratch sound (high-pitch pulmonic sound similar to pericardial rub)

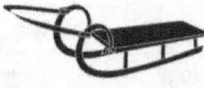

- Give the complications of hyperthyroidism.

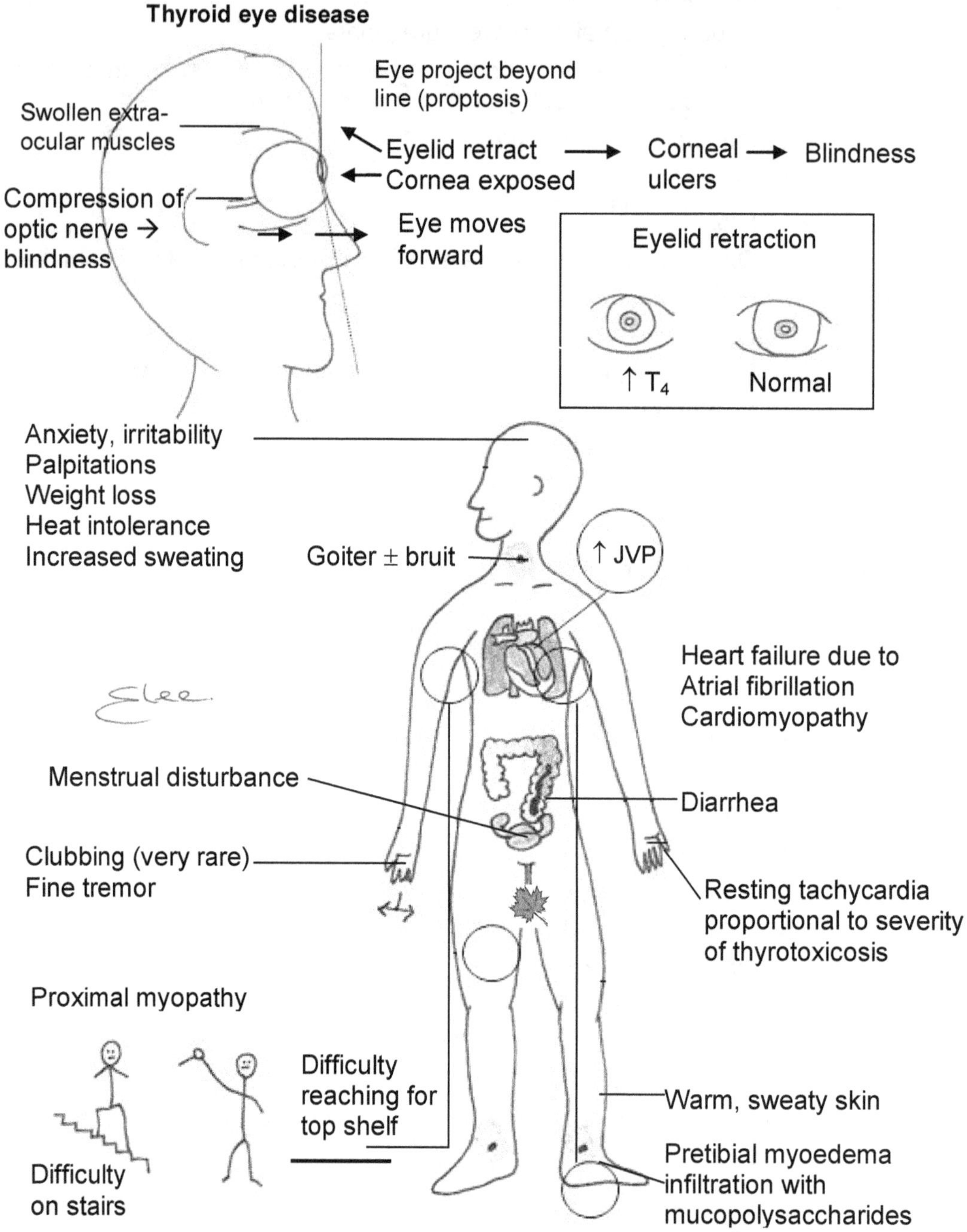

Thyroid eye disease

Swollen extra-ocular muscles

Eye project beyond line (proptosis)

→ Eyelid retract → Corneal → Blindness
← Cornea exposed   ulcers

Compression of optic nerve → blindness

Eye moves forward

Eyelid retraction	
↑ T_4	Normal

Anxiety, irritability
Palpitations
Weight loss
Heat intolerance
Increased sweating

Goiter ± bruit

↑ JVP

Heart failure due to
Atrial fibrillation
Cardiomyopathy

Menstrual disturbance

Diarrhea

Clubbing (very rare)
Fine tremor

Resting tachycardia
proportional to severity
of thyrotoxicosis

Proximal myopathy

Difficulty
reaching for
top shelf

Warm, sweaty skin

Difficulty
on stairs

Pretibial myoedema
infiltration with
mucopolysaccharides

Adapted from: Davey P. *Wiley-Blackwell* 2006, page 278.

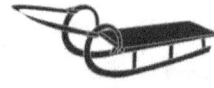

Useful background: **Wayne diagnostic index** for hyperthyroidism

Symptoms of recent onset or increased severity	Present	Signs	Present	Absent
o Dyspnea on effort	+1	o Palpable thyroid	+3	-3
o Palpitations	+2	o Bruit over thyroid	+2	-2
o Tiredness	+2	o Exophthalmos	+2	
o Preference for heat	-5	o Lid retraction	+2	
o Preference for cold	+5	o Lid lag	+1	
o Excessive sweating	+3	o Hyperkinetic movements	+4	-2
o Nervousness	+2	o Fine finger tremor		
o Appetite increased	+3	o Hands:	+1	-2
o Appetite decreased	-3	– Hot	+2	-1
o Weight increased	-3	– Moist	+1	
o Weight decreased	+3	o Casual pulse rate:		
		– Atrial fibrillation	+4	
		– <80, regular	-3	
		– 80-90, regular	0	
		– >90, regular	+3	

Wayne index	Sensitivity (%)	Specificity (%)	PLR
o <11 points	1-6	13-32	0.04
o 11-19 points	12-30	…	NS
o >20 points	66-88	92-99	18.2

Abbreviation: PLR, positive predictive value

Source: McGee SR. *Saunders/Elsevier* 2007, Box 22-4, page 268.

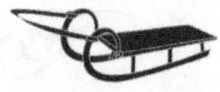

➢ Diagnostic imaging

• Give the diagnostic imaging of hyperthyroidism.

Cause	Comments
o Graves disease	– Due to thyroid-stimulating immunoglobulins activating the TSH receptor
	– Most common cause of hyperthyroidism
	– Patients frequently have eye disease and possibly pretibial myxedema.
	– RAIU is elevated and thyroid scan with pertechnetate or ^{123}I shows a diffuse pattern.
o Subacute thyroiditis	– Scan poorly defines the gland – RAIU is very low
o Postpartum thyroiditis	– Scan poorly defines the gland – RAIU is very low (not recommended if patient is lactating)
o Toxic nodule	– Thyroid scan shows hot area
o Toxic multinodular goiter	– Scan shows multiple hot areas. – RAIU is slightly elevated.
o Iodine excess	– Usually in setting of multinodular goiter
	– RAIU is low.
o Iatrogenic	– Due to over-treatment with thyroid hormones – Scan shows no thyroid; 0% RAIU
o Struma ovarii	– Very rare – Thyroid hormone production in ectropic sites – RAIU is 0% – Body scan will show thyroid tissue in ovary.

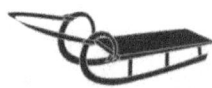

Cause	Comments
o Metastatic thyroid cancer	– With large tumor burden
o TSH-producing pituitary adenoma	– TSH elevated
o Stimulation of TSH receptor (by excessive human chorionic gonadotropin)	– Hydatidiform mole – Hyperemesis gravidarum – Other tumors

Abbreviations: RAIU, radioactive iodine uptake; TSH, thyroid-stimulating hormone

Reproduced with permission: Therapeutics Choices. Sixth Edition. Ottawa, Canada: *Canadian Pharmacist Association* 2012, Table 1, page 368.

Buzz Words

In the context of hyperthyroidism and MCQs, give the likely diagnosis.

Buzz words	Think of diagnosis on MCQ
o Autoimmune conditions	– Grave disease
o Family history	
o Viral illness, tender / painful neck	– de Quervain (subacute thyroiditis)
o Atrial fibrillation (AF)	– Look to see if amiodarone was used for treatment of AF → amiodarone induced thyrotoxicosis
o Nurse / MD, small thyroid, I* ↓/* uptake	– Surreptitious ingestion of thyroxine
o Radiocontrast containing iodine, or ↑ oral intake of iodine	– Toxic multinodular goiter, or toxic adenoma

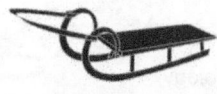

- Give the performance characteristics of physical findings for hyperthyroidism.

Finding		PLR
o Pulse	- Pulse > 90 beats/min	4.4
o Skin	- Moist and warm	6.7
o Thyroid	- Enlarged thyroid	2.3
o Eyes	- Eyelid retraction	31.5
	- Eyelid	17.6
o Neurologic	- Fine finger tremor	11.4

Adapted from: McGee SR. *Saunders/Elsevier* 2007, Box 22-4, page 268.

➤ Diagnostic imaging

The uptake of radiolabelled iodine (I^*) into the thyroid is obtained with a thyroid scan.

- Give the diagnosis of thyrotoxicosis associated with conditions giving low or high ^{131}I uptake on thyroid scan, or low/high flow on Doppler colour ultrasound.

	Uptake on I^* scan or Doppler ultrasound	Diagnosis
^{131}I uptake	↓	Surreptitious intake
	↑	Thyroiditis
Flow Doppler		Thyroiditis

➤ Laboratory

To make the diagnosis of hyperthyroidism, measure TSH, T3 (triiodthyronine and fT4 (free thyroxine).

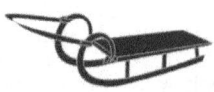

- Based on the following measurements, give the **type of hyperthyroidism**.

TSH	T3	f T4	Type of hyperthyroidism
↑	↑	↑	○ Hyperthyroidism secondary to a pituitary tumor (central, or secondary hyperthyroidism)
↓	↑	↑	○ Primary hyperthyroidism
↓	↑	N	○ T3 toxicosis, primary hyperthyroidism
↓	N	N	○ Subclinical hyperthyroidism

Abbreviation: N, normal

Note: If an acutely ill patient has ↓ TSH, ↓ T3, ↓ / N fT4, and no symptoms / signs of hyperthyroidism, suspect ESS (euthyroid sick syndrome)

Clinical Challenge

A patient presents with mild fatigue. Psychological assessment as well as all investigations are normal (T4, T3, I^{131} uptake), except for a reduced TSH concentration.
- Give the management of this patient with **subclinical hyperthyroidism**.
  - ○ Monitor patient for development of
    - – Symptoms of hyperthyroidism
    - – Laboratory thyroid test
  - ○ If TSH < 0.3 mU/L (0.3 µ U/mL)
    - – Treat to prevent atrial fibrillation
  - ○ If TSH 0.1 mU/L (0.1 µU/mL)
    - – Treat to prevent other cardiac disorders, as well as adverse effects on CNS and bones

- Give the thyroid disorder which may cause poor glycemic control in a diabetic.
  - ○ Hyperthyroidism, increasing hepatic production of glucose.

- Give the explanation for the patient with clinical thyrotoxicosis having a ↓ I^{131} uptake.
  - ○ Thyroiditis
  - ○ Intake of L-thyroxine (exogenous thyroid hormone replacement therapy, which suppress thyroid activity, so I^{131} uptake is low.

Look It Up: In any patient with thyroid disease, use a reference source to look up medications which may cause thyroid dysfunction. For example, see MSKAP 15, Endocrinology and Metabolism, 2009, page 34.

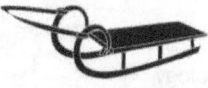

➢ Treatment

The treatment of hyperthyroidism includes drugs (methymazole, PTU [propylthiouracil], ^{131}I (radioactive iodine), or surgery (thyroidectomy).

- The following conditions, understanding the drugs may be used as bridging therapy to ^{131}I a surgery causing hyperthyroidism. Give the usually recommended therapy for 5 of the conditions.

Condition	First-line Therapy
○ Toxic multinodular goiter, or toxic adenoma	– ^{131}I or surgery, with methimazole bridging
○ Graves disease	– Methimazole or surgery, or corticosteroids followed by ^{131}I
○ de Quervain thyroiditis	– Corticosteroids or NSAIDs
○ Surreptitious ingestion	– Stop thyroxine, psychotherapy
○ Pregnancy	– PTU; T2/T3, methimazole
	– Do **not** give ^{131}I
○ Malignant nodule	– Confirm diagnosis by fine needle aspiration / biopsy thyroidectomy
○ ↑ sympathetic activity	– B-blocker (atenolol or propranolol)
○ Thyroid storm	– B-blocker (atenolol or propranolol)
	– PTU (propylthiouracil)
	– KI (iodine-potassium solution)
	– Corticosteroids

Graves Disease

➢ Definition
- ○ Hyperthyroidism caused by an autoimmune process leading to antibodies to the TSH receptor stimulating autonomous production of increased T4 and T3.
- ○ Graves disease may be subclinical

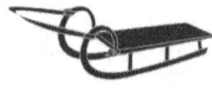

- ➢ Clinical

- • Give factors associated with the clinical presentation of Graves disease.

  - o Family history of Graves disease
  - o Patient
    - – Autoimmune disease
    - – Stress (severe, recent)
    - – Tobacco use
    - – Virus infection

- • Give the **unique clinical presentation** of Graves disease and octogenarian thyrotoxicosis.

  - o Graves disease
    - – Goiter
    - – Ophthalmopathy
      - ▪ Proptosis
      - ▪ Chemosis
      - ▪ Extraocular muscle paralysis
    - – Pretibial myxedema
  - o Old age hyperthyroidism
    - – Depression
    - – HF (heart failure)
    - – AF (atrial fibrillation)

- • Perform a focused physical examination for Graves disease.
  - o Diffuse goiter
  - o Pretibial myxedema
    - – Local thickening of the skin due to infiltration of lymphocytes, other inflammatory cells, as well as mucopolysaccharides
    - – May be itchy
    - – May be pigmented
  - o Thyroid ophthalmopathy
    - – Exophthalmos
    - – Proptosis (> 18mm forward protrusion of the age) (bilateral in 95%)

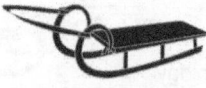

- Congestion
    - Conjunctivitis
    - Chemosis
    - Periorbital edema
    - Papilledema
    - Optic atrophy
- Ophthalmoplegia
    - Medial rectus
    - Inferior rectus
    - Amblyopia ↓ gaze upwards ↓ convergences
    - Double vision
    - ↓ usual acuity ↓ blinking
    - Tremor of upper eyelids when eyes are closed
    - Brown pigment on eyelids
  - Association with other autoimmune disorders
    - Hyper-/ hypopigmentation (vitiligo)
    - Premature greying (!)
  - Miscellaneous - Plummer nails
    - Separation of the nail from the nailed (onycholysis)
    - Separation is usually in the 4th digit

Pretibial myxedema is not caused by hyperthyroidism; i.e. is not related to the active thyroid; PM is only an association.

A bruit auscultated over a goiter is highly suggestive of Graves disease, (↑ vascularity), but not for other causes of hyperthyroidism.

- Give 4 causes of a bruit in the neck.
  - Graves thyrotoxemia
  - Venous hum
  - Carotid bruit
  - Aortic stenosis/ sclerosis

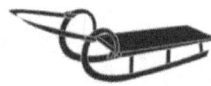

77

ENDOCRINOLOGY

- Perform a focused physical examination to distinguish between Graves disease from other causes of a diffuse enlargement of the thyroid gland and evidence of hyperthyroidism.
  - o Pretibial myxedema
    - Local infiltration of the skin
    - May be pigmented or pruritic
  - o Ophthalmopathy (exophthalmos)
    - Proptosis/ strabismus (involvement of medial and inferior rectus muscles)
    - Amblyopia
    - ↓ convergence
    - ↓ visual fields
  - o Thyroid bruit
  - o Signs of autoimmune disorders
    - Vitiligo
    - Premature graying
    - Hyperpigmentation
  - o Onycholysis (Plummer nails: may be seen in other causes of hyperthyroidism)

- ➤ Treatment
  - o Beta-blockers
    - Anti-thyroid drugs (6 to 18 mon)
      - Propylthiouracil (PTU)
        - -Drug-free remission ~ 40% at 1 year
        - Role of hepatic damage agranulocytosis
        - PTU may be used in first trimester of pregnancy
    - Methimazole
  - o I^{131} treatment
    - Avoid in presence of severe opthalmopathy

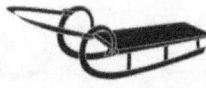

- Surgery
  - – L. thyroxine replacement therapy for associated and resulting hypothyroidism
  - – Ophthalmopathy worsened by I^{131}
  - – Large goiter
  - – Nodules of concern

Clinical Quiz

In a patient with Graves disease Ohthalmopathy presents 3 year after I^{131} treatment and associated hypothyroidism treated with L-thyroxine.

- Give the mechanism responsible for the late onset of eye changes in Graves disease
  - Persistence of the TSH receptor antibodies after I^{131} treatment leads to the opthalmopathy.

A patient with thyrotoxicosis from Grave disease experiences a worsening of adrenergic symptoms as well as a tender thyroid 2 weeks after I^{131} treatment.

- Give the mechanisms for the development of

  I^{131} causes radiation thyroiditis with neck pain and tenderness
  - Performed thyroxine is released, worsening symptoms

- Give the mechanism of the **fetal thyroid dysfunction** which may develop in the third trimester of pregnancy of a mother with Graves disease
  - Antibodies to the TSH receptor cross the placenta and may affect the fetus

A patient who smokes and has a family history of Graves ophthalmopathy fails to respond to local measures for their exophthalmous, proptosis, conjuctional redness and periorbital edema. They develop diplopia and reduced visual acuity.

- Give the **urgent therapy** for severe opthamopathy involving the extraocular muscle and optic nerve.
  - Corticosteroids
  - Irradiation of the eye
  - Urgent surgical decompression of the orbit

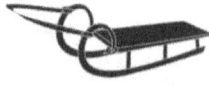

Trick Questions!

- Give the signs of Grave disease, which are not due to the associated hyperthyroidism.
  - Pretibial myxedema
  - Exophthalmos

- Give which two functional thyroid disorders are associated with pretibial myxedema.
  - Graves disease
  - Hypothyroidism

Thyroid Storm

➢ Causes

- Give **precipitating causes** of thyroid storm.
  - May be associated with Graves syndrome
    - CVS
      - MI
    - Lung
      - PE (pulmonary embolus)
    - Endocrine
      - DKA (diabetic ketoacidosis)
      - Childbirth
      - Iodine
      - I^{131} therapy
      - ASA (salicylates)
      - Pseudoepinephrine
    - Infection / sepsis
    - Trauma / surgery

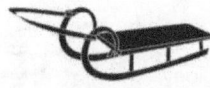

➤ Clinical

 o Suspect thyroid storm when a clinical picture of hyperthyroidism occurs with systemic **decompensation**, such as

  – Fever

  – CNS symptoms (agitation, confusion, coma)

  – CVS (tachycardia, HF, AF)

  – GI/H (nausea/vomiting, pain, diarrhea, jaundice).

 o Scoring scales are available to establish the diagnosis.

Abbreviations: AF, atrial fibrillation; CNS, central nervous system; CVS, cardiovascular system; GI / H, gastroenterology / hepatology; HF, heart failure;

➤ Treatment

 o ↓ core temperature

  – Cooling blankets

   ▪ Acetaminophen

 o B-blocker

 o PTU (propylthiouracil)

 o I^{131}

 o Treat participants and complications

➤ Prognosis

 o Mortality rate 15-20%

The Eyes in Hyperthyroidism

• Perform a focused physical examination for thyroid **ophthalmopathy**.

 o Eyelid   – Retraction

          – Upper eyelid lag on downward gaze

          – Tremor (closed eyelid)

          – ↓ blinking

 o Conjunctiva   – Edema

          – Hyperemia

 o Cornea   – Erosion / ulceration

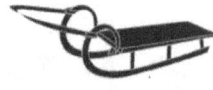

- o Orbit — Oxophthamos (aka proptosis)

- o Optic nerve — Visual loss (optic nerve edema and compression)

- o Extraocular motility — Impaired

Source: Mangione S. *Hanley & Belfus* 2000, pages 81 and 82.

➤ Clinical

- Perform a focused physical examination of the eye in a patient with thyrotoxicosis.
  - o Eyelids
    - Retraction (Dalrymple sign) – sclera visible above the upper limbus of the cornea
    - Lag – with movement, the lid lags behind the eyeball (von Graefe sign)
    - ↓ blinking (Stellway sign)
    - Tremor of closed eyelids (Rosen bach sign)
    - ↑ pigmentation of eyelid margins (Jellink sign)
    - Upper eyelid difficult to (Gifford sign)
    - Upper eyelid difficult to move downward (Grove sign)
    - ↑ fullness of eyelid (Enroth sign)
    - Sclera - visible between the lower eyelid and lower limbs of cornea
  - o Eyeball
    - Exophthalmos
    - When eyeball looking down, the eyelid stops moving down (Boston sign)
    - When looking up, upper lids move upwards faster than eyeball (Kocher sign)
  - o Pupils
    - Jerky contraction to consensual light (Cowen sign)
    - Unequal dilation (Knie sign)
  - o Cornea
    - ↓ strength of one or more extraocular muscles (Ballet sign)

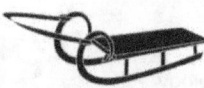

- o Optic nerve
  - – ↓ vision
  - – Paralysis (Jendrassik sign)
  - – ↓ fixation on lateral gaze (Suker sign)
- o Muscles
  - – ↓ movement of eyeball due to extraocular muscle involvement
  - – ↓ convergence (Mobius sign)
- o Forehead muscle
  - – ↓ wrinkling on quickly gazing upward (Joffroy sign)

- • Give the causes of **exophthalmos**.

  - o Bilateral
    - – Graves disease
  - o Unilateral
    - – Cavernous sinus thrombosis
    - – Tumors of the orbit, (e.g. dermoid, optic nerve glioma, neurofibroma, granuloma)
    - – Pseudotumors of the orbit
    - – Graves disease

Source: Talley NJ, et al. *Maclennan & Petty Pty Limited* 2003, Table 9.4, page 316.

Thyrotoxicosis

Remember, thyrotoxicosis may be due to
- o Graves disease – diffuse hyperplasia of thyroid gland
- o Toxic nodule (adenoma, single or multiple)

Remember – the clinical symptoms of hyperthyroidism do not necessary correlate with serum concentration of ↓ TSH.

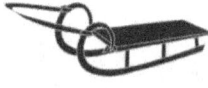

- Perform a focused physical examination to distinguish between Graves disease (GD) and Toxic Nodular Goitre (TNG).

Sign	GD	TNG
o Age	– Younger	Older
o Thyroid	– Diffuse goiter	Nodular, enlarged thyroid gland
o Eye signs	– Common	Rare
o Atrial fibrillation	– Rare	Common (~40%)
o Associated autoimmune disease	– Common	Rare

Adapted from: Baliga RR. *Saunders/Elsevier* 2007, page 369.

Destructive Thyroiditis

➢ Definition
  o Destruction of the thyroid follicles, thereby releasing T4

➢ Causes / associations
  o Subacute painfall "de Quervain" thyroiditis, possibly related to viral infection
  o Silent thyroiditis
    – Autoimmune, painless
  o Drugs
    – Amiodarone, type II

  o Postpartum
    – 5% of pregnancies
    – Recurs with future pregnancies
  o Familial
    – HLA haplotype associated thyroiditis

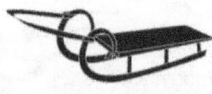

- Give the phases of changes in thyroid function tests in destructive thyroiditis.
  - Initially
    - Hyperthyroid phase: ↑ T4, ↓ TSH, ↓ I^{131} uptake
  - Then
    - Hypothyroid phase: ↓ T4, ↑ TSH, ↑ I^{131}, uptake
  - Finally
    - Euthyroid: some patients may be permanently hypothyroid

➢ Treatment
  - Beta-blockers, L-thyroxine if late phase is permanent hypothyroidism
  - For neck pain from deQuervain destructive thyroiditis
    - NSAIDs or
    - Corticosteroids

Drug-Induced Thyrotoxicosis

➢ Causes / associations
  - Lithium (more common than hyper-, lithium causes hypothyroidism)
  - Interferon –α
  - Interleukin-2
  - Iodine loading
  - Amiodarone
    - Type I
      - Hyperthyroidism (iodine-induced from amiodarone-associated iodine [15 mg / tablet!]
      - Rx thyroid drugs
    - Type II
      - Hypothyroidism: destructive thyroiditis
      - ↓ blood flow, negative Doppler
      - Rx prednisone

Note: These medications may also cause hypothyroidism

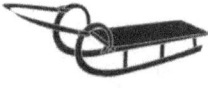

➢ Laboratory

• Give the value of T3 measurements to distinguish type I from type II **amdiodarone-induced thyroid disease**.

  o Limited: amiodarone reduced the production of T3 from T4, so the expected ↑ or ↓ reflecting thyroid function may be minimized.

Clinical Challenge

Hypothyroidism is common in patients with **celiac disease**.

• Give the reason why the patient with celiac disease, may be resistant to therapy early in the course of their disease.

  o The hypothyroidism associated with celiac disease is treated with L-thyroxine.

  o L-thyroxine is poorly absorbed in untreated disease, and higher doses must be given.

  o Once the abnormal histology of the small intestine is revised by a gluten-free diet, the absorption of L-thyroxine will become normal, and the usual doses may be used.

  o If a patient with hypothyroidism requires large doses of L-thyroxine, suspect celiac disease, or intake of L-thyroxine with food.

• Give the most likely explanation why a patient with proven hypothyroidism fails to respond to appropriate doses of compliantly taken L-thyroxine.

  o The absorption of L-thyroxime is reduced by food, and the drug must be taken 1 hour before or 1-2 hr after meals.

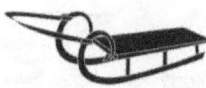

Gem and Pearls

- o FNA (fine needle aspiration) is > 90% sensitive for a thyroid malignancy, especially when < 3 cm in size, and with a papillary thyroid cancer.

- o FNA is not adequate to diagnose a follicular cancer, because a biopsy is necessary to determine if there is invasion of the blood vessels or capsule of the nodule.

- o Some guidelines suggest taking a biopsy from a non-toxic thyroid nodule, even if it is small < 1 cm, and even if the patient has no high rate factors.

- o A thyroid nodule which is found incidentally should be investigated in the usual manner (cancer risk 5% to 10%), except when the in cidentaloma is found by [18]FDG PET, in which the cancer risk is 14-50%, if the [18]FDG PET has diffuse uptake, it is usually benign, whereas focal uptake suggests cancer, including metastatic disease from a melanoma, or cancer of the breast or thyroid.

Simple Goiters

➤ Definition

- o An enlarged thyroid gland without nodules

➤ Management

• Give sufficient L-thyroxine to ↓ TSH to low-normal concentrations.

- o Measure thyroid antibodies (tPO and TG) if Hashimoto thyroiditis suspected

- o Remember – in Hashimoto thyroiditis there is an ↑ risk of lymphoma

Abbreviation: TG, thyroglobulin antibody; TPO, anti-thyroid peroxidase antibody

Pregnancy and the Thyroid

- o ↑ estrogen concentration in pregnancy leads to
    - – ↑ thyroxine-binding globulin
    - – ↓ TSH LLN (T1)
    - – ↑ T4 1.5 x ULN
    - – ↓ free T4 LLN
- o ↑ gonadotropin

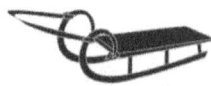

- o ↑ L-thyroxine to normalize free T4 (↑ dose 35-50% in T1 and T2)
- o Note: goiter does not normally occur during pregnancy in iodine-sufficient areas, whereas in iodine-deficient areas, there may be a ~ 30% increase in size of the thyroid during pregnancy.

Abbreviations: LLN, lower-limit of normal; ULN, upper-limit of normal

- Give the important considerations for treating the **pregnant patient** with thyroid disease.
  - o Certain thyroid studies cannot be done safely in pregnancy (scans, uptake studies with I^{131}).
  - o Suspect Graves disease in pregnancy if there is
    - – Goiter (especially in iodine sufficient area)
    - – Ophthalmopathy
    - – Antibodies to TSH-receptor
  - o Give enough PTU (safe in pregnancy) to keep TSH LLN and free T4 ULN
  - o Do not use beta-blockers (→ fatal bradycardia)
  - o Surgery is rarely needed.

Abbreviations: LLN, lower limit of normal; ULN, upper limit of normal

ADRENAL DISEASE

➤ Definition

  - o Disease of the adrenal glands leads to primary adrenal insufficient (AI) of corticosteroids (cortisol), Aldosterone, DHEA (dehydroepiandrosterone) and DHEA sulfates
  - o Loss of ACTH secretion leads to central or secondary adrenal insufficiency of the ACTH-dependent corticosteroid cortisol, DHEA and DHEA-sulfate.

➤ Causes

  - o The commonest cause of primary AI is autoimmune adrenalitis, whereas the most common cause of secondary AI is the intake of exogenous sterids, which suppresses the HPA (hypothalamic-pituitary-adrenal) axis, leading to ↓ ACTH.

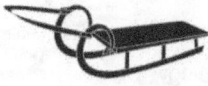

Addison disease

➢ Causes / associations

- Give a systematic approach to the causes of Addison disease.

  o Idiopathic atrophy of adrenal cortical tissue

  o Sudden withdraw/ of therapeutic use of steroids

  o Infiltration
    - TB amyloid
    - Sarcoidosis
    - Hemorrhage

  o Infarction

➢ Clinical

- Take a directed history for the causes of hypoadrenalism (Addison disease).

  o Acute
    - Septicemia (especially meningococcal)
    - Adrenalectomy
    - Any stress in a patient with chronic hypoadrenalism or abrupt cessation of prolonged high-dose steroid therapy

  o Chronic
    - Primary
      ▪ Acute or chronic gland destruction
        - Idiopathic atrophy (Addison's disease)
        - Infection: TB, fungal
        - Infiltration: metastasis, amyloidosis, etc.
        - Hemorrhage (especially Waterhouse-Friderichsen syndrome)
      ▪ Surgery
        - Metabolic failure
        - Virilizing hyperplasia, e.g. C21-hydroxylase deficiency
        - Enzyme inhibitors, e.g. metopirone
        - Drugs, e.g. OPDDD (cytotoxic)
        - Drugs (warfarin)
    - Secondary
      ▪ Hypopituitarism
      ▪ Suppression of hypothalamic-pituitary axis
        - Exogenous glucocorticoids
        - Endogenous glucocorticoids, e.g. Cushing's syndrome following tumor removal

Adapted from: Talley NJ, et al. *Maclennan & Petty Pty Limited* 2003, page 327; Davey P. *Wiley-Blackwell* 2006, page 290.

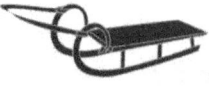

A patient has salt craving and postural dizziness.

- Perform a focused physical examination for hypoadrenalism (Addison disease).

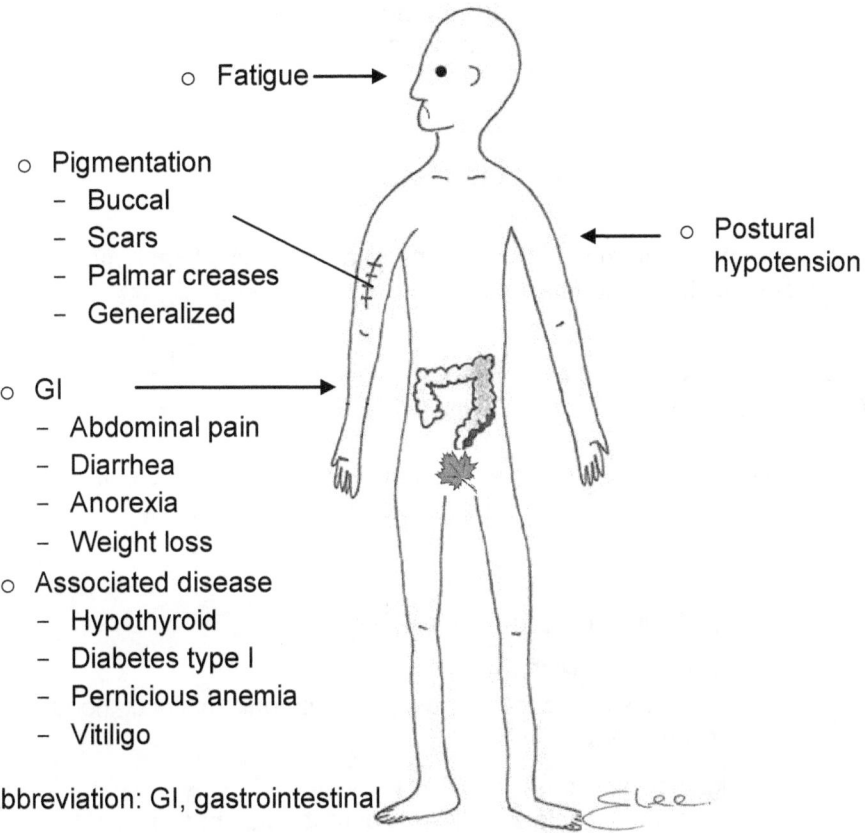

o Fatigue

o Pigmentation
  - Buccal
  - Scars
  - Palmar creases
  - Generalized

o Postural hypotension

o GI
  - Abdominal pain
  - Diarrhea
  - Anorexia
  - Weight loss
o Associated disease
  - Hypothyroid
  - Diabetes type I
  - Pernicious anemia
  - Vitiligo

Abbreviation: GI, gastrointestinal

Adapted from: Davey P. *Wiley-Blackwell* 2006, page 290.

o General	- Weight loss
	- Depression
o Skin	- Pigmentation
	• Hands
	• Mouth & hips
	• Covered areas (e.g. collars, nipples, ring)
	• Scars
	- Vitiligo

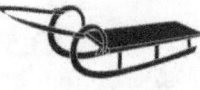

- o Hair — ↓ pubic & axillary hair

- o CVS — ↓ BP, postured hypotension
  - Small heart

- o Causes — TB
  - HIV
  - Metastases

- o Associated autoimmune conditions (e.g. thyroiditis [Hashimoto], B12 deficiency [pernicious anemia])

XXXXXXXXXXXXXXXXXXXXXXXXXXXXXXXXXXXXXXXXXXXXXXXXXX

SO YOU WANT TO BE ENDOCRINOLOGIST!

In the context of Addison disease (AD), give what are the Schmidt, polyglandular and Allgrove syndromes.

- o Schmidt syndrome
  - AD plus hypoparathyroidism

- o Polyglandular (PGS), type I
  - AD, plus hypoparathyroidism, plus chronic mucocutaneous candidiasis

- o Allgrove syndrome
  - AD* plus Achiolasia, plus alacrima, plus neurological disease

*AD; AD from loss of adrenal sensitivity to ACTH
Abbreviation: T_1DM, type I diabetes mellitus

- • Perform a focused physical examination for disorders associated with hyperpigmentation.

- o General — Hereditary (racial)

- o Liver — PBC (Primary biliary cirrhosis)
  - Hemochromatosis, hereditary

- o Kidney — Uremia

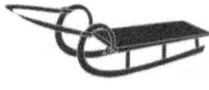

o Intestinal/ nutritional	– Malabsorption – Carotenemia – Protein-caloric malnutrition – Alcoholism
o Metabolic	– Porphyria cutanea tarda – Ectopic ACTH

Adrenal Insufficiency (AI)

- Take a directed **history** and perform a focused **physical examination** in the patient with adrenal insufficiency to determine if the condition is primary or secondary. Indicate differences in lab' measurements.

Features	Primary AI	Secondary AI
o Symptoms	– Salt craving – Postural dizziness	No symptoms of aldosterone deficiency
o Signs	– ↑ pigmentation – Hypovolemia / dehydration – Hypotension	- - -
o Laboratory	– ↓ basal (AM) cortisol (< 148 mmol/L [5.0 µg/dL])	√
	– ↓ response to cosyntropin (< 511 nmol/L [< 18.5 µg/dL]) (dose, 250 µg or 1 µg)	√
	– ↓ DHEA and DHEA-s	√
		N
	– ↑ K^+_s (hyperkalemia)	N
	– ↑ renin	N / ↓
	– ↑ ACTH	N
	– ↓ aldosterone	

Abbreviations: √, same as; N, normal; DHEA-S, dehydroepiandrosterone-sulfate

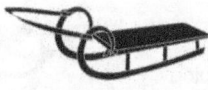

➢ Laboratory

A Pearl and a Gem

- The interpretation of the meaning of the total serum cortisol concentration as a surrogate measure of the free cortisol level depends on the binding proteins.

Conditions	Binding protein	Total serum cortisol	Free (non-protein bound) serum cortisol
o Pregnancy, estrogen, OCP	↑	↑ (falsely high)	N
o Hypoproteinemia	↓	↓ (falsely low)	N

- Taking into account the variable levels of binding protein, - useful suggestion: measure cortisol in saliva or urine.

Abbreviation: OCP, estrogen-containing oral contraceptive pill

---

- From the assessment of serum electrolytes, give how to suspect if **adrenal insufficiency** is primary or secondary.

  - o Primary disease of adrenal glands
    - ACTH-normal
    - ↓ cortisol
    - ↓ mineralocorticoids → hyperkalemia (↑ K^+)
    - ↓ ACTH
    - ↓ cortisol
    - Normal mineralocorticoids (controlled by renin-angiotension system) – normal K^+

  - o Adrenal insufficiency secondary to adrenal disease

ACTH-deficiency from pituitary disease, leading to secondary adrenal deficiency

Site of disease	ACTH	Cortisol	Mineralocorticoids
1° adrenal	N	↓	↓ (K^+ ↑)
1° pituitary (central) 2° adrenal	↓	↓	N (K^+N)

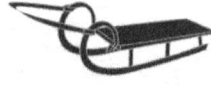

ACTH-deficiency from pituitary disease, leading to secondary hypothyoidism

	TSH	Free T4	T3
1° thyroid	↓		N
1° pituitary, 2° thyroid	N / ↑ (↓ bioactivity)	↓	
Euthyroid sick syndrome			↑

Provocative Testing

- o When the levels of hormone usually produced by an endocrine gland are high, provocative testing is focused on suppressing the elevated levels.
- o For example, if the serum or cortisol 24 hr urine concentration are increased, give 1 mg dexamethasone (dexamethasone suppressant).
- o A positive dexamethasone test is represented by the serum cortisol failing to fall to < 5 micrograms / dL (i.e., the dexamethasone should reduce the serum control to < 5 micrograms / dL, and failure to achieve the suppression [inadequate suppression] represents a positive test).
- o A positive dexamethasone suppression test suggests Cushing syndrome.

- Give causes of false-positive 1 mg dexamethasone suppression test.
  - o Alcoholism
  - o Obesity
  - o Psychological disease

Useful reminder: don't forget
- o Commonest cause of
  - – Cushing syndrome
    - Exogenous use of corticosteroids
  - – Cushing disease (central)
    - ACTH secreting pituitary tumor
- o Commonest cause of
  - – Primary adrenal insufficient
    - Autoimmune adrenalitis
  - – Secondary adrenal insufficiency
    - Pituitary disease (hypothalamic-pituitary suppression)

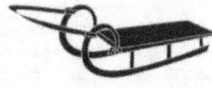

- Give the reason why secondary adrenal insufficiency, caused by pituitary disease, is not associated with aldosterone deficiency, whereas primary adrenal insufficiency is associated with aldosterone deficiency.

  o Secondary insufficiency (pituitary disease) is due to ↓ ACTH

  o Synthesis of aldosterone is not dependent upon ACTH, so aldosterone levels are normal.

  o In primary disease of the adrenal glands, there will be deficiency of cortisol, adrenal androgens, as well as aldosterone.

MCQ Trick

- Give the dose of dexamethasone recommended to treat Addison disease.

  o Got ya: trick question!

    – Remember that the dexamethasone test for Cushing syndrome: dexamethasone suppresses serum cortisol – not what you want in Addison disease.

"Great thoughts speak only to the thoughtful mind, but great actions speak to all mankind."

Emily P. Bissell

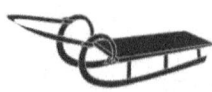

➤ Treatment

Clinical Challenge

- Give the reason why the **duration of suppression** of the HPA axis is more prolonged when a course of exogenous steroids is given in the evening than in the morning.

There is a morning peak in the circadian rhythmic concentration of endogenously secreted cortisol which will be suppressed by giving bedtime prednisone.

o AM dosing	– Exogenous plus endogenous cortisol, including AM endogenous pea
o PM dosing	– Exogenous plus endogenous cortisol without AAM peak, leading to lower overall cortisol concentration
o AM plus PM dosing	– Exogenous plus very low amounts of endogenous cortisol from inhibition of ACTH release throughout the day, leading to more marked suppression of the HPA axis, lasting 9-12 months after stopping exogenous steroids

---

- Give the treatment of adrenal insufficiency (AI).

o 1° / 2° AI	– Hydrocortisone 15 mg to 25 mg / day, in divided doses e.g. 8 am, 7.5-12.5 mg; 12:00 noon, 5.0-7.5 mg), 6:00 pm, 2.5-5.0 mg
	– "stress doses" up to 150 mg to 200 mg/d IV in four divided doses (in septic shock, this high dose treats both AI plus the systemic inflammatory response)
o 1° AI	– Also use mineralocorticoid replacement (fludrocortisone) plus

Remember: Adrenal insufficiency due to use of exogenous corticosteroids may be associated with reduced

- o Cortisol concentration
- o ACTH (adrenocorticotropic hormone)

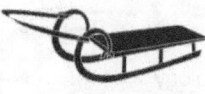

Hyperadrenalism (Cushing Syndrome)

➢ Causes

- o The hypercortisolism of Cushing Syndrome (CS) may be endogenous and ACTH-dependent (~75%) or ACTH-independent (~25%)

- o The administration of exogenous cortisol, or synthetic steroids, or other drugs affecting serum corticol concentrations is overall the commonest causes of CS (exogenous CS)

- o ACTH-dependent endogenous CS is usually caused by an ACTH-secreting pituitary adenoma, and less commonly tumors causing ectopic ACTH or CRH secretion.

- o ACTH-independent endogenous CS is usually caused by an adrenal adenoma or carcinoma.

- • Give the causes of Cushing syndrome.

  - o Adrenocorticotropic hormone (ACTA) dependent

  - o Exogenous administration of excess steroids or ACTH (most common)

  - o Adrenal hyperplasia (with or without increased pituitary ACTH)
    - – Secondary to increased pituitary ACTH production (Cushing disease)
      - ▪ Microadenoma
      - ▪ Macroedema
      - ▪ Pituitary-hypothalamic dysfunction
    - – Secondary to ACTH-producing tumors (e.g. small cell lung carcinoma)

  - o Adrenal neoplasia
    - – Adenoma
    - – Carcinoma (rare)

  - o Pituitary adenoma (Cushing's disease) (70%) F>M
    - – Ectopic ACTH (14%)
    - – Bronchial carcinoma
    - – Carcinoid- lung, gastrointestinal tract, thymus

  - o ACTH independent
    - – Adrenal adenoma (10%)
    - – Adrenal carcinoma (5%)
    - – Adrenal hyperplasia (1%)

Adapted from: Talley NJ, et al. *Maclennan & Petty Pty Limited* 2003, Table 9.9, page 324; Davey P. *Wiley-Blackwell* 2006, page 290.

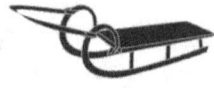

➢ Clinical

● Perform a focused physical examination for Cushing's syndrome.

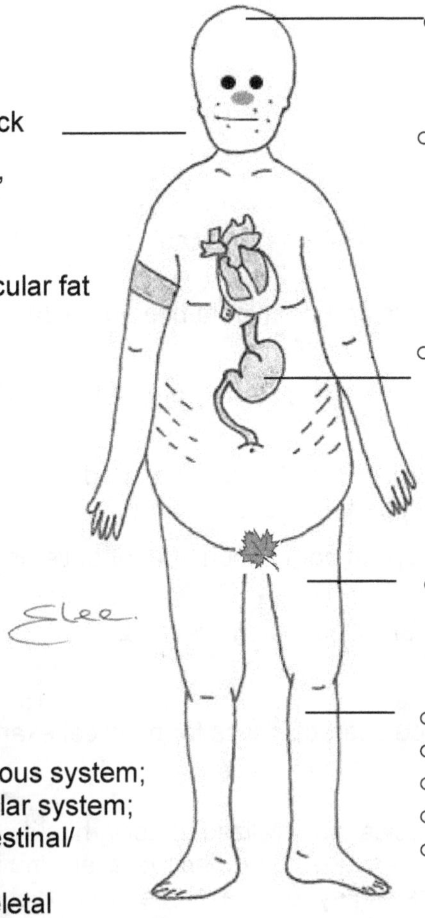

○ CNS
  - Depression
  - Psychosis

○ CVS
  - Premature ischemic
    heart disease
  - Hypertension

○ Head and neck
  - Thin hair
  - 'Moon face'
  - Acne
  - Hirsutism
  - Supraclavicular fat
    pad

○ GI / GU
  - Peptic ulcer
  - Dysmenorrhea
  - Impotences

○ MSK
  - Proximal hypopathy

Abbreviations:
CNS, central nervous system;
CVS, cardiovascular system;
GI/ GU, gastrointestinal/
genitourinary;
MSK, musculoskeletal

○ Skin
○ Central obesity
○ Striae
○ Thin
○ Easy bruising

Adapted from: Davey P. *Wiley-Blackwell* 2006, page 290; and McGee SR. *Saunders/Elsevier* 2007, Table 12-1, page 110.

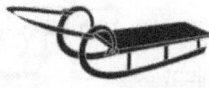

- Give the distribution of adipose tissue in Cushing syndrome.

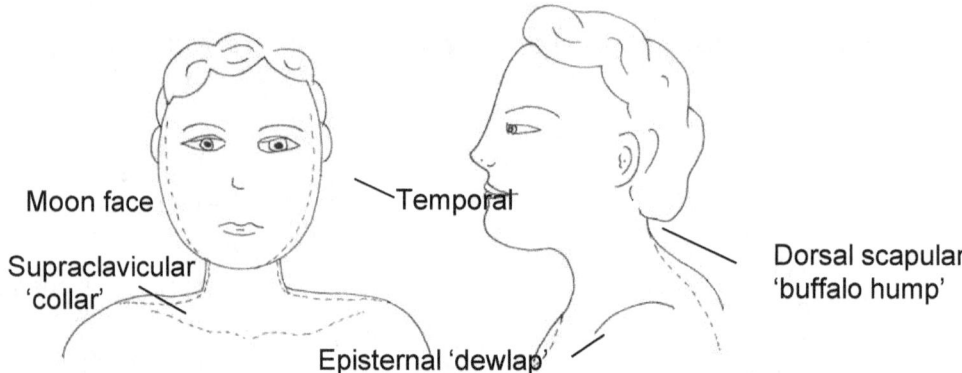

Moon face

Temporal

Supraclavicular 'collar'

Dorsal scapular 'buffalo hump'

Episternal 'dewlap'

- o Rounding of cheeks and prominent bitemporal fat produces the characteristic 'moon facies'.

- o Fat also may accumulate bilaterally above the clavicles ('supraclavicular collar').

- o In front of the sternum (episternal area), and over the back of the neck (dorsal cervical fat pad, or 'buffalo hump').

- o The dotted line depicts normal contours of patients without Cushing Syndrome.

Adapted from: McGee SR. *Saunders/Elsevier* 2007, Figure 12-1, page 111.

- Give the performance characteristics for physical examination for Cushing syndrome.

- o Although moon facies, generalized obesity, hirsutism (in women), striae, proximal muscle weakness, and peripheral edema have been suggested to be signs of Cushing syndrome, these are in fact either non-significant or have positive likelihood ratios (PLR) < 2.

Finding		PLR
o Vital signs	- Hypertension	2.3
o Body habitus	- Central obesity	3.0
o Skin findings	- Thin skinfold	115.6
	- Plethora	2.7
	- Ecchymoses	4.5
	- Acne	2.2

Adapted from: McGee SR. *Saunders/Elsevier* 2007, page 114.

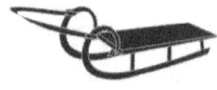

SO YOU WANT TO BE AN ENDOCRINOLOGIST!

- Give the distinction between Cushing disease, Cushing syndrome and pseudo-Cushing syndrome

  o Cushing disease
    - Caused by pituitary adenoma
    - ↑ ACTH levels
    - ↑ adrenal production of steroids
  o Cushing syndrome is
    - Caused by increased steroids from any cause:
    - Steroids, including adrenocorticotropic hormone (ACTH)
    - Pituitary adenoma (Cushing disease)
    - Adrenal adenoma
    - Adrenal carcinoma
    - Ectopic ACTH (usually from small cell carcinoma of the lung)
  o Pseudo-Cushing syndrome
    - Chronic alcoholics
    - Depressed persons
    - ↑ urinary steroids
    - No diurinal variation in serum steroids
    - Positive over-night dexamethasone test
    - All of these abnormalities which return to normal when causative factors abate

SO YOU WANT TO BE AN ENDOCRINOLOGIST!

The prevalence of denial is of epidemic proportions in persons with increased body mass (aka "obesity"). Give the endocrine causes that you consider when a patient claims "doctor, it's my glands.

  o Hypothyroidism
  o Hypogonadism
  o Cushing syndrome
  o Insulinoma
  o Stein- Leventhal syndrome

In the same context, give the meaning of Nelson syndrome.

  o Bilateral adrenalectomy leading to increased
    - ↑ ACTH levels
    - Pituitary adenoma
    - Hyperpigmentation

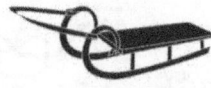

➢ Laboratory

• Give the laboratory methods used to make a **diagnosis** of Cushing syndrome.

  ○ ↑ serum corticol
    – 24-hr measurements
    – Loss of AM↑
    – Loss of suppression with dexamethasone (repeat with dexamethasone if normal dose result is equivocal)
    – Caution
      ▪ Interpret in light of possible ↑ CBG or ↓ albumin
    – Dynamic testing may also be done with vasopressin or CRH

  ○ ↑ salivary

  ○ ↑ urinary cortisol
    – Especially 24-hr urine free cortisol / expression

  ○ ACTH
    – Central (primary, e.g. pituitary adenoma) – N/P
    – Peripheral (secondary, e.g. adrenal adenoma) - ↓

Abbreviation: CRH, corticotropin-releasing hormone

Clinical Gem:

• Give the **"best" tests** for diagnosing Cushing Syndrome.
  ○ A 24-hr urine free cortisol excretion, plus
  ○ 1 mg overnight dexamethasone suppression test.

Clinical Caution:
  ○ The ACTH concentration is elevated in ACTH-secreting conditions such as pituitary adenoma and is usually suppressed by high-dose dexamethasone.
  ○ In contrast, ACTH-dependent ectopic ACTH secretion by tumors is not; however, the converse can also be observed.
  ○ The administration of CRH and measurements of ACTH from blood sampled from bilateral IPS (inferior petrosal sinus) catheterization should be done only in highly subspecialized facilities.

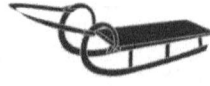

SO YOU WANT TO BE AN ENDOCRINOLOGIST!

- Give the reasons which the diagnosis of Cushing Syndrome / Disease may be difficult in pregnancy.
  - In pregnancy there is
    - A normal increase in serum cortisol as well as 24-hr free cortisol
    - The normal suppression if cortisol levels by dexamethasone is impaired in pregnancy

➢ Diagnostic imaging

  - Imaging MI of sella turcica shows ~ 50% of pituitary adenomas

  - If MRI is negative, in the presence of hypercortisolism plus ↓ ACTH
    - Perform CT scan of adrenal glands (adrenal adenoma or caner)

Please see diagnostic algorithms in resources such as MKSAP 15, Endocrinology and Metabolism, 2009, Figure 9, page 42.

➢ Treatment

  - Pituitary adenoma   − Adenomectomy, with gamma knife irradiation for recurrent disease corticosteroid replacement for adrenal deficiency

  - Adrenal-adenoma   − Laparoscopic adrenallectomy
    - Replacement therapy with corticosteroids plus mineralocorticoids

  - Carcinoma   − Laparoscopic adrenaletomy
    - Adjuvant therapy
    - Mitotane (adrenal cytotoxic)
    - Replacement hormone therapy

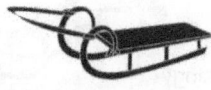

- o Ectopic ACTH
  secretion

- Control hypercortisolism
  - ↓ synthesis
    - Ketoconazole
    - Metyrapone
  - ↓ effects
    - Mifepristone
  - Cytotoxic
    - Mitotane
- Finding primary site of ACTH-secreting tumor
  - CNS
    - Neuroblastoma
    - Paragangloma
    - Gangioma
  - Thymus
    - Carcinoid
  - Thyroid
    - Medullary carcinoma
  - Lung
    - Small cell tumor
    - Bronchial carcinoid
  - Adrenal
    - Pheochromocytoma
  - Pancreas
    - Carcinoid
    - Islet cell tumor

Adrenal Incidentaloma

- o Is the lesion benign or malignant:
  - Suggestions that lesion is malignant
    - > 6 cm (25% are malignant)
    - Irregular borders
    - Areas of necrosis

- o Is the lesion primary or secondary (metastatic)
  - Suggestions that lesion is metastatic
    - ↑ attenuation on CT
    - ↑ vascularity
    - Often bilateral (M)
    - MRI, T2-weighted ↑ intensity
  - Is the lesion functioning or non-functioning
    - Catecholamines
    - Cortisol
    - Aldosterone
    - If functioning → surgery

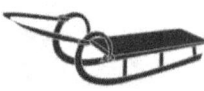

METABOLIC BONE DISEASE, PARATHYROID AND CALCIUM DISORDERS

Hypercalcemia And Hypercalciuria

➢   Causes / associations

- Give a systematic approach to the causes of hypercalcemia and hypercalciuria.
  - o Hypercalcemia
    - – Hyperparathyroidism
      - ▪ Adenoma
      - ▪ Hyperplasia
      - ▪ Carcinoma (rare)
    - – Tumor
      - ▪ Malignancy (with or without metastases, eg breast cancer)
      - ▪ Myeloma
      - ▪ Reticulosis
    - – Vitamin D
      - ▪ Increased intake (eg milk-alkali syndrome)
      - ▪ Increased sensitivity to vitamin D (eg sarcoidosis)
    - – Increased release of Ca^{2+} from bone
      - ▪ Steroid withdrawal
      - ▪ Immobilization
      - ▪ Paget disease
  - o Hypercaluria
    - – Hypercalcemia
    - – Idiopathic
    - – Osteoporosis
      - ▪ Renal tubular acidosis (RTA)
      - ▪ Fanconi syndrome

Clinical Gem and Pearl

  - o Hypercalciuria occurs with all causes of hypercalcemia as long as renal function is normal.

  - o Causes of hypercalciuria without hypercalcemia include osteoporosis and renal tubular acidosis (RTA), idiopathic.

Adapted from: Talley NJ, et al. *Maclennan & Petty Pty Limited* 2003, Table 9.13, page 328; Table 9.14, page 329; Burton JL. *Churchill Livingstone* 1971, page 99.

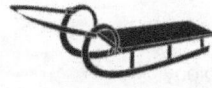

Non-PTH-mediated Hypercalcemia ($\uparrow Ca^{2+} \rightarrow \downarrow$ PTH)

- Give causes Non-PTH-mediated Hypercalcemia.

  - Malignancy
  - Granulomatous disease
    - TB (tuberculosis)
    - Sarcoidosis
  - Endocrine disease
    - Hyperthyroidism
    - 1° adrenal insufficiency
    - Pheochromocytoma
  - ↓ mobilization
  - Paget disease of bone
  - Drugs
    - Antacids
    - Thiazide diuretics
    - Vitamin A, D
    - Lithium
  - Genetics
    - Benign familial hypocalciuric hypercalcemia

Malignancy-associated hypercalcemia may be related to tumor production of PTH-related protein, ↑ 1, 25 dihydroxy vitamin D and ↑ calcitrol (e.g. B-cell lymphoma), and local osteolytic hypercalcemia (e.g. multiple melanoms, breast cancer, lymphoma).

- Give a **classification** of the tumors causing humoral hypercalcemia of malignancy.

  - Squamous
    - Mouth, larynx
    - Esophagus
    - Bronchus
    - Vulva, cervix

  - Adenocarcinoma
    - Breast
    - Ovary

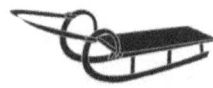

- o Other types of tumor
  - − Hepatocellular
  - − Islet cell
  - − Multiple myeloma
  - − Renal cell
  - − T cell lymphoma
  - − Transitional cell

- Give the multiple **mechanisms of hypercalcemia** in lymphoma, myeloma or breast cancer.

  - o Lymphoma
    - − PTH-related protein
    - − Local osteolytic jypercalcemia
    - − ↑ 1, 25 −dihydroxy vitamin D

  - o Myeloma, breast cancer
    - − PTH-related protein
    - − Local osteolytic hypercalcemia

➤ Pathophysiology

- Give the **mechanisms** for the hypercalcemia which develops in 3 non-malignant endocrine conditions.

  - o Thyrotoxicosis
    - − ↑ turnover of bone
  - o 1° adrenal insufficiency
    - − ↓ vascular volume
    - − ↓ Ca^{2+} clearance
  - o Pheochromocytoma
    - − PTH-related protein
  - o Steroid-induced bone disease
    - − ↑ bone resorption

➤ Clinical

- Take a directed history for the causes of hypo- and hypercalcemia.

Causes	Hypocalcemia	Hypercalcemia
o Parathyroid	− Hypoparathyroidism − Pseudohypo- parathyroidism	▪ Primary hyperparathyroidism

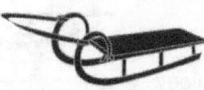

	Hypocalcemia	Hypercalcemia
o Thyroid	– After thyroidectomy, idiopathic	▪ Thyrotoxicosis ▪ Hypothyroidism in infants
o Gut	– Malabsorption – Deficiency of vitamin D – Magnesium deficiency	▪ Milk – alkali syndrome
o Pancreas	– Acute pancreatitis	
o Kidney	– Chronic renal failure	▪ Associated with renal failure (e.g. severe secondary hyperparathyroidism)
o Drugs		▪ Thiazide diuretics ▪ Vitamin D excess ▪ Milk-alkali syndrome ▪ Steroid withdrawal syndrome
o Malignancy	– Hypocalcemia of malignant disease (with or without metastases)	▪ Carcinoma (bone metastases or humoral mediators) ▪ Excessive intake production of vitamin D metabolites ▪ Vitamin D sensitivity Sarcoidosis ▪ Multiple myeloma ▪ Reticulosis
o Inactivity		▪ Prolonged immobilization or space flight ▪ "steroid withdrawal syndrome"
o Miscellaneous		▪ Paget disease ▪ Infantile hypercalcemia

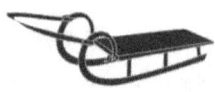

➤ Treatment

- Give the **treatment** of hypercalcemia from any cause.
  - IV fluids to achieve urine output of > 250 mL/h
  - Bisphosphonates ($\downarrow$ bone resorption)
    - Calcitonin
    - Gallium
    - Mithramycin (aka plicamycin)
  - Peritoneal / hemodialysis
  - Corticosteroids
  - $\downarrow Ca^{2+}$ intake
  - Phosphate-containing drugs
  - Controversial role of diuretics (furosemide)

➤ Laboratory

- Give the causes of hypercalcemia and the associated changes in PTH and serum concentrations of urine calcium (Ca2+) and phosphate (PO4) concentrations.

Condition	PTH	PO_4	$\uparrow Ca^{2+}_u$
Primary hyperparathyroidism			
Associated vitamin D deficiency	$\uparrow$ (80%) / N (20%)	$\downarrow$	$\uparrow$
Familial hypocalciuric hypercalcemia	$\uparrow$		$\downarrow$
Malignancy-related hypercalcemia	$\downarrow^1$	N/$\downarrow$	
Local osteolytic hypercalcemia	$\downarrow$		$\downarrow$
Multiple myeloma	$\downarrow$		$\downarrow$
Multiple myeloma	$\downarrow$	$\uparrow$	
Sarcoidosis, TB, lymphoma	$\downarrow$	$\uparrow$	
Milk alkali syndrome	$\downarrow$	$\uparrow$	
Hyperthyroidism	N^2	N	N

[1] malignancy-related hypercalcemia may have $\uparrow$ PTH-related protein

[2] The hypercalcemia of hyperthyroidism may be an incidental finding due to thyroxine stimulating bone osteoclasts and releasing Ca^{2+}

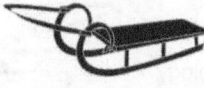

SO YOU WANT TO BE A ENDOCRINOLOGIST!

- Give the way to distinguish hypercalcemia, which is and is not mediated by PTH.
  - PTH-mediated (hyperparathyroidism [$\uparrow$ PTH, $\uparrow$ Ca^{2+}])
  - Non-PTH-mediated ($\downarrow$ PTH, $\uparrow$ Ca^{2+})

Hypoparathyroidism

➢ Causes / associations
- Idiopathic
  - Dysembryogenesis (DiGeorge syndrome)
- Iatrogenic
  - Radioactive iodine therapy
  - External neck irradiation
  - Damage during thyroid or neck surgery
- Infiltration
  - Metastatic disease (breast, lung, lymphoproliferative disorder)
- Corticosteroids
- Immune
  - Polyglandular autoimmune syndrome (PGA type 1; aka autoimmune polyendocrinopathy-candidiasis-ectodermal dystrophy [APECD])
- Metabolic
  - Hemochromatosis, hereditary
  - Wilson deficiency

Adapted from: Baliga RR. *Saunders/Elsevier* 2007, page 380.

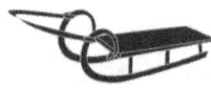

SO YOU WANT TO BE AN ENDOCRINOLOGIST!

- On the basis of just the physical examination as well as the serum calcium (Ca) and phosphate (PO₄) concentrations, and their response to PTH, distinguish between the following three variations of hypoparathyroidism:

Test	Hypo-parathyroidism	Pseudo-hypoparathyrodism*	Pseudo-pseudo-hypoparathyroidism
Ca	↓	↓	N
PO₄	↑	↑	N
Response to TSH	Yes	No	No
Skeletal changes		Yes **	Yes

*conceptualize as "end-organ non-responsiveness

** Typical skeletal changes

- ○ Short neck
- ○ Short fingers
- ○ Less than 5 fingers

Hyperparathyroidism

➢ Causes

- Give the causes of hyperparathyroidism.

  - ○ Primary
    - – Adenoma (80%)
    - – Hyperplasia
    - – Carcinoma (rare)
    - – ↑ PTH

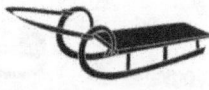

- o Secondary
  - – Hyperplasia associated with chronic renal failure
  - – $\downarrow Ca^{2+} \rightarrow \uparrow$ PTN
  - – $\downarrow$ vitamin D
  - – Chronic renal disease
- o Tertiary
  - – Autonomous hyperparathyroidism is a complication of secondary hyperparathyroidism
  - – In chronic renal disease, $\uparrow Ca^{2+}$ causes parathyroid hyperplasia, which leads to autonomous PTH secretion
- o Parathyroid adenoma
  - – Single 85%
  - – Double ~5%
  - – Multigland (MEN 1 and 2a, hyperparathyroidism in > 95% and ~ 50%, respectively) 10%
  - – Carcinoma < 1%

Source: Talley NJ, et al. *Maclennan & Petty Pty Limited* 2003, Table 9.12, page 328.

➢ Diagnostic imaging

- • Give the causes of radiographic punctate translucencies in skull.
  - o Malignancy
    - – Myelomatosis
    - – Metastatic deposits
  - o Metabolic
    - – Hyperparathyroidism
    - – Cushing disease
  - o Hematological
    - – Sickle-cell anemia
    - – Leukemia
    - – Histiocytosis X

Adapted from: Burton JL. *Churchill Livingstone* 1971, page 99.

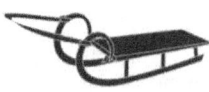

SO YOU WANT TO BE AN ENDOCRINOLOGIST!

- Give radiological signs for hyperparathyroidism.

  o Subperiosteal erosions
    - Femoral necks
    - Fingers, middle phalanges
    - Fragmental cortex of phalanges

  o Multiple bone cysts (aka osteitis fibrosa cystic; von Reckling hausen disease)
    - May project from surface of affected bone
    - Often affects the jaw))

  o Loss of lamina dura around teeth

  o Punctuate translucencies of the skull ("mottling" or "pepper-pot skull")

Source: Davies IJT. *Lloyd-Luke (medical books) LTD* 1972, pages 222 and 223.

- Give the effects of renal osteodystrophy.

  o Secondary hyperparathyroidism

  o Osteoporosis

  o Osteomalacia

➢ Diagnosis
o Biochemical
  - ↑ urine Ca^{2+}
  - ↑ serum $PO_4^{=}$
  - Hyperchloremic metabolic acidosis (↑ renal excretion of HCO_3^{-}
  - 25-OH-vitamin D normal
  - 1, 25-OH-vitamin D ULN or ↑

o Diagnostic imaging
  - Ultrasound
  - MRI
  - Scintigraphy with Tc 99-m (technetium)
  - Correct vitamin D levels before considering surgery
  - Hydration
  - Normal intake of Ca^{2+}
  - Avoid thiazide diuretics

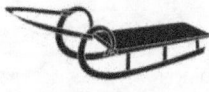

Condition	Serum Calcium	Serum Phosphate	Parathyroid hormone Infusion, response
o Hypoparathyroidism	↓	↑	Marked
o Pseudo-hypoparathyroidism	↓	↑	None
o Pseudo- pseudo-hypoparathyroidism			None

Source: Burton JL. *Churchill Livingstone* 1971, page 100.

SO YOU WANT TO BE AN ENDOCRINOLOGIST!

- Give the neurological changes associated with hyperparathyroidism.
  - o Cataracts
  - o Papilloedema
  - o Basal ganglia defects
  - o Benign intracranial hypertension

Source: Burton JL. *Churchill Livingstone* 1971, page 81.

➤ Treatment

SO YOU WANT TO BE A PARATHYROIDOLOGIST!
- Give the **guidelines** for parathyroidectomy (with implantation of gland into muscles of forearm) in an asymptomatic patient with hyperparathyroidism.

The patient must have the following

- o Patient
  - – < 50 yrs
  - – Medical surveillance not possible or deserved
- o Calcium > 0.25 mmol/L (1 mg/dL) above the ULN (upper limit of normal)
- o Creatinine clearance < 60 mL/min (1 mL/ sec)
- o Dexascan: ↓ bone mineral density (femoral neck, lumbar spine, distal radius) T-score < -2.5)

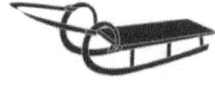

METABOLIC BONE DISEASE

➢ Useful background

  o The serum calcium (Ca^{2+}) concentration is tightly regulated (2.3 to 2.6 mmol/L [9.0-10.5 mg/dL]) by PTH, vitamin D and calcitonin.

  o About half of the serum [Ca^{2+}] is free (ionized).

  o When there is ↓ serum ionized Ca^{2+}, there is less Ca^{2+} bound to the calcium-sensing receptor (caSRs) on the membrane of the parathyroid cells.

  o ↓ Ca^{2+} bound to CaSRs leads to preformed PTH released from the parathyroid cells.

  o PTH acts on kidney, GI tract and bone.

  – Kidney
  - ↑ tubular reabsorption of Ca^{2+}
  - ↑ renal excretion of HCO_3^- → hyperchloremic metabolic acidosis
  - ↓ renal Ca^{2+} excretion (↑ renal excretion of phosphate, so the product of serum Ca^{2+} x $PO_4^=$ remains constant)
  - ↑ renal 1α-hydoxylase → ↑ 1, 25-dihydroxy vitamin D

  – GI
  - ↑ 1, 25-dihydroxy vitamin D → ↑ absorption of Ca^{2+}

  – Bone
  - ↓ osteoblast function
  - ↑ osteoclast resorption of bone

"It's not your perfection that makes you an angel;
it's your intention."

Alberto Agraso and Mony Dojeiji

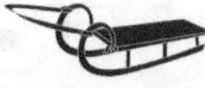

Calcium Homeostasis and Bone Disease

➤ Useful background

- o When $\downarrow Ca^{2+}_s \rightarrow \uparrow$ PTH; $\uparrow Ca^{2+}_s \rightarrow \downarrow$ PTH

- o In primary hyperparathyroidism (1° $\uparrow$ PTH), then there will be $\uparrow Ca^{2+}_s$ and $\uparrow Ca^{2+}_u$

- o In 1° hyperparathyroidism plus vitamin D deficiency; $\uparrow$ PTH, $\downarrow Ca^{2+}_s$ and $\downarrow Ca^{2+}_u$

- o PTH is (inappropriately) normal when $\uparrow Ca^{2+}_s$, suspect hyperparathyroidism

- o If $\uparrow$ PTH, $\uparrow Ca^{2+}_s$ but $\downarrow Ca^{2+}_u$, suspect familial hypocalciuric hypercalcemia, not hyperparathyroidism

Abbreviations: Ca^{2+}_s, serum; Ca^{2+}_u, urine calcium

Osteoporosis

➤ Definition

- o Osteoporosis ≥ -2.5

- o Osteopenia < -1.0 to 2.5

- o Normal > -1

Abbreviations: DEXA, dual-energy x-ray absorptiometry; SD, standard deviation

– T score	▪ Number of standard deviations above or below mean BMD (bone mineral density) of young healthy adult
– Z-score	▪ Number of SD by which the patient differs from the mean for his or his age group

- o $\uparrow$ risk of fracture

  Translating each 1 SD below age-adjust mean

Risk of fracture	RR
– Lumber spine	2.3
– Hip	2.6

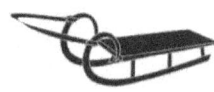

- Pre-existing vertebral features, post-menopausal women ↑RR 4x
  - As above, plus ↓ BMD
  - ↑ risk of vertebral fractures, as well as fractures at other sites
- Hip fracture ↑ risk
  - ↓ BMI
  - History of mother having hip fracture
  - Age
  - Falls
  - Previous fractures
  - Estrogen deficiency

➢ Causes

  o Be prepared to give list of causes of secondary osteoporosis, using reference sources such as MKSAP 15, Endocrinology and Metabolism 2009, Table 31, page 63.

➢ Clinical

• Take a directed history to determine the cause of osteoporosis.

  o Gender
    - Female

  o Life style
    - Smoking
    - Malnourished
    - Alcohol abuse

  o Inherited
    - Osteogenesis imperfect
    - Turner syndrome
    - Klinefelter syndrone

  o Ideopathic (young persons)

  o Immobility
    - Senilty
    - Local or generalized

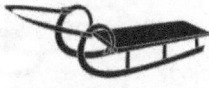

- o Immune
  - Rheumatoid arthritis
  - Other chronic inflammatory conditions, such as Crohn disease
- o Infiltration
  - Systemic mastocytosis
  - Multiple myeloma
- o Endocrine
  - Deficiency of
    - Estrogen
    - Androgen
    - Protein
    - Vitamin C
    - Calcium
  - Hyperthyroidism
  - Diabetes mellitus
  - Acromegaly
  - Glucocorticoid therapy
  - Hyperparathyroidism
  - Cushing syndrome
  - Hyperprolactinemia
  - Hypogonadism
  - Osteomalacia
- o Blood
  - Hemolytic anemia
    - Sickle-cell disease
    - Thalassemia minor
  - Polycythemia
  - Malignancy
    - Leukemia
    - Lymphoma
    - Myeloma
- o Musculoskeletal (MSK) disorders
  - Homocystinuria
  - Osteogenesis imperfecta

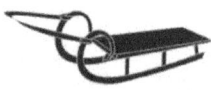

- o Drugs
  - – Corticosteroids
  - – Anti-counvulsants
  - – Heparin
- o Liver
  - – Chronic cholestasis
  - – Steroid use
  - – Glycogen storage disease
  - – Cirrhosis in children
- o Kidney
  - – Azotemic osteodystrophy
  - – Chronic renal failure
  - – Renal tubular acidosis (RTA)

Adapted from: Burton JL. *Churchill Livingstone* 1971, page 100.

- • Give the likelihood ratios for physical examination maneuvers suggesting presence of osteoporosis or spinal fracture.

	PLR	NLR
o Weight < 51 kg	7.3	0.8
o Wall-occiput distance > 0 cm	3.8	0.6
o Rib- Pelvis distance < 2 fingerbreadths	3.8	0.6
o Tooth count < 20	3.4	0.8
o Height loss > 3 cm	3.2	0.4
o Self reported humped back	3.0	0.85

Adapted from: Simel DL, et al. McGraw-Hill Medical *2009, table 36.5 and 36.6, page 483.*

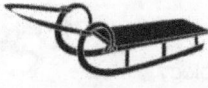

➢ Prevention and Treatment

- o Lifestyle
  - – ↓ smoking
  - – ↓ BMI
  - – ↓ caffeine
  - – Exercise

- o Medications
  - – Calcium plus vitamin D
  - – Bisphosphonates

- o Treat underlying causes

Curious things about Bisphosphonate

- o Bisphosphonates are effective for the pain in CRPS (complex regional pain syndrome, even in the absence of osteoporosis.

- o Bisphosphonates should not be combined with teriparatide (recombinant human PTH [parathyroid hormone])

- o Bisphosphonate must not be given to persons with
  - – CRD (chronic renal disease)
  - – Erosive esophagitis (gastroesophageal reflux disease)

- o If bisphosphonates cannot be tolerate, use raloxifen unless the patient has ↑ risk of TED (thromboembolic disease)

- o IV bisphosphonate therapy is convenient, but warn the patient about the ↑ risk of osteonecrosis of the jaw in persons with cancer

- o Only risedronate and zoledronate are indicated for both prevent and treatment of post-menopausal on for steroid-induced osteoporosis, as well as for treatment of osteoporosis in men

- o If bisphosphonate fail or are contraindicated, consider

- o Raloxifene or teriparatide (recombinant human parathyroid hormone)

- o Raloxifene (a selective modulator of the estrogen) is indicated for prevention and treatment of post-menopausal osteoporosis, but has a second important indication

- o ↓ risk if invasive breast cancer in post-menopausal women with or without osteoporosis

- o Men with prostate cancer may be treated with anti-androgen therapy, and this androgen deprivation as associated with ~5% / yr of ↓ BMD of the spine and hip, and a risk of ~19% fracture over 5 years

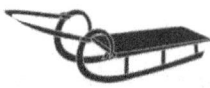

- o Bisphosphonates given to men with prostate cancer who are on anti-androgen therapy have a lower decline in bone loss or even an ↑ BMD, but unfortunately their bone fracture rate is unchanged

- o The dose and duration of corticosteroids influences the risk for ↓ BMD / fractures, and for any given BMD, the risk of fractures is increased further by taking steroids.

In the woman with osteoporosis who has not suffered a bone fracture, give the laboratory test (other than DEXA scan) which is most likely to be abnormal.

- o In the absence of fractures, there are no laboratory abnormalities in primary osteoporosis.

Osteomalacia

➢ Definition

- o Osteomalacia is defective mineralization of bone due to deficiency of calcium or phosphorus, with or without associated deficiency of vitamin D.

- o Reduced osteoid mineralization due to deficiency of calcium or phosphate.

➢ Pathophysiology

- Give the **site of the inadequate osteoid mineralization** in rickets and in osteomalacia.

    - o Growth plate
        - – Rickets
    - o Bone surface
        - – Osteomalacia

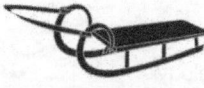

➤ Causes / associations

• Take a directed history to determine the causes of osteomalacia (Ruckets in children).

Urine calcium ↓

- o ↓ intake/ absorption of calcium
- o Vitamin D deficiency
  - Hyperparathyroidism
  - Renal acidosis
- o ↑ requirements
  - Multiple pregnancies
  - Pigmented skin
  - Prematurity
  - Prolonged breast feeding
  - ↓ UV light
- o GI
  - Malabsorption
  - Malnutrition deficiency of vitamin D
  - Post-gastrectomy (probably dietary)
- o Renal
  - Chronic renal failure
  - Fanconi syndrome
  - Hypo-phosphatasia
  - Idiopathic hypercalcuria
  - Tubular acidosis
- o Secondary to hyperparathyroidism.

Adapted from: Burton JL. *Churchill Livingstone* 1971, page 98.

➤ Laboratory

- o Urine
  - Calcium, normal
    - ▪ ↑ Phosphate
  - Renal tubular acidosis
  - Fanconi syndrome
  - Uremia

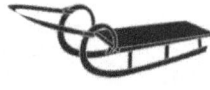

- Give the clinical **distinction** between osteoporosis and osteomalacia.

Clinical	Osteoporosis	Osteomalacia
Proximal myopathy	-	+
Bone pain	+	+
Site, common	Lumbar spine	Pelvis
	Hip	Medial side of femur

➢ Treatment

A 70 yr old woman falls in her nursing home and breaks her leg. She has been taking supplements of vitamin D, but the bone X-ray suggests mild osteoporosis. Curiously, the X-ray also shows bands running perpendicular to the surface of the bone.

- Give the amount of vitamin D to which her dose should be increased.

  o The bands perpendicular to the surface of the bone likely represent Looser zones from osteomalacia

  o Osteomalacia required treatment with calcium, phosphate plus magnesium if it is deficient

  o In old persons who have an atraumatic fall leading to bone fracture, ↓ mineralization of bone needs to be suspected, as well as osteoporosis.

Clinical Curiosity

Note: While the mechanism is unknown, it is fascinating to be reminded that giving regular supplements of vitamin D to older persons with vitamin D deficiency actually reduces their frequency of falls (as well as fractures).

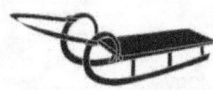

Phosphate Deficiency Osteomalacia

➢ Causes / aociationss

  o Usually due to ↑ renal excretion of $PO_4^=$

  o Congenital
    – X-linked hypophosphatemic rickets
    – Autosomal dominant hypophosphatemic rickets

  o Malignancy

➢ Laboratory

  o Non-PTH-mediated (↓ PTH, ↑ Ca^{2+})Laboratory
    – Unlike calcium associated osteomalacia, where serum calcium and vitamin D (25-OH or 1, 25 diOH vitamin D) are ↓ / N, in phosphate deficiency osteomalacia these are usually normal, but serum phosphate is low and urinary phosphate is high (unless there is treatment-associated secondary hyperparathyroidism).

Paget Disease

➢ Definition: "……. a focal disorder of bone remodeling that leads to greatly accelerated rates of bone turnover, disruption of the normal architecture of bone, and sometimes gross deformities of bone (enlargement of the skull, bowing of the femur or tibia".

Board Basics 2013, page 92.

➢ Clinical

  o Eyes   –   Angioid retinal streaks

  o CNS / PNS   –   CNS compression syndromes
                  –   Spinal stenosis
                  –   Nerve root syndromes

  o Heart   –   High-output heart failure (HF)

  o Bone   –   Pain, heat
                  –   Fractures

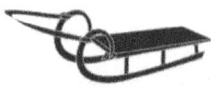

➢ Diagnostic imaging

You are shown a skull x-ray of an elderly patient with bone pain. You are expecting to see lytic lesions from metastases, or sclerotic lesion from multiple myeloma. You see a "cotton wool" appearance of the skull.

- Give the likely diagnosis, and state your next steps of action.

    o Paget disease is suspected

    o Measure serum alkaline phosphatase, which you anticipate to be increase

    o Order a bone scan to localize sites of accelerate bone turn over

---

Words to the Wise

o While calcitonin is secreted by thyroid parafollicular C cells, its physiological action is weak, and its effects on Ca^{2+} levels is seen only when used in pharmacological doses.

o Vitamin D3 diet, effect of sunlight on skin $\xrightarrow{\text{liver}}$ 25-OH-V_D $\xrightarrow[\text{(under control of PTH)}]{\text{kidney}}$ 1,25-V_D

HYPERURICEMIA

- Give the causes of secondary hyperuricemia.

    o Nutrition
    - Obesity
    - Increased purine ingestion

    o Tumor
    - Myeloproliferative disorders
        - Polycythemia, primary or secondary
        - Myeloid metaplasia
        - Chronic myelocytic leukemia
    - Lymphoproliferative disorders
        - Chronic lymphocytic leukemia
    - Plasma cell proliferative disorders
        - Multiple myeloma
    - Disseminated carcinoma and sarcoma

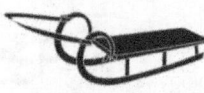

- o Anemia
  - Sickle cell anemia
  - Thalassemia
  - Chronic hemolytic anemia

- o Skin
  - Psoriasis

- o Infections
  - Infectious mononucleosis

- o Kidney
  - Chronic renal insufficiency of diverse causes
  - Saturnine gout (lead nephropathy)

- o Drugs / toxins
  - Cytotoxic drugs
  - Drug-induced
    - Cyclosporine
    - Ethacrynic acid
    - Ethambutol
    - Furosemide
    - Laxative abuse
    - Levodopa
    - Low-dose aspirin
    - Nicotinic acid
    - Pyrazinamide
    - Thiazide diuretics

- o Endocrine
  - Adrenal insufficiency
  - Bartter syndrome
  - Diabetic ketoacidosis
  - Ethanolism
  - Glycogen storage disease type I
  - Hyperparathyroidism
  - Hypoparathyroidism
  - Hypothyroidism
  - Lactic acidosis
  - Nephrogenic diabetes insipidus
  - Pseudohypoparathyroidism
  - Starvation

- o Genetic

- o Other causes
  - Sarcoidosis
  - Down syndrome
  - Beryllium disease

Adapted from: Ghosh AK. *Mayo Clinic Scientific Press* 2008, page 1004.

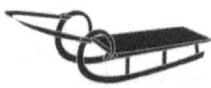

HYPOCALCEMIA AND HYPERPHOSPHOTEMIA

Hypocalcemia

There are numerous causes of hypocalcemia (please see reference source, such as MKSAP 15, Endocrinology and Metabolism 2009, Table 29, page 61.

Thinking about the many causes of hypocalcemia may be simplified by considering the mechanisms.

➢ Causes / mechanisms

- Give the **mechanisms and causes** of hypocalcemia.

o Vitamin D	–	Deficiency
		Sunlight
		Diet
		Malabsorption
		Liver disease
		Kidney disease (1α-hydroxylase deficiency Vitamin D dependent rickets type I
	–	Resistance
		↓ Mg^{2+} (hypomagnesemia)
		Vitamin D dependent rickets type II
	–	Altered metabolismdomyolysis
		Drugs
o PTH	–	Hypoparathyroidism
	–	Pseudohypoparathyroidism (PTH resistance)
o Bone	–	↓ resorption – bisphosphonate
	–	Hungry-bone syndrome
o GI tract	–	↓↓ intake / absorption of vitamin D, calcium
o Extracellular deposition	–	Pancreatitis
	–	Rhabdomyolysis
	–	Tumor lysis syndrome
	–	Osteoblastic metastasis
	–	Sepsis
	–	Acute respiratory alkalosis
	–	Artifactual hypoglycemia with hypoalbuminemia

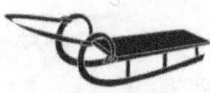

➢ Laboratory

• Give the changes in PTH, $PO_4^=$, 25-OH Vitamin D and 1, 25 diOH Vitamin D in causes of hypocalcemia.

Condition	$PO_4^=$	PTH	25-OH Vitamin D	1, 25 diOH
o Vitamin D deficiency	↓	↑	↓	↓
o Vitamin D-dependent rickets typeII	↓	↑		↑
o Hypoparathyroidism	↑	↓/N		
o PTH resistant pseudohypoparathyroidism	↑	↑	N	
o Medications altering vitamin D metabolism, or causing intravascular			↓	↓
o Extravascular deposition	↑ / ↓			
o Sepsis		↓		↓

Adapted from MKSAP 15, Endocrinology and Metabolism 2009, page 61.

• In the patient with hypocalcemia such as from vitamin D deficiency, give the reason why more useful information comes from finding ↓ 25-OH vitamin D than finding ↓ 1, 25-DiOH vitamin D.

o ↓ 25-OH vitamin D
– ↓ sun exposure to vitamin D
– ↓ intake or absorption of vitamin D
– Intake of phenytoin
– Nephrotic syndrome (↓ vitamin D binding protein)
– Hepatobiliary cholestatic disorders

o ↓ 1, 25- diOH vitamin D
– Yet N/↑ 25-on vitamin D
– Renal disease
– ↓ renal 1α-hydroxylase
– Hypoparathyroidism

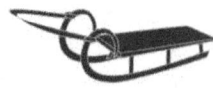

- ○ ↑ 1, 25-diOH vitamin D
  - – Hereditary vitamin D-resistant rickets
  - – The ↓ Ca^{2+} from vitamin D deficiency leads to ↑ PTH
  - – ↑ PTH stimulates renal conversion of 25-OH vitamin D to 1, 25-diOH vitamin D
  - – Measurement of 25-OH vitamin D give the best assessment of body stores of vitamin

Based on the metabolism of vitamin D, give the rationale for using various analogs for management of deficiency.

- ○ 25-hydroxylation → liver

- ○ 1-hydroxylation → kidney

- ○ In liver disease, give 25-OH vitamin D, since this step is defective in liver disease

- ○ In renal disease, give 1, 25-di OH vitamin D, since the 1-hydroxylation step is impaired

- ○ Neither liver nor kidney disease, give cholecalciferol (D3) or ergocalciferol (D2)

A patient is found to have hypocalcemia and hyperphosphatemia. On the basis of their PTH and vitamin D measurements, give the likely cause of the hypocalcemia.

Condition	PTH	Vitamin D
○ Hypoparathyroidism	↓	
○ Pseudohypoparathyroidism (PTH resistance)	↑	N
○ Chronic renal disease	↑	↓1, 25-dihydroxy vitamin D

There may be numerous causes of hypocalcemia (please see reference source, such as MKSAP 15, Endocrinology and Metabolism 2009, Table 29, page 61.

- – Thinking about the many causes of hypocalcemia may be simplified by considering the mechanisms.

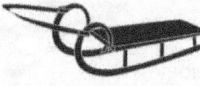

Clinical Pearl

In the patient with hypocalcemia, always check to see if the serum magnesium level (Mg^{2+}_s) is reduced. Give the reason why

- ↓ Mg^{2+}_s - ↓ PTH release
                   - ↑ PTH resistance

➤ Diagnostic imaging

A 60-year old patient is subject to prolonged metabolized in bed for a pelvic fracture. You monitor their serum calcium concentration, anticipating hypercalcemia of immobilization. Although the patient has been eating adequate amounts of calcium and vitamin D, they become hypocalcemic.

- Give the diagnostic imaging study which is likely to give the explanation for the unexpected rise in their serum calcium concentration.
    - The patient likely has Paget disease, with bone turnover, leading to hypercalcemia, above scan would be sensitive to detect the sites of bone disease which would need to be treated with a bisphosphonate.

➤ Prevention and Treatment
    - Lifestyle   – ↓ smoking
                                – ↓ BMI
                                – ↓ caffeine
                                – ↑ exercise

    - Medications   – Calcium plus vitamin D
                                – Bisphosphonates

    - Treat underlying
      causes

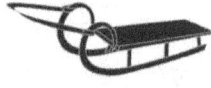

MALE REPRODUCTIVE DISORDERS

➢ Useful background

o There is pulsative release of GnRH (gonadotropin-releasing hormone) from the supraoptic nucleus of the hypothalamus

o GnRH acts on the pituitary to releasing
- ↑ LH to act on the Leydig cells of the testes for the production of testosterone
- FSH from the pituitary to act on cells for the maturation and release of sperm (spermatogenesis)

o Some testosterone is converted to dihydrotestosterone or estradiol.

o Testosterone, dihydrotestosterone and estradiol inhibit pulsatile release of LH and GnRH

o Sertoli cells produce inhibit B which inhibit FSH.

o Testosterone is bound weakly to albumin, and strongly to SHBG (sex hormone-binding globulin)

o Changes in SHBE
- ↑ old men
- ↓ obesity

o Before deciding on the clinical implication of a low-normal serum testosterone, the concentration of free testosterone must be assessed

Gynecomastia

➢ Causes / associations

o ↑ estrogen production
- Leydig cell tumor
- Adrenal carcinoma
- Bronchial carcinoma (human chorionic gonadotrophin)
- Liver disease (increased conversion of androgens to estrogens)
- Starvation

o ↓ androgen production (hypogonadal states)
- Klinefelter syndrome

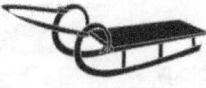

- Secondary testicular failure
    Orchitis
    Castration
    Trauma
  - o Testicular feminization syndrome
  - o Drugs
    - Estrogen receptor binders
      - Estrogen
      - Digoxin
      - Marijuana
    - Antiandrogens
      - Spironolactone
      - Cimetidine

* Gynecomastia does not regress, but mammaplasia (enlarged male breast) does regress

- Take a directed history and perform a focused physical examination to determine the causes of gynecomastia.

  - o Congenital
    - Hermaphrodite
    - Male pseudohermaphrodite
    - Kleinfelter syndrome

  - o Physiological
    - Neonate
    - Puberty
    - Old age

  - o Hermaphroditism or pseudo- hermaphroditism

  - o Endocrine
    - Diabetes
    - Hypo-/ hyperthyroidism
    - Acromegaly
    - Cushing disease
    - Addison disease
    - Tumors of testicle and adrenal glands

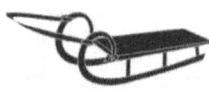

- o Systemic diseases
  - – Heart
    - ▪ Failure
  - – Blood
    - ▪ Leukemia
    - ▪ Lymphoma
  - – Kidney
    - ▪ Failure
    - ▪ Cancer
  - – Lung
    - ▪ Bronchial cancer
    - ▪ Obstructive sleep apnea
  - – GI
    - ▪ Ulcerative colitis
    - ▪ Starvation
    - ▪ Cirrhosis
  - – CNS
    - ▪ Paraplegia
  - – MSK
    - ▪ Rheumatoid arthritis
- o Drugs
  - – Heart
    - ▪ Digitalis, methyldopa, reserpine, spironolactone, INH, amphetamine
  - – Hormones
    - ▪ Estrogens, androgens
  - – GI
    - ▪ Prokinetics (metocloprimide, H2 blockers)
    - ▪ Steroids
  - – Stimulants

Adapted from: Burton JL. *Churchill Livingstone* 1971, page 94; Talley NJ, et al. *Maclennan & Petty Pty Limited* 2003, Table 9.16, page 334.

"Absence of evidence is not
Evidence of absence."

Grandad

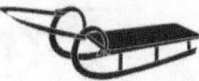

Male Hypogonadism

➤ Definition

  ○ Serum total testosterone (T)
    – Male hypogonadism
      ▪ < 200 ng/dL
    – Shades of grey
      ▪ 200-350 ng/dL

  ○ If ↓ T, measure LH, FSH, prolactin
    – ↑ LH, FSH, prolactin   (primary) testicular failure
    – ↓ LH, FSH, prolactin   (secondary) pituitary hypothalamic failure

• Give the causes and features of male hypogonadism.

  ○ Primary testicular failure (usually associated with infertility)
    – Congenital
      ▪ Chromosome 46, XXY karyotype
      ▪ Klinefelter syndrome
    – Drugs / chemicals
      ▪ Chemotherapy
    – Trauma / surgery
    – Infiltration

  ○ Primary testicular   – ↓ testosterone
    failure   – Small gonads
                              – ↑ gonadotropins
    (Klinefelter   – Eunechoid proportions ↓
    syndrome)   – Gynecomastia
                              – Diagnose by determining karyotype

  ○ Secondary   – ↓ hypothalamic +/- pituitary dysfunction (in men)
                              – Hyperprolactinemia → ↓ gonadotropins: look for
                                pituitary tumor
                              – Drugs
                                ▪ Steroids
                                ▪ Narcotics
                                ▪ Alcohol
                              – Nutrition
                                ▪ Malnutrition
                                ▪ Obesity
                              – Chronic illness

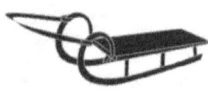

➢ Diagnosis

  o ↓ testosterone, normal LH and prolactin → ADAM (androgen deficiency in the aging male) syndrome

  o ↓ LH and N/↓ prolactin → suggests
    - Intake of androgens, estrogens, narcotics
    - Hemochromatosis
    - Kallman syndrome (congenital disorders of GnRH production)

  o ↓ LH and ↑ prolactin → suspect pituitary disease

- Give drugs which can cause secondary pituitary / hypothalamic failure leading to male hypogonadism (↓ T; ↓ LH, FSH, prolactin).

  o Corticosteroids

  o Opiates

Androgen Deficiency in the Aging Male (ADAM)

➢ Pathogenesis
  o ↓ pulses of GnRH, LH
  o ↑ conversion of free testosterone → estradiol (causing ↓ free testosterone)
  o ↑ SHBG (causing ↓ free cholesterol)

➢ Clinical
  o Testosterone
    - ↓ libido, +/- ED (erectile dysfunction)
    - Osteoporosis
    - ↓ cognitive function
    - ↓ muscle strength

➢ Diagnosis
  o Suspect if screening testosterone < 12.2 mmol/L (350 mg/dL)
  o ↓ free testosterone
    - Liquid chromatography and tanden mass spectrometry
    - Immunoassay and chromatography
  o Normal LH and prolactin (plus ↓ testosterone)

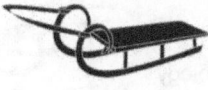

SO YOU WANT TO BE A GENERAL INTERNIST!

We know who was "Adam" of Adam and Eve fame. In the context of male hypogonadism, what is the "Adam syndrome".

The androgen deficiency in the aging male syndrome, aka Adam syndrome, is comprised of

- o Age < 60 yr
- o Testosterone 150-300 ng/dL
- o LH and prolactin
  - – Normal

SO YOU WANT TO BE A HEPATOLOGIST DISTINGUISHED AS AN ENDOCRINOLOGIST!

Testosterone replacement may be effectively achieved with injections, patches, gels and lozenges.
Give the relative **contraindications** for TRT (testosterone therapy).

o GU	– Prostate Ca
	▪ Hypertrophy
o Endocrine	– Dyslipidemia (↓ HDL cholesterol)
o Respiratory	– OSA (obstructive sleep apnea)
o Blood	– Polycythemia
o GI / liver	– Cirrhosis

Testosterone may be given safely to men with BPH / benign prostatic hypertrophy). Give the role of measuring PSA in mark on testosterone.

- o If PSA increases ≥ 2x, or
- o If PSA continues to increase after 6 mon of assess for prostate Ca

---

A Pearl and a Gem

Hypogonadotropic hypogonadism may be associated with OCA (obstructive sleep apnea), and may be effectively treated with continuous positive-airway pressure.

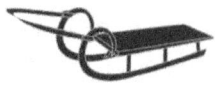

Anabolic Steroid Abuse in Males

- Give clinical features which would suggest anabolic steroid abuse in males.
  - o Muscular hypertrophy
  - o Gynecomastia
  - o Testicular atrophy
  - o Deep / hoarse voice
  - o Acne
  - o Irritability
  - o Evasive speech

Tricky Treatment

- o If a man has hypogonadism plus infertility, treat the infertility with HCG (human chorionic gonadotropin) injection or infusion pump to provide pulsatile delivery of GnRH
    - – Klinefelter syndrome
    - – Consider adding FSH if hypogonadism is severe.

➢ For adverse effects
  - o Gynecomastia   – Tamoxifen
    -                 – Aromatase inhibitor
  - o Acne   – Tretinoin

➢ For suspecting self-administration of
  - o Growth hormone   – ↑ serum IGF-1 (insulin-like growth factor I)
  - o Androgens   – ↓ LH
    -                 – ↓ FSH

➢ Tricky Question

- Give reasons why treatment of male fertility **fails with testosterone** treatment.
  - o Effects of testosterone intake
    - – ↓ LH and FSH
    - – ↓ testosterone production by Leydig cells
    - – ↓ spermatogenesis by Sertoli cells

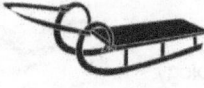

> Tricky Associations:
  - Hypogonadism, ↓ FSH, ↓ LH, ↑ prolactin → think of possible pituitary tumor
  - Hypopituitary following head injury: assess HPA axis: cortisol; if low, then metyrapone or cosyntropin (1 µg) stimulation test.
  - Osteoporosis in a young man
    - Think hypogonadism, and treat osteoporosis with TRT (testosterone replacement therapy)
  - Hypopituitarism, first hormone to replace is
    - Corticosteroids
  - Hypogonadism plus chronic use of steroids
    - Think ↓ GnRH, ↓ LH, ↓ FSH (common features of exo- or endogenous Cushing Syndrome

FEMALE REPRODUCTIVE DISORDERS

> Useful background
  - GnRH pulses stimulate release of LH and FSH from pituitary
  - LH acts on theca cell of ovary synthesize antrostenedione and testosterone.
  - LH inhibits GnRH (negative feedback inhibition)
  - FSH acts on granular cells of ovary to
    - Synthesize estradiole
    - To activate aromatase activity
    - To produce inhibitin B
  - Aromatase transforms androstenedione and testosterone to estradiole
  - Estradiole triggers ovulation
  - Inhibitin B inhibits FSH (negative feedback inhibition)
  - After ovulation the granulosa cells forms a corpus luteum.
  - The corpus luteum synthesizes progesterone.
  - Withdrawal of progesterone leads to menstruation.

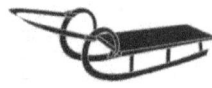

Amenorrhea

➢ Definition

  o Primary

Secondary sexual characteristics	Absence of spontaneous menses by age (yr)
Yes	16
No	14

  o Secondary

    – "Absence of menses for 3 or more consecutive months in a woman who previously has menstruated"

MKSAP 15, Endocrinology and Metabolism, 2009, page 53.

SO YOU WANT TO BE AN ENDOCRINOLOGIST!

In the setting of the woman with secondary amenorrhea, give the meaning of the **Asherman syndrome**.

  o The Asherman syndrome is secondary amenorrhea arising from scarring of the endometrium following a D & C (dilation and curettage)

• Take a directed history and perform a focused physical examination to determine the cause of amenorrhea.

➢ Congenital

  o Intersexual states

    – Hermaphrodite: testicular plus ovarian elements in gonads

    – Male pseudohermaphrodite have tests, but are feminized because of end-organ non-responsiveness

    – Female pseudohermaphrodites: have ovaries, but are musculinized due to

      ▪ Congenital adrenal hyperplasia

      ▪ Virilizing condition in mother

      ▪ Mother given androgens during pregnancy

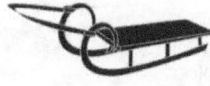

- ➢ Physiological
  - ○ Prepuberty
  - ○ Menopause
  - ○ Pregnancy
  - ○ OCP (oral contraceptive pill)
  - ○ Pre-pubertal
  - ○ Pregnancy
  - ○ Infarction or pituitary apoplexy
  - ○ Menopausal
  - ○ "Functional"
    - – Change in environment
    - – Emotional upset
    - – Rapid change in weight
    - – Aggressive training
  - ○ Anatomical defects

- ➢ Head
  - ○ Mid brain tumor
  - ○ Trauma
  - ○ Surgery radiation infection
    - – Pelvic TB
    - – Systemic infection

- ➢ Endocrine
  - ○ Hyperthyroidism
  - ○ Hypopituitarism
  - ○ Mid brain tumor
  - ○ Congenital adrenogenital syndrome
  - ○ Androgen
    - – Secreting tumor
      - ▪ Hyperplasia
      - ▪ Adenoma
      - ▪ Carcinoma
- ➢ Systemic disease
- ➢ Malnourishment (e.g. anorexia nervosa, Crohn disease)

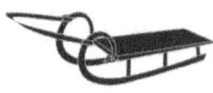

- ➢ Uterus
    - o Uterine anomaly
    - o Hysterectomy
- ➢ Ovary/ adrenal - ↑ estrogen/ progesterone
    - o Stein-Leventhal syndrome, tumors, e.g. arrhenoblastoma, hilus-cell
    - o Oophorectomy
    - o Follicular or lutein retention cyst
    - o Granulosa cell tumor
    - o Irradiation
    - o Ovarian failure
        - – Surgical removal of ovary / uterus
        - – Asherman syndrome
        - – Systemic illness
        - – Malnutrition / rapid weight loss / anorexia nervosa
        - – Turner syndrome
        - – Agenesis of Mullerian duct
        - – Congenital hypopituitary
    - o Chronic anovulation, estrogen level
        - – Normal
            - ▪ PCOS (polycystic overy syndrome)
            - ▪ Cushing syndrome
            - ▪ Mild 21-hydroxylase deficiency
            - ▪ Hyperprolactinemia
    - – Hypothalamic causes
        - ▪ Tumor
        - ▪ Lymphoma
        - ▪ Sarcoidosis
        - ▪ Chemotherapy

- ➢ Drugs
    - o Estrogen, progesterone, testosterone
    - o Glucocorticoids, spironolactone

Adapted from: Burton JL. *Churchill Livingstone* 1971, page 97.

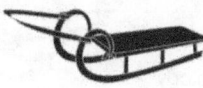

> Diagnosis
  - ○ ↑ FSH
  - ○ Progestin withdrawal challenge
    - – Menstruation
    - – Normal production of estrogen and normal outflow tract
  - ○ No menstruation
    - – ↓ estrogen +/-
    - – Abnormal outflow tract

- Give absolute contraindications to estrogen and progestin therapy.

  - ○ Estrogen therapy
    - – Undiagnosed vaginal bleeding
    - – Active liver disease
    - – Active thromboembolic disease
    - – Known or suspected carcinoma of the breast or other estrogen-sensitive tumors
    - – Pregnancy
    - – The risk of recurrence of breast cancer or thrombosis following estrogen therapy is unknown.
    - – Caution is recommended in women with cardiovascular disease.
  - ○ Progestin therapy
    - – Undiagnosed vaginal bleeding
    - – Known or suspected carcinoma of the breast
    - – Pregnancy

Reproduced with permission: Therapeutics Choices. Sixth Edition. Ottawa, Canada: *Canadian Pharmacist Association* 2012, Table 1, page 946.

"The difference between how a person treats the powerless versus the powerful is as good a measure of human character as I know."

Robert Sutton

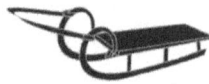

Polycystic Ovary Syndrome

➢ Clinical
- o Hirsuitism (hyperandrogenism)
- o Amenorrhea / ovulatory dysfunction
- o Galactorrhea
- o Bruising
- o May progress to metabolic syndrome diabetes

- Give the features necessary to make a diagnosis of POS (2 of the following 3).
  - o Polycystic ovaries on ultrasound
  - o Dysfunction of ovulation
  - o Hyperandrogenism
  - o Note: In the woman who is overweight or obese, and who has insulin resistance, POS (polycystic ovary syndrome) will be suspected if she has hirsutism and oligomenorrhea.

➢ Laboratory
- o Measure serum testosterone in suspected POS to exclude
  - – Cushing syndrome
  - – Androgen-producing tumor
  - – 21-hydroxylase deficiency
- o ↑ testosterone → abdominal / pelvic CT scan looking for ovarian tumor
- o Note: Laboratory testing for testosterone, DHEAS (dehydroepiandrosterone sulfate) and LH (luteinizing hormone) and FSH (follicle-stimulating hormone) for calculation of LH / FSH > 2 is not necessary unless there is suspicion of an androgen-secreting tumor.

➢ Treatment
- o Achieve ideal body weight
- o Correct insulin resistance
- o Fertility not desired (correct hirsutism)
  - – Oral contraceptives
- o Fertility (ovulation) desired
  - – Clomiphene
  - – Metformin

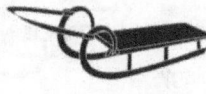

Hirsutism

➢ Causes / associations

- Give the causes of hirsutism.
  - o Racial, familial
  - o Ovarian
    - – Tumor
    - – Stein-Leventhal syndrome
    - – Polycystic ovary syndrome (commonest cause)
  - o Endocrine
    - – Adrenal
      - ▪ Cushing syndrome
      - ▪ Congenital adrenal hyperplasia
      - ▪ Androgen secreting tumor (more often a carcinoma than an adenoma)
      - ▪ Acromegaly
  - o Porphyria cutanea tarda
  - o Drugs
    - – Anabolic steroids
    - – Diazoxide
    - – Minoxidil
    - – Phenytoin
    - – Streptomycin

TIC TAC TOE

Would you like to play ("X's, O's, Y's")

o Turner syndrome	XO
o Kleinfelter syndrome	XXY
o Supermale	XXY
o Superfemale	XXX

Adapted from: Talley NJ, et al. *Maclennan & Petty Pty Limited* 2003, Table 9.15, page 333.

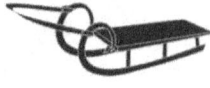

HYPOTHALAMIC DISEASE

➢ Causes / associations

• Give **causes** of hypothalamic disease.

  o Genetic

  o Tumor

  o Sarcoidosis

  o Trauma

  o Irradiation

  o Subarachnoid hemorrhage

  o Infarction (Sheehan syndrome)

  o Empty sella syndrome

  o Metabolic

    – Hemochromatous

    – Anorexia nervosa

    – Critical illness

  o Lymphocytic hypophysistis

➢ Suspicions

  o Hypopituitary plus diabetes insipidus → suspect craniopharyngioma

  o Hypopituitary plus diabetes insipidus and hyperprolactinemia → suspect hypothalamic causes

  o During / after pregnancy, mass effect (lymphocytic infiltration), ACTH / cortisol deficiency → think lymphocytic hypophysitis

  o Pregnancy, bleeding and infarction of pituitary

• Give the short-term **adverse effects of growth hormone deficiency** which can be prevented by initially using low dose replacement therapy.

  o Joint pain

  o Carpal tunnel syndrome

  o Peripheral edema

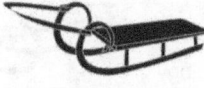

PITUITARY TUMORS

➢ Types
- o Microadenomas < 10 mm
- o Microadenomas > 10 mm
  - – Defects in usual fields
  - – Cranial nerve palsy (invasion of cavernous sinus)

Non-functioning Pituitary Adenomas: **Incidentalomas**

- o Assess for hypercortisolism and for pheochromocytoma
- o If there is hypercortisolism, pheochromocytoma and hypertension, measure the aldosterone / plasma renin to determine if the ratio is increased.
- o Treat any associated hormone production increase or decrease visual field defects
- o Enlargement of incidentulomas over time
  - – Microadenomas 10%
  - – Macroadenomas 24%

Prolactinoma

➢ Definition
- o ↑ serum prolactin from pituitary adenoma

➢ Causes / associations

• Give causes of **hyperprolactinemia.**

- o Pituitary
  - – Pituitary disease, especially prolactinomas
  - – Hypothalamic disease
  - – Sellar and parasellar disease
- o CNS
  - – Neurogenic disease of spinal cord disease of chest wall
- o Liver
  - – Chronic liver disease (cirrhosis)

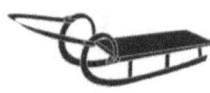

- o Kidney
  - – Chronic renal failure
- o Breast
  - – Lesion stimulation
- o Pregnancy
- o Endocrine
  - – Acromegaly
  - – Hypothyroidism
- o Idiopathic
- o Drugs
  - – Metoclopramide
  - – Verapamil
  - – Tricyclic antidepressants (TCA)
  - – Phenothiazines
  - – H2-receptor antagonist (cimetidine)

➢ Pathophysiology

- Give the **mechanism** of hyperprolactinemia in three of the following conditions.

o Suprasella lesions	– Compression of
	  ▪ Hypothalamus
	  ▪ Pituitary stalk

o Pregnancy	– High estrogen levels
	  ▪ Lactotroph hyperplasia
	  ▪ Hyperprolacctinemia

o Disease of liver, kidney, thyroid	– Abnormal metabolism and excretion
o Acromegaly	– Coproduction of growth-hormone (GH) secreting pituitary adenoma
o Non-functioning adenoma	– Ectopic production of GH-releasing hormone – Adenoma-dysfunction of the hypothalamus or stalk of the pituitary may cause mild hyperprolactinemia in the patient with a so-called "non-functioning" pituitary adenoma

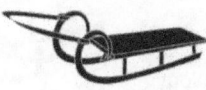

➢ Clinical

• Give the typical symptoms of hyperprolactinemia.

- o Breast
  - – Galactorrhea
- o Reproductive organs
  - – Amenorrhea
  - – Oligomenorrhea
  - – ↓ libido
  - – ↓ fertility
  - – Gynecomastia
  - – Erectile dysfunction
- o Bone
  - – Osteopenia

➢ Laboratory

• Give the caution about measurements of serum prolactin.

- o Falsely low
  – Very high serum concentration may measure normal or low because the antibodies used to measure the prolactin levels become saturated ("hook effect")
  - ▪ Solution: dilute the serum

- o Macroprolactinemia
  – Prolactin dimers or prolactin aggregates with immunoglobulins
  - ▪ Causes falsely positive higher level of prolactin
  - ▪ Magnitude of effect may become bigger during pregnancy

A Gem and a Pearl:

Men who have experienced high levels of prolactin for a prolonged period may develop damage to the gonadal axis, which persists even after the hyperprolactinemia was been corrected; these men will need **TRT** (testosterone replacement therapy).

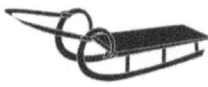

➢ Treatment

- Give the **treatment of prolactinomas.**
  - o Medical therapy of prolactinomas
    - – Dopamine agonist
      - ▪ Bromocriptine
      - ▪ Caborgoline (use doses < 3 mg/d to avoid development of cardiac valve abnormalities
      - ▪ ↓ tumor size by 50% in 80-90% of patients
      - ▪ Stop during pregnancy and restart over breastfeeding is finished
  - o Conception desired – dopamine agonist (e.g. bromocriptine)
  - o Contraception not desired
    - – Bromocriptive plus OCP (estrogen replacement)

Note – bromocriptine will not shrink a pituitary adenoma which is non-functioning

---

A Gem: In acute hypopituitarism with apoplexy, immediately give stress doses of hydrocortisone (50 mg q 8 h)

  - o Other than prolactinomas, surgical techniques
    - – Endoscopic endonasal approach
    - – Sublabial transsphenoidal approach
      - ▪ Initial remission rate:
    - – Microadenoma 70-80%
    - – Macroadenoma 25-40%
    - – Surgery with irradiation
  - o Radiation without surgery
    - – Gamma knife
    - – Sterrotactic radiotherapy (for non-responders to medical or surgical therapy

Note: follow the patient having irradiation of pituitary adenoma for development of hypopituitarism

- Give the mechanism of failure of correction of fatigue and reduced libido with correction of massive hyperprolactinemia.
  - o ↑↑ prolactin → ↓ GnRH → ↓ LH, ↓ FSH (irreversible damage from ↑↑ prolactin), so testosterone is needed for treatment.

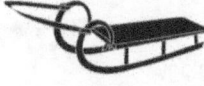

ACROMEGALY

➢ Clinical

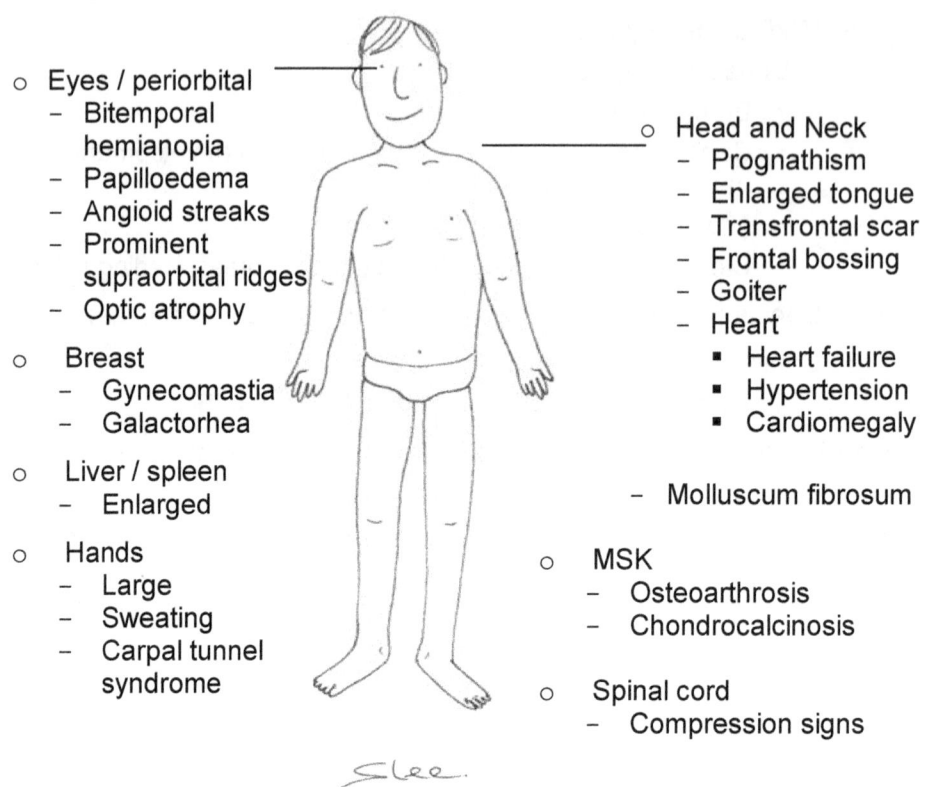

o Eyes / periorbital
  - Bitemporal hemianopia
  - Papilloedema
  - Angioid streaks
  - Prominent supraorbital ridges
  - Optic atrophy

o Breast
  - Gynecomastia
  - Galactorhea

o Liver / spleen
  - Enlarged

o Hands
  - Large
  - Sweating
  - Carpal tunnel syndrome

o Head and Neck
  - Prognathism
  - Enlarged tongue
  - Transfrontal scar
  - Frontal bossing
  - Goiter
  - Heart
    ▪ Heart failure
    ▪ Hypertension
    ▪ Cardiomegaly

  - Molluscum fibrosum

o MSK
  - Osteoarthrosis
  - Chondrocalcinosis

o Spinal cord
  - Compression signs

Adapted from: Talley NJ, et al. *Maclennan & Petty Pty Limited* 2003, page 321.

• Perform a focused physical examination for acromegaly.

  o General
    - Hyperhidrosis
  o Eyes
    - Prominent supraorbital ridges
    - Bitemporal hemianopia
    - Optic atrophy
    - Papilledema
    - Angiod streaks

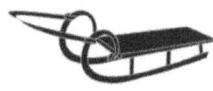

- o Nose & lips
  - – Large
- o Jaws
  - – Prognathia (large protruding lower jaw)
  - – Macroglosia
- o Neck
  - – Goiter
- o Axillae
  - – Skin tags (molluscum fibrosum)
  - – Acanthosis nigrans
- o Hands
  - – Large hands
  - – Sweating
- o Breasts
  - – Gynecomastia
  - – Galactorrhea
- o Heart
  - – Cardiomegaly
  - – Hypertension
  - – Heart failure
- o Abdomen
  - – Hepatosplenomegaly
  - – Abdominal mass (colon cancer)
- o MSK
  - – Carpal tunnel syndrome signs
  - – Chondrocalcinosis
  - – Kyphosis
  - – Large ring finger
  - – Osteoarthrosis (hands, hips, knees, feet)
- o Spinal cord
  - – Compression signs
  - – Spinal stenosis
- o Endocrine
  - – Signs of hypopituitarism
  - – Signs of diabetes mellitus

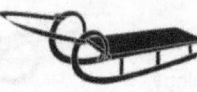

- Based on the ↑ risk of various conditions in acromegaly, give suggestions for a screening / surveillance program
  - Colonoscopy for adenomas and colorectal cancer
  - Blood sugar and HgA1C for diabetes
  - Measurement of blood pressure
  - Assessment of cardiac risk

➢ Laboratory

- Give the season why a single, measurement of insulin-like growth factor-1 is more likely to be abnormal than GH in acromegaly.
  - GH is released intermittently (in pulse) in acromegaly.
  - IGF-1 reflects integrated release of GH.
  - Diagnose autonomous secretion of GH by showing suppression of GH during a GTT (glucose tolerance test)
  - In pregnancy, the placenta produces a form of GH, so the true value of GH in the mother can best be determined after pregnancy.

➢ Diagnostic imaging

SO YOU WANT TO BE ENDOCRINOLOGIST!

- Give the typical X-ray changes in the hands and feet of a person with acromegaly.
  - "tufting" of terminal phalynx of fingers & toe
  - ↑ thickness of heal pad

➢ Treatment

- Give the treatment of acromegaly.
  - Medical
    - Cabergoline (dopamine agonist)
    - Somatostatin analogs
      - Octreotide
      - Lanreotide
    - Pegvisomant

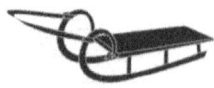

- Stop when pregnancy is planned or is diagnosed
- Somatostatin receptors in placenta and some fetal tissues
  - First line, but successful in only 10-20%
  - May have additive effect when combined in the somatostatin analog, normalized GH, IGF-1 in 60%
  - Normal tumor size in most
  - GH analogue which prevents GH binding to GH receptor
  - Normalizes ↑ IGF-1 levels in 90%, but no effect on size of tumor
- o Surgery, transsphenoidal
  - Normalizes ↑ GH and ↑ IGF-1
    - Microadenomas 80-90%
    - Macroadenomas 30-40%
- o Indication
  - For poor response to medical or surgical therapy

➢ Prognosis

- o The 2-3 fold ↑ mortality rate in acromegaly may be reverse when therapy is successful.

PITUITARY DISEASE

Hypopituitarism

➢ Causes and

• Give the causes of hypopituitarism.

- o Infiltration
  - Pituitary tumor (non-secretory or secretory)
  - Other tumors
    - Craniopharyngioma
    - Sarcoma
- o Infection
  - Granulomata (e.g. sarcoid, tuberculosis)
- o Idiopathic

Adapted from: Talley NJ, et al. Maclennan & Petty Pty Limited 2003, page 320.

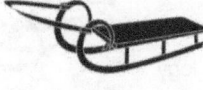

➢ Practical tip

  o While the following laboratory results will make you think of pituitary tumors causing prolactinoma, acromegaly and Cushing disease,

    – ↑ prolactin and galactorrhea, amenorrhea, impotence

    – ↑ GH, ↑ IGF-1, enlarged facial features, hands, feet

    – ↑ ACTH, 24-hr urine cortisol

    – ↓ Na^+_s (diabetes insipidus)

  o Don't forget to exclude non-prolactinoma causes of hyperprolactinemia.

    – Pregnancy (HCG)

    – Hypothyroidism (↑TSH)

    – Drugs

● Give examples of provocative tests used in the **investigation of hypopituitarism**.

  o Acromegaly

    – ↑ GH, ↓ IGF-1

      ▪ Failure of GTT (oral glucose tolerance test) to ↓ the ↑ GH stimulation

      ▪ ↓ response of arginine and GH-releasing hormone

  o Cushing disease

    – ↓ ACTH, ↓ cortisol concentration

      ▪ ↑ cortisol with 1 µg ACTH metyrapone → ↓ response of cortisol and 11-deoxycortisol

  o Diabetes insipidus

    – ↓ ADH (vasopressin)

      ▪ Water deprivation → failed ↑ U_{osm} (urine < 200 mOsm/kg H_2O, and fails to become more concentrated)

      ▪ Desmopressin challenge → ↑ U_{osm} indicating central DI

➢ Treatment

  o Tricky, probably needs specialist team approach

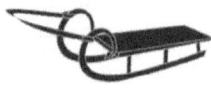

Size of adenoma	Symptoms	Treatment
< 10 mm (microadenoma)	Menses normal	Follow-up
> 10 mm (macroadenoma)	Yes	Cabergoline (somatostatin analog), or bromocriptine

- o When MRI no longer shows adenoma and prolactin is normal, following-up (recurrence 50%)
- o Surgery
  - – Secreting adenomas
    - ▪ GH
    - ▪ TSH
    - ▪ ACTH
  - – Mass effect
    - ▪ Visual fields (bitemporal hemiporal hemianopia)
    - ▪ Hypopituitarism
  - – Prolactinomas
    - ▪ Not responding to dopamine agonist
- o Radiation
  - – Non-surgical candidates
  - – Secreting tumors which persist after surgery
  - – Tumor persisting after surgery

A 50-yr patient has symptoms of hypothyroidism, with ↓ T3 and ↓fT4. However, the TSH is also reduced and central hypothyroidism due to a central cause, and MRI confirms a pituitary adenoma. Accordingly, it was planned to begin therapy with L-thyroxine 100 microgram per day, and to follow the TSH levels until they normalize.

- • Give any additional suggestions related to medical management.
  - o Check the ACTH levels for possible associated adrenal insufficiency from associated hypopituitarism, and use corticosteroid replacement **before** thyroxine therapy to prevent adrenal crisis.
  - o The laboratory value to follow when treating secondary / central hypothyroidism is serum fT4, **not** TSH

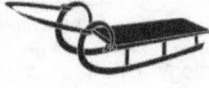

PHEOCHROMOCYTOMA

➢ Clinical

• Give the characteristic "H"s of pheochromocytoma.

  o Headache

  o Hypertension

  o Hypotension
    – Postural
    – During induction of anesthesia

  o Hypermetabolism

  o Hypermetabolism

  o Hyperglycemia

  o Hypokalemia

• Perform a focused physical examination for pheochromocytoma (catecholamine-secreting tumor).

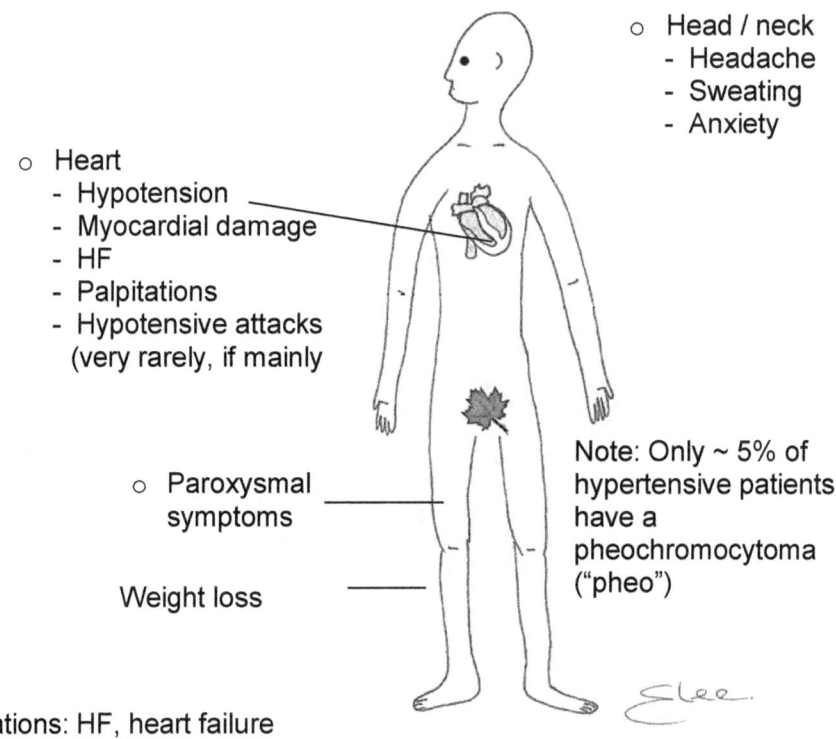

o Head / neck
  - Headache
  - Sweating
  - Anxiety

o Heart
  - Hypotension
  - Myocardial damage
  - HF
  - Palpitations
  - Hypotensive attacks
    (very rarely, if mainly

o Paroxysmal symptoms

Weight loss

Note: Only ~ 5% of hypertensive patients have a pheochromocytoma ("pheo")

Abbreviations: HF, heart failure

Adapted from: Davey P. *Wiley-Blackwell* 2006, page 290.

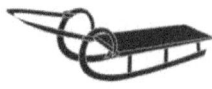

- Give the mechanism of postural (orthostatic) hypotension associated with pheochromocytoma.

    o The excess excretion from the adrenal medulla of norepinephrine, epinephrine and dopamine cause vasoconstriction-related volume depletion, which predisposes the patient to orthostatic hypotension.

➤ Causes / associations

    o Familial
        – 25%

    o Asymptomatic
        – 10%

    o Malignant
        – 10%

    o Location
        – Adrenal medulla 90%
        – Along the symptomatic chain 10%

➤ Laboratory

- Give the profile of the hypertensive patient who requires **genetic testing** for possible familial pheochromocytoma.

    o Patient   –   Family history of pheochromocytoma
                        –   Young person with other tumors

    o Tumor   –   Bilateral adrenal location
                        –   Extra-adrenal location
                        –   Recur after surgery

- Give the methods of **diagnosis** of pheochromocytoma.

    o Plasma   –   Catecholamines
                            ▪ Epinephrine + norepinephrine
                        –   Clonidine suppression test (↓ total catecholamines after 0.3 mg clonidine
                            ▪ In persons with ↑ catecholamines for reasons other than pheo', e.g. stress, 1° hypertension
                        –   ↑ metabolites
                            ▪ Metanephrine, normetanephrine

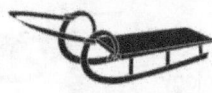

- o Urine   – ↑ metaneprines, normetanephrines, vanillylmandelic acid (sensitivity only 65%, but specificity for pheo' of 95%, as long as dietary sources of vanilylmandelic acid are excluded)

Note: Antihypertensive medications do not interfere with the measurement of catecholamine (the exception is labetalol)

Pheo' and Tricks

- • Give the reasons why **not all** patients with pheochromocytoma have hypertension.
  - o The hypertension may be intermittent
  - o If the tumor secretes mostly epinephrine rather than norepinephrine, they may present with the hypotension.

- • Give the reason why the patient treated with beta-blockers for hypertension due to unrecognized pheochromocytoma have worsening of their hypertension.
  - o The B-blockers remove the B-stimulation, but α-stimulation remains, and blood pressure rises

---

➢ Diagnostic imaging
  - o Confirm pheochromocytoma biochemically, then identify site of tumor
  - o CT /MRI
  - o ^{131}I
    - – MIBG scan (iodine-131-meta iodobenzylguanidine)
    - – Use when CT or MRI is negative, or
    - – To distinguish positive with pheo' negative with metastasis to adrenal

---

Recall Reminder: The three adrenal causes of hypertension include
  - o Hypercortisolism (Cushing syndrome)
  - o Hyperaldosterronism
  - o Pheochromocytoma

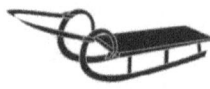

➢ Treatment

• Give the **preoperative management** of the patient scheduled for laparoscopic adrenal resection for a proven pheo'.

o Alpha blockage	–	Prazosin 2 mg to 5 mg tis
	–	Doxazosin 2 mg to 8 mg od
	–	Terazosin 2 mg to 5 mg od
	–	Phenoxybenzamine now outdated

o Control of hypertension
- Calcium channel blockers
  - Verapamil
  - Amlodipine
- Avoid B-blockers
  - If patient's preop BP is high: BB → ↑ BP
  - If patient's preop BB is normal BB → ↑ BP during manipulation of adrenal
- IV fluid infusion, as needed
  - Nitroprusside IV during surgery

o Malignant pheochromocytoma
- Radiation
  - External
  - Targeted ^{131}I – MIBG
- Follow-up ~ 15% of pheo' recur after resection, so follow patient for at least 10 year

• Give the principles of managing the patient with pheochromocytoma in the **perioperative** interval.

o α-adrenergic blockage
- Phenoxybenzamine
- Doxazosin

o B-adrenergic blockage
- Nicardipine

o Adequate IV 0.9% saline

o For intraoperative hypertensive crisis
- Nitroprusside
- Phentolamine

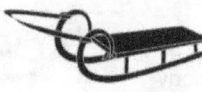

PRIMARY HYPERALDOSTERONISM

➤ Definition

  o "Primary hyperaldostesteronism is characterized by excessive and autonomous aldosterone production by the adrenal zona glomerulosa independent of its physiologic system" (MKSAP 15, Endocrinology and Metabolism, page 46)

➤ Cause / associations

  o Primary
    – Solitary adenoma
    – Unilateral / bilateral hyperplasia
    – Carcinoma

A Pearl and a Gem

• Give the clinical profile of the patient with hypertension due to primary hyperaldosteronism.

  o Hypertension is difficult to control

  o Hypokalemic acidosis (↑ aldosterone → ↑ renal excretion of K^+, H^+)

---

  o Both pheochromocytoma and primary hyperaldosteronism may be associated with
    – Hypokalemia
    – Hard-to-treat hypertension
    – Family history

➤ Laboratory

• Give the laboratory testing, in addition to hypokalemia, which suggests primary hyperaldosteronism.

  o Plasma aldosterone > 15 ng/dL

  o Plasma aldosterone / renin activity > 20

  o High salt diet or IV salt load
    – Failure to suppress plasma aldosterone < 5 ng/dL (↑ salt load normally ↓ aldosterone)

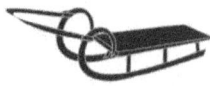

Note: In order for the above lab criteria to be interpretable, the patient must not be on spironolactone or eplerenone, aldosterone antagonists.

- Give the methods to **diagnose** primary hyperaldosteronism.

  - o Blood
    - – ↑ aldosterone
    - – ↓ renin
    - – ↑ aldosterone / renin > 20

  - o Diagnostic imaging
    - – CT scanning

      If aldosterone is ↑ and renin is ↓, proceed with a "salt load test"

      ↑ Na po or IV → ↓ aldosterone concentration in normal, but remain high in primary autonomous hyperaldosterone, due to ↓ production aldosterone

---

A trick in diagnosing primary hyperaldosteronism

- o In the patient already treated with ACE inhibitor or the ARB ratio of aldosterone / renin > 10

- o The aldosterone concentration would not be as high in patient with primary hyperaldosteronism treated with ACEI or ARB, and the renin would not be as low, so the ratio would not be > 20, as would be the case of a patient with primary hyeraldosteronism not treated with ACE-I or ARB.

- o In the patient on spironolactone, the blood aldosterone will be reduced, renin will not be as reduced, and the ratio aldo' / renin will not be as high. WHAT TO DO – make measurements when patient of spironolactone or eplerenone.

- o Having trouble distinguishing cause of single adenoma vs. bilateral hyperplasia?
    - – Refer for selective venus sampling of catheterized samples for aldosterone.

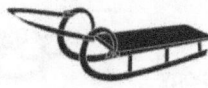

➢ Treatment

- Give the treatment of primary hyperaldosteronism.
  - ○ Single adenoma laparoscopic resection if affected adrenal gland
  - ○ Bilateral hyperplasia
    - – Aldosterone antagonist
      - ▪ Spironolactone
      - ▪ Eplerenone
    - – Objective: correct
      - ▪ Hypertension
      - ▪ Hypokalemic alkalosis
      - ▪ Hyperaldosteronism

- Give the reason why some patients with **bilateral adrenal hyperplasia** develop adverse effects and must be switched to eplerenone.

  - ○ Spironolactone inhibits both the aldosterone as well as the androgen receptor, so the patient may develop adverse effects
    - – Gynecomastia
    - – Impotence
    - – ↓ libido
    - – Menstrual irregularities
  - ○ Eplerenone is more selective for just the aldosterone receptor

"Success strategies for implementing quality improvement."

James Calvin

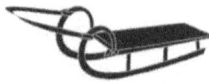

PARANEOPLASTIC SYNDROMES

- Perform a focused physical examination for paraneoplastic syndromes and hormone producing cancers.

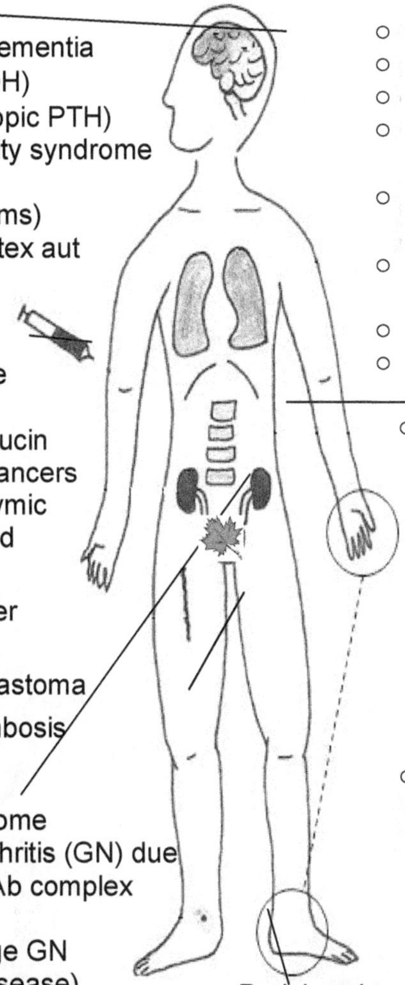

  o CNS
    - Confusion/Dementia
    - $\downarrow$ Na+ (SIADH)
    - $\uparrow$ Ca2+ (ectopic PTH)
    - Hyperviscosity syndrome (myeloma, Waldenstroms)
    - Cerebral cortex aut antibodies
  o Hematology
    - Anemia
      - Autoimmune haemolytic anaemia- mucin producing cancers
      - Aplasia: Thymic tumor related
    - Polycythemia
      - Renal cancer
      - Cerebellar hemangioblastoma
  o Deep vein thrombosis
  o Cachexia
  o Nephrotic syndrome
    - Glomerulonephritis (GN) due to tumor Ag-Ab complex deposition
    - Minimal change GN (Hodgkin's disease)
    - Membranous GN (many cancers)
    - Membranoproliferative GN (non-Hodgkin's lymphoma)

  o Muscle weakness
  o Fatigue
  o Cachexia
  o Polymyositis/ dermatomyositis
  o $\downarrow$ K+ (2^0 to ectopic ACTH production)
  o $\uparrow$ Ca2+ (2^0 to ectopic PTH production)
  o Eaton-Lambert syndromes
  o Guillain – Barre syndrome

  o Spinal cord syndromes
    - Myelitis, often in thoracic region, $\rightarrow$ rapid paralysis + death
    - ALS (=motor neuron disease) 5-10% are cancer related

  o Hypertropic pulmonary osteoarthropathy

  o Hypercalcaemia
    - Estopic PTH secretion
    - PTH related hormone syndromes

Peripheral neuropathy

Adapted from: Davey P. *Wiley-Blackwell* 2006, page 361; Talley NJ, et al. *Maclennan & Petty Pty Limited* 2003, Table 9.16, page 339

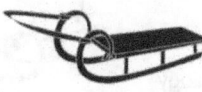

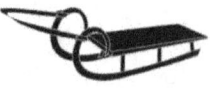

INDEX

Note: Page number followed by f and t indicates figure and table respectively.

 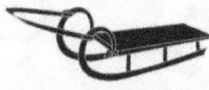

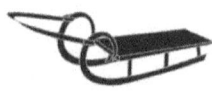

C
Calcium homeostasis, 117
Cushing disease, 96, 99, 102, 113, 135, 157
Cushing syndrome
  adipose tissue in, 101, 101f
  causes, 99–100
  vs. Cushing disease, 102
  diagnostic imaging, 104
  laboratory, 102–104
  performance characteristics for, 101t
  physical examination for, 100f
  in pregnancy, 104
  vs. pseudo-Cushing syndrome, 102
  treatment of, 104–105

D
Dawn phenomenon, in diabetes mellitus, 19
Destructive thyroiditis
  causes of, 85
  definition, 86
  thyroid function tests in, 87
  treatment, 87
Diabetes insipidus
  causes, 35
  diagnosis of, 36
  types, 35
Diabetes mellitus
  classification
    type 1, 4
    type 2, 6
  clinical, 7–9
  dawn phenomenon in, 19
  definition, 4–5
  diabetic foot
    clinical caution, 14
    clinical tests for, 13t
    definition, 12
    limb-threatening infection, 14
    management of, 13
    physical examination of, 12
  diabetic ketoacidosis (DKA)
    definition, 19
    pathogenesis of, 20
    treatment, 20–22
  diabetic nephropathy
    terms, 23

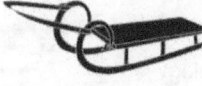

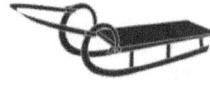

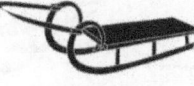

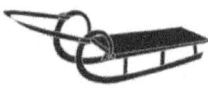

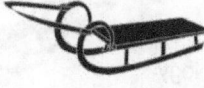

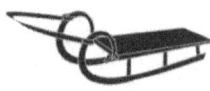

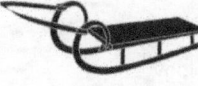

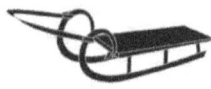

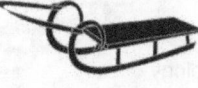

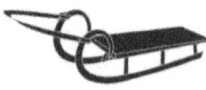

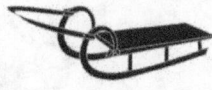

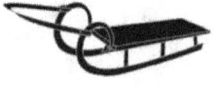